FOURTH EDITIC

MW01000915

Clinical Nurse Leaders Beyond the Microsystem

A Practical Guide

FOURTH EDITION

Clinical Nurse Leaders Beyond the Microsystem

A Practical Guide

James L. Harris, PhD, APRN-BC, MBA, CNL, FAAN

Professor and Coordinator, Clinical Nurse Leader Track
University of South Alabama
College of Nursing
Mobile, Alabama

Linda A. Roussel, PhD, RN, NEA-BC, CNL, FAAN

Nursing Education Consultant

Patricia L. Thomas, PhD, RN, NEA-BC, ACNS-BC, CNL, FACHE, FNAP, FAAN

Associate Dean, Nursing Faculty Affairs
Associate Professor
Wayne State University
College of Nursing
Detroit, Michigan

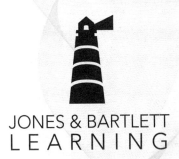

JONES & BARTLETT
LEARNING

World Headquarters
Jones & Bartlett Learning
25 Mall Road, 6th Floor
Burlington, MA 01803
978-443-5000
info@jblearning.com
www.jblearning.com

Jones & Bartlett Learning books and products are available through most bookstores and online booksellers. To contact Jones & Bartlett Learning directly, call 800-832-0034, fax 978-443-8000, or visit our website, www.jblearning.com.

Substantial discounts on bulk quantities of Jones & Bartlett Learning publications are available to corporations, professional associations, and other qualified organizations. For details and specific discount information, contact the special sales department at Jones & Bartlett Learning via the above contact information or send an email to specialsales@jblearning.com.

Production Credits
VP, Product Development: Christine Emerton
Director of Product Management: Matt Kane
Product Manager: Tina Chen
Manager, Content Strategy: Carolyn Pershouse
Project Manager: Jessica deMartin
Project Specialist: Erin Bosco
Digital Project Specialist: Rachel DiMaggio
Senior Marketing Manager: Jennifer Scherzay

Product Fulfillment Manager: Wendy Kilborn
Composition: S4Carlisle Publishing Services
Project Management: S4Carlisle Publishing Services
Cover Design: Michael O'Donnell
Senior Media Development Editor: Troy Liston
Rights Specialist: Benjamin Roy
Cover Image (Title Page, Part Opener, Chapter Opener):
    © Voinalovych Mykola/Shutterstock
Printing and Binding: CJK Group Inc.

Library of Congress Cataloging-in-Publication Data
Names: Harris, James L. (James Leonard), 1956- editor. | Roussel, Linda,
    editor. | Thomas, Patricia L., 1961- editor.
Title: Clinical nurse leaders beyond the microsystem : a practical guide /
    [edited by] James L. Harris, Linda A. Roussel, Patricia L. Thomas.
Other titles: Initiating and sustaining the clinical nurse leader role.
Description: Fourth edition. | Burlington : Jones & Bartlett Learning,
    [2022] | Revision of: Initiating and sustaining the clinical nurse
    leader role. 2018. Third edition. | Includes bibliographical references
    and index.
Identifiers: LCCN 2021021107 | ISBN 9781284227277 (paperback)
Subjects: LCSH: Nurse practitioners. | Nurse administrators. | Leadership.
    | BISAC: MEDICAL / Nursing / General
Classification: LCC RT82.8 .I555 2022 | DDC 610.7306/92--dc23
LC record available at https://lccn.loc.gov/2021021107
6048

Printed in the United States of America
25 24 23 22 21   10 9 8 7 6 5 4 3 2 1

Brief Contents

Preface   **xvi**

Acknowledgments   **xvii**

Chapter Contributors   **xviii**

Exemplar Contributors   **xx**

Reviewers   **xxvi**

CHAPTER 1   **The Clinical Nurse Leader Footprint Across the Healthcare Landscape** 1

CHAPTER 2   **Clinical Nurse Leaders in the Global Community** 19

CHAPTER 3   **The Prominence of CNL Microsystem Leadership for High-Reliability and Value-Added Outcomes** 37

CHAPTER 4   **CNLs Creating a Culture of Quality, Safety, and Value** 63

CHAPTER 5   **Improvement and Implementation Sciences: Links to Innovation, Effectiveness, and Safety** 103

CHAPTER 6   **How Communication Improves Care and Builds Alliances** 127

CHAPTER 7   **The Imperative for Collaboration and Interprofessional Team Improvement** 139

CHAPTER 8   **Networking and Community Advocacy** 169

CHAPTER 9   **Preparing Preceptors for CNL Immersions** 193

CHAPTER 10   **Creative and Meaningful Clinical Immersions** 215

CHAPTER 11   **Using Evidence to Guide CNL Project and Clinical Outcomes** 227

CHAPTER 12   **Using Project Management Basics for Sustained Improvement** 251

CHAPTER 13   **Collecting, Analyzing, and Managing Projects and Improvement Data** 271

CHAPTER 14   **Using Informatics and Healthcare Technologies to Guide CNL Practice** 289

CHAPTER 15   **Transitions in Care** 313

CHAPTER 16   **The CNL's Role in Population Health and Management** 345

CHAPTER 17   **Achieving Excellence in CNL Practice** 361

CHAPTER 18   **The CNL Engagement in Health Policy** 383

CHAPTER 19   **CNL Certification and Professional Development** 395

CHAPTER 20   **Creating a Culture of Health and Wellness: A Catalyst for Sustaining the CNL's Role** 407

Index   **425**

Contents

Preface xvi

Acknowledgments xvii

Chapter Contributors xviii

Exemplar Contributors xx

Reviewers xxvi

CHAPTER 1 The Clinical Nurse Leader Footprint Across the Healthcare Landscape 1

James L. Harris, Linda A. Roussel, and Patricia L. Thomas

Introduction 2

CNL Footprint Past and Present. 3

Future Implications for CNL Education and Practice 5

From Evolution to a Peaceful Revolution 6

Summary 7

CHAPTER 2 Clinical Nurse Leaders in the Global Community 19

Gordana Dermody and Patricia L. Thomas

Introduction 20

The Challenges of Using Best Practice in the Global Community ... 22

Humanitarian and Health Crisis 22

Models and Frameworks to Facilitate CNL
    Praxis in the Global Community 23

Leveraging Digital Health to Overcome Global Health Problems ... 24

CNL Praxis in Global Communities 24

Application of CNL Competencies in the Global Community 25

Conclusion 28

Summary 29

**CHAPTER 3 The Prominence of CNL Microsystem
Leadership for High-Reliability and Value-Added
Outcomes** **37**
Patricia L. Thomas

Introduction 38
The CNL's Role 39
    High-Reliability Organizations 40
    Process Excellence 42
    Evidence-Based Practice 42
Process Excellence Training 43
Healthcare Economics 44
Risk Management 45
Conclusion 46
Summary 46

**CHAPTER 4 CNLs Creating a Culture of Quality,
Safety, and Value** **63**
James L. Harris and Patricia L. Thomas

Introduction 64
Background 66
Supporting a Culture of Safety 67
Risk Anticipation, Risk Assessment, and Risk Management 68
Quality Improvement, Evidence-Based Practice,
    and the CNL Role 69
Philosophical Elements
    of Quality Improvement 70
Defined Aim or Purpose 71
Review of the Literature 71
Resources to Facilitate Improvement 72
Mapping Current Processes 72
Design Thinking 72
Root-Cause Analysis 73
Selecting Appropriate Tools 73
Selecting Measures and Metrics 73
Rapid Cycle Review 74
Relevance of the Microsystem 74
Assessment of the Microsystem for Selection of Quality
    Improvement Projects 75

Systematic and Purposeful Identification of Quality
  Improvement Initiatives 75
Structure for Monitoring Quality Improvement Projects 76
Team Leader Tools for Success 76
Linking Quality Improvement to the Clinical Immersion
  Experience and the Daily Life of a CNL 77
The Spectrum of Value Related to Quality Immersion Projects 78
Conclusion 78
Summary 79

CHAPTER 5 Improvement and Implementation Sciences: Links to Innovation, Effectiveness, and Safety 103

Kathleen R. Stevens

Introduction 104
Background 104
The Importance of Improvement Science 105
The Need for Priorities in Improvement and
  Implementation Research 108
Priorities in Improvement Science 109
Research Priorities in Implementation Science 111
Point 1: Discovery Research 113
Point 2: Evidence Summary 114
Point 3: Translation to Guidelines 114
Point 4: Integration 115
Point 5: Evaluation 118
Growing CNL Capacity in Evidence-Based Quality Improvement 120
Summary 120

CHAPTER 6 How Communication Improves Care and Builds Alliances 127

James L. Harris, Patricia L. Thomas, and Shanda Scott

Introduction 128
Effective Communication 128
Building Alliances with Others 130
Using Clinical Decision Support Tools to Communicate Plans
  and Outcomes 132
Meeting the Triple and Quadruple Aims: The CNL's Contribution . . . 133
Summary 133

CHAPTER 7 The Imperative for Collaboration and Interprofessional Team Improvement.................**139**
James L. Harris and Charlene Myers

Introduction 140
Synergistic Interprofessional Teams 141
Value and Interprofessional Team Collaboration 143
Interprofessional Competency Development and Team
  Effectiveness.. 144
Emotional Intelligence and Interprofessional Teams 145
Summary 145

CHAPTER 8 Networking and Community Advocacy..**169**
Linda A. Roussel and Lonnie K. Williams

Introduction 170
Preparation of the CNL 171
Community Networks and Ambulatory Care................ 171
Leadership and Interdisciplinary
  Team Building....................................... 172
Complexity and Community
  Networking.. 173
Tools and Models for the CNL's Role
  in Networking and Advocacy 173
    Discharge Planning.................................174
    Transition Care Model 175
    Networking and Interprofessional Team Building.....175
    The Epidemiological Triad 175
    The Natural History of Disease Model...............176
    Mind Maps..177
    The Use of Story: Messages to Innovate Team Collaboration.............177
Community Assessment 179
Summary 181

CHAPTER 9 Preparing Preceptors for CNL Immersions **193**
Rebekah Barber, Kristen Noles, and Keaton Lloyd

Preceptor and Preceptee Roles and Core Competencies
  for Each.. 194
    The Preceptor.....................................194
    The Preceptee.....................................196
The CNL Clinical Immersion and Requirements
  for a Successful Immersion Experience............... 197

Learning Environment
and Lifelong Learning 199
Developing Meaningful and Sustainable Clinical
Immersion Projects 200
    Identifying and Selecting a Project Plan 201
    Set Measurable and Attainable Goals 204
    Develop a Step-by-Step Time Line 205
    Summarize Findings and Results 206
Examples of Clinical Immersion Projects and Impact on
the Healthcare System. 206
Summary 207

**CHAPTER 10 Creative and Meaningful
Clinical Immersions. 215**

Patricia L. Thomas, James L. Harris, and Linda A. Roussel

Introduction: Intention of the Immersion—Value Added
for the Organization 216
Using Data and Resources to Identify Needs to Craft
Meaningful Clinical Immersions 217
Applying the Business Model to CNL Clinical Immersions 220
The Usefulness of Portfolios. 221
Performance Contracts. 222
Measurement of CNL Success 222
Summary 224

**CHAPTER 11 Using Evidence to Guide
CNL Project and Clinical Outcomes 227**

Clista C. Clanton, Linda A. Roussel, and Patricia L. Thomas

Introduction 228
EBP Core Competency: Systematically Conducts
an Exhaustive Search for External Evidence to Answer
Clinical Questions. 230
EBP Core Competency: From Multiple Sources,
Locate Evidence Summary Reports for Practice
Implications in Context of EBP 231
EBP Core Competency: Using Existing Standards,
Critically Appraise Evidence Summaries for Practice
Implications in the Context 234
EBP Competency: Assemble Evidence Resources
from Multiple Sources on Selected Topics into Reference
Management Software. 240
Summary 241

**CHAPTER 12 Using Project Management
Basics for Sustained Improvement**......................**251**

Patricia L. Thomas

Introduction 252
Interprofessional and Organizational Team Leaders
    in Project Management 253
Conducting Microsystem Assessments 254
The 5 P Assessment 255
Examples of a SWOT After the Microsystem Assessment
    Is Completed.. 258
    Tool Selection for Quality Improvement and Project Management 259
Evaluation of the Improvement Plan 262
Conclusion 262
Summary 263

**CHAPTER 13 Collecting, Analyzing,
and Managing Projects and Improvement Data** **271**

James L. Harris, Patricia L. Thomas, and James M. Smith

Introduction 272
Improvement and Timely Implementation.................. 273
Causation 274
Process and Solution.................................... 274
Additional Consideration................................ 276
Analyzing Data: Tests of Statistical Significance 278
Analyzing Data: Correlations............................ 280
Presenting Data 283
    Types of Charts...................................... 284
Summary 285

**CHAPTER 14 Using Informatics and Healthcare
Technologies to Guide CNL Practice**......................**289**

Julia Stocker Schneider

Introduction 290
Nursing Informatics..................................... 290
Role of IT in Healthcare................................. 291
Electronic Health Record 291
Barriers to Health IT Adoption 291
HITECH Act... 292
Meaningful Use 292
EHR Maturity 293

Emerging Health IT Tools and Applications 293
   Tablets 293
   Patient Education and Engagement. 294
   Telehealth. 294
   mHealth 294
   Algorithms/Machine-Learning Models 295
Informatics Competencies 295
CNL Informatics Competencies 295
Core Healthcare Informatics Knowledge, Skills, and Abilities
   for CNL Practice. 296
CNL Informatics Competency Themes 297
   Use of Technology to Support Patient Care. 297
   Clinical Decision Support. 297
   Understanding and Evaluating Data 298
   Communicating and Disseminating Healthcare Information. 298
   Patient Safety, Risk Management, and Care Improvement 299
   Systems Life Cycle 299
   Privacy and Security 300
Summary 301

CHAPTER 15 Transitions in Care. 313

Linda A. Roussel

Introduction 314
Distinction Between Transitional Care and Transitions
   of Care. 318
Transitions in Care and Their Impact on Quality and Safe
   Patient Outcomes. 318
Root Causes of Ineffective Transitions of Care 320
Transitions of Care Models: Major Components of the
   Most Commonly Used Frameworks 321
Summary 323

**CHAPTER 16 The CNL's Role in Population Health
and Management 345**

Margaret Moore-Nadler, Linda A. Roussel, and Patricia L. Thomas

Population Health 346
Health Promotion and Illness Prevention: Overview. 347
Understanding the Larger Perspective Through the Lens
   of *Healthy People 2020* and *2030* 347
Context for Public Health and Health
   of Communities: Policy and Action. 348
Promoting the Foundational Capabilities of Population Health. . . . 350
Summary 351

CHAPTER 17 **Achieving Excellence in CNL Practice** **361**

James L. Harris, Linda A. Roussel, and Patricia L. Thomas

Introduction 362
Science of Innovation. 362
The Need for Clinical Leadership. 364
Clinical Leadership Behaviors 365
Information Management, Technology, and Analysis:
   A Core Skill to Lead Change 366
Engagement, Teams, Satisfaction, and Outcomes
   Necessary to Lead 367
Contemporary Leadership Theories. 367
   Servant Leadership. 367
   Listening. 368
   Empathy. 368
   Healing. 368
   Awareness. 368
   Persuasion 368
   Conceptualization. 368
   Foresight 368
Stewardship 369
Commitment to the Growth of People 369
   Building Community 369
   Transactional and Transformational Leadership 369
Microsystem Partnerships and Clinical Leadership
   Through Team Science. 371
CNLs in Action 371
Conclusion 371
Summary 372

CHAPTER 18 **The CNL Engagement in Health Policy** **383**

James L. Harris, Linda A. Roussel, and Patricia L. Thomas

Introduction 384
Health Policy, Engagement, and Advocacy Defined 384
Unintended Consequences of Health Policy: CNLs Respond. 387
Trends and Impacts of Health Policy 388
Summary 390

CHAPTER 19 **CNL Certification and Professional
Development.** **395**

Linda A. Roussel, James L. Harris, and Patricia L. Thomas

Introduction 396
CNL Certification 396

Professionalism 397
CNL Transition to Practice 398
Professional Development 402
The CNLA 403
Summary 404

**CHAPTER 20 Creating a Culture of Health
and Wellness: A Catalyst for Sustaining
the CNL's Role** **407**
Linda A. Roussel, James L. Harris, and Patricia L. Thomass

Introduction 408
National and International Initiatives Supporting
    Healthy Workplaces 410
IHI Joy in the Workplace 410
American Nurses Association's Healthy Nurse,
    Healthy Nation Campaign 411
AACN Healthy Work Environments 412
WHO's Healthy Workplace Framework and Model 413
Resiliency 413
Approaches to Building Resiliency 414
Resiliency Tools 416
Storytelling Activity 416
The Upside of Stress Activity 416
Perform Acts of Kindness Activities 416
Gratitude Activities 417
Body Scan Activities 417
Measuring Resilience 418
Connor-Davidson Resilience Scale (CD-RISC) 418
Resilience Scale for Adults (RSA) 419
Net Promoter Score (NPS) 419
Brief Resilience Scale (BRS) 419
Daily Visual Measure 420
Maintaining Healthy Work Environments During a Pandemic 420
Summary 420

Index **425**

Preface

The need for clinical nurse leaders (CNLs) has been consistent, but the requirements to be effective in today's healthcare environment have progressively changed. The multiple challenges confronting healthcare facilities have extended beyond the bedside and created new care horizons amid competition, reduced capacity, and a demographic shift in the demand for community and telehealth services. With any challenge comes opportunities for boundless innovation to respond and be forward thinking. CNLs are prepared to contribute to meeting the challenges of healthcare, leading interprofessional improvement teams, advocating for change, and utilizing a myriad of skills that promote meaningful and sustainable outcomes for patients, communities, and healthcare agencies regardless of the setting.

The Fourth Edition provides a different narrative for administrators, educators, and CNLs to view the role through a new lens, create a vision that embraces the role while recognizing its value as an agent for change, innovation, and contribution to the health and well-being of a global society. Using evidence-based content, case exemplars, and reflective learning opportunities, this textbook offers a visionary approach that captures the value and essence of the CNL during a turbulent marker in healthcare history. The CNL of today and in the future will lead, guide, champion change, innovate, and be a significant contributor to the next generation of health care.

James L. Harris
Linda A. Roussel
Patricia L. Thomas

Acknowledgments

Commitment to advancing professional nursing is a marker of a point in time. Since the introduction of the CNL, many improvements in healthcare delivery have occurred through the energies of dedicated leaders, educators, and practicing CNLs. What began as a collaborative effort initiated by the American Association of Colleges of Nursing (AACN) has evolved into a powerful force of administrators, educators, and professionals dedicated to a purposeful goal, exceptional care and teamwork, and continuous improvement. The editors of this textbook recognize the enduring efforts of Dr. Joan Stanley, CNL graduates, educators, and numerous leaders who have forged lasting partnerships. Advancing any journey is never easy, but the efforts are acknowledged nationally and internationally as health disparities are identified and addressed.

James L. Harris
Linda A. Roussel
Patricia L. Thomas

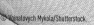

Chapter Contributors

Rebekah Barber, DNP, RN, CNL, LSSGB
RN-Sepsis Coordination
UAB Hospital
Birmingham, AL

Clista C. Clanton, MSLS
Biomedical Library
University of South Alabama
Mobile, AL

Gordana Dermody, PhD, MSN, RN, CNL
Edith Cowan University
Joondalup, Western Australia

James L. Harris, PhD, APRN-BC, MBA, CNL, FAAN
Professor and Coordinator, Clinical
   Nurse Leader Track
University of South Alabama
College of Nursing
Mobile, AL

Keaton Lloyd, MSN, RN, CNL
Nursing Professional Development
   Specialist
UAB Hospital
Birmingham, AL

Margaret Moore-Nadler, DNP, RN
Associate Professor
University of South Alabama
College of Nursing
Mobile, AL

Charlene Myers, DNP, RN, ACNP-BC
Associate Professor
University of South Alabama
College of Nursing
Mobile, AL

Kristen Noles, DNP, RN, CNL
Quality and Process Improvement
USA Health
Mobile, AL

Linda A. Roussel, PhD, RN, NEA-BC, CNL, FAAN
Nursing Education Consultant

Shanda Scott, DNP, RN, CRNP, ANP-BC
Assistant Professor
University of South Alabama
College of Nursing
Mobile, AL

James M. Smith, PhD
Consultant
LaGrangeville, NY

Kathleen R. Stevens, EdD, MS, RN, ANEF, FAAN
Professor and Director, Academic
   Center for Evidence-Based Practice
University of Texas Health Sciences
   Center at San Antonio
Improvement Science Research
   Network
San Antonio, TX

Julia Stocker-Schneider, PhD, RN
University of Detroit Mercy
Detroit, MI

**Patricia L. Thomas, PhD, RN,
NEA-BC, ACNS-BC, CNL, FACHE,
FNAP, FAAN**
Associate Dean, Nursing Faculty
   Affairs
Associate Professor
Wayne State University
College of Nursing
Detroit, MI

Lonnie K. Williams, MSN, RN
Consultant
Washington, DC

Exemplar Contributors

Jennifer Acken, RN
Texas Department of Criminal Justice
Galveston, TX

Kristi Alexander, RN
MD Anderson Cancer Center
Houston, TX

Ericia Arnold, MSN, RN, CNL, CHFN
UAB Medical Center
Birmingham, AL

Patricia Baker, MSN, RN-BC, CNL
Formerly at South Texas Veterans
    Health Care System
San Antonio, TX

Glemen Banaglorioso, RN
MD Anderson Cancer Center
Houston, TX

Darla Banks, MS, RN, CNL
Fort Worth, TX

Yorshikka Barringer, MSN, RN, CNL, GRN, CMSRN
Atrium Health's Carolinas Medical
    Center
Charlotte, NC

Toy Bartley, MSN, RN, CNL, CCRN
Sparrow Hospital and Health System
Lansing, MI

Miriam Bender, PhD, MSN, RN, CNL
Associate Professor and Associate Dean
    for Academic and Student Affairs
University of California, Irvine
Irvine, CA

Barbara Bonnah, MSN, RN, CNL
Hunterdon Medical Center
Flemington, NJ

Susan Blumstein, MT, CIC, CPHQ
UAB Medical Center
Birmingham, AL

Denise Bourassa, MSN, RNC, CNL, CNE
University of Connecticut School of
    Nursing
Storrs, CT

Tru Byrnes, DNP, RN-BC, CNL, CMRSN
Central Division Geriatric
    CNL/NICHE Coordinator
Atrium Health's Carolinas Medical
    Center
Charlotte, NC

Lihui Cao, MSN, RN-BC, CNL
MD Anderson Cancer Center
Houston, TX

Heidi Chappell, MSN, RN-BC, CNL, CHPN
Atrium Health's Carolinas Medical
    Center
Charlotte, NC

Cathy Coleman, DNP, RN, OCN, CPHQ, CNL
University of San Francisco
Assistant Professor
San Francisco, CA

Cassie Crauswell, MSN, CNRN, CNL
Texas Health Resources
Fort Worth, TX

Patricia Davis, DNP, RN-BC, MS, NEA-BC, CNL
CNL Track Coordinator
University of Texas Medical Branch
Galveston, TX

Catherine Delanoix, MS, RN, CNL, ONC
MD Anderson Cancer Center
Houston, TX

Gordana Dermody, PhD, MSN, RN, CNL
Edith Cowan University
Joondalup, Western Australia

Megan T. Dickinson, BSN, RN
CNL Student, University of South
    Alabama College of Nursing
USA Health
Mobile, AL

Jessica R. Driscoll, MSN, RN
Tampa, FL

Lucila Duarte, RN
Texas Health Resources
Fort Worth, TX

Patricia Eagan, MS, RN-BC
University of Connecticut
Storrs, CT

Courtney D. Edwards, MSN, RN
University of Alabama at Birmingham
Birmingham, AL

Lisabeth Emley, MSN, RN, CNL, CNE
Instructor
University of South Alabama College
    of Nursing
Mobile, AL

Ann Eubanks, MSN, RN, CNL
Mobile, AL

Madalyn Frank-Cooper, MS, RN, CNL
Winthrop University Hospital
Mineola, NY

Heather Galang, MSN, RN-BC, CNL
UAB Medical Center
Birmingham, AL

Samantha Gillam, MSN, RN
Saucier, MS

Meridith Gombar, MSN, RN, CNL
Atrium Health's Carolinas Medical
    Center
Charlotte, NC

Bridget Graham, MSN, RN-BC, CNL
Mercy Health, Mercy Saint Mary's
    Grand Rapids Campus
Grand Rapids, MI

Bethel Guk-Ong, MS, RN, CNL, ONC
MD Anderson Cancer Center
Houston, TX

Nicholas Hall, MSN, RN
Nursing Professional Development
    Specialist
UAB Hospital
Birmingham, AL

Melanie Hamilton, MSN RN
Atlanta, GA

Melanie Hanes, RN, CCRN
Texas Health Resources
Fort Worth, TX

Sharon Hayes, MSN, RN
UAB Medical Center
Birmingham, AL

Lauren Hardin, MSN, RN-BC, CNL
Director Cross Continuum
    Transformation
National Center for Complex Health
    and Social Needs, Camden Coalition
    of Healthcare Providers
Camden, NJ

Mary Harnish, MSN, RN, CDE, CNL
Mercy Health, Mercy Saint Mary's
 Grand Rapids Campus
Grand Rapids, MI

Valerie Heinl, MSN, RN, CNL
USA Health
Mobile, AL

Kevin Hengeveld, MSN, RN, CNL
Mercy Health, Mercy Saint Mary's
 Grand Rapids Campus
Grand Rapids, MI

Neetha Jawe, MSN, RN, CNL
MD Anderson Cancer Center
Houston, TX

Amanda Johnson, BSN, RN
Infection Control and Disease
 Prevention Coordinator
USA Health Children's and Women's
 Hospital
Mobile, AL

Carla Johnson, MSN, RN, CNL, CCRN
MD Anderson Cancer Center
Houston, TX

Minami Kakuta, MSN, RN, CNL
Saint Anthony College of Nursing
Rockford, IL

Jennifer Kareivis, MSN, RN, CNL
Hunterdon Medical Center
Flemington, NJ

Susan E. Koons, MSN, RN, CNL
Pine Rest Christian Mental Health
 Services
Grand Rapids, MI

Jessie Kyles, RN
Texas Health Resources
Fort Worth, TX

Kenia Latin, MSN, RN-BC, CPN, ONC, CNL
Texas Department of Criminal Justice
Galveston, TX

Leah Carnick Ledford, MSN, RN-OB, CNL, CCE, SAGE
Atrium Health's Carolinas Medical
 Center
Charlotte, NC

Katrina Lindsay, MSN, RN, CMSRN, CNL
Atrium Health's Carolinas Medical
 Center
Charlotte, NC

Sharon K. Lizer, PhD, APRN, FNP-BC, FAANP
Saint Anthony College of Nursing
 Health Sciences Center
Rockford, IL

Keaton Lloyd, MSN, RN, CNL
Nursing Professional Development
 Specialist
UAB Hospital
Birmingham, AL

Christina Lupo, MSN, RN, CCRN, CNL
Texas Health Resources
Fort Worth, TX

Myrna Martinez, MS, RN, ONC, CNL
MD Anderson Cancer Center
Houston, TX

Lyzanne Mason, MSN, RN, CCRN-CSC
MD Anderson Cancer Center
Houston, TX

Kristin Mast, MSN, RN, CNL, CNRN, SCRN
Mercy Health, Mercy Saint Mary's
 Grand Rapids Campus
Grand Rapids, MI

Amy McRae, MHA, RN, JD
Director of Quality Management
USA Health Children's and Women's
 Hospital
Mobile, AL

Donna Meador, MSN, RN
Akron, OH

Noel Mendez, MS, RN-BC, ONC, CNL
MD Anderson Cancer Center
Houston, TX

Brandie Messer, DNP, RN, PCOE
Saint Anthony College of Nursing
  Health Sciences Center
Rockford, IL

Lisa Mestas, MSN, RN, CORN
Chief Nursing Officer
USA Health
Mobile, AL

Toby Meyers, MSN, RN, ONC, CNL
MD Anderson Cancer Center
Houston, TX

Sharon Mills, MSN, RN
UAB Medical Center
Birmingham, AL

David C. Mulkey, DNP, RN, CPHQ, CCRN, CHSE
Denver Health
Denver, CO

Gladis Mundakal, RN
Texas Health Resources
Fort Worth, TX

Alex Nava, MSN, RN, CNL, PCCN, CMSRN
Texas Health Resources
Fort Worth, TX

Brunella Neely, RN, CNL
Texas Health Resources
Fort Worth, TX

Ann Nguyen, MSN, RN, WCC
University of San Francisco
San Francisco, CA

Kristen Noles, DNP, RN, CNL
Quality and Process Improvement
USA Health
Mobile, AL

Tommie Norris, DNS, RN, CNL
University of Tennessee Health
  Sciences Center
Memphis, TN

Kylia Parker
Sterile Processing Department
  Manager
USA Health Children's and Women's
  Hospital
Mobile, AL

Megan Pashnik, MSN, RN, CNL
Mercy Health, Mercy Saint Mary's
  Grand Rapids Campus
Grand Rapids, MI

Beverly Phillips, RN, CWOCN
Hunterdon Medical Center
Flemington, NJ

Leslie Phillips, MSN, RN, CNL
St. Joseph Mercy Health System
St. Joseph Mercy Hospital
Ann Arbor, MI

Rebecca Pomrenke, MSN, RN, CNL
USA Health
Mobile, AL

Sarah Pratt, MSN, RNC-OB, CNL
Atrium Health's Carolinas Medical
  Center
Charlotte, NC

Sarah A. Price, MSN, RN, CNL, SCRN
Atrium Health's Carolinas Medical
  Center
Charlotte, NC

Kaisa Qutermous, MSN, RN-BC, CNL
Atrium Health's Carolinas Medical
  Center
Charlotte, NC

Christine Radzinski Raby, MSN, RN, CMSRN, CNL
Atrium Health's Carolinas Medical
  Center
Charlotte, NC

Veronica Rankin, DNP, RN-BC, CNL, CMSRN, CNL
Atrium Health's Carolinas Medical Center
Charlotte, NC

Lisa Rasimowicz, BSN, RN, CIC
Infection Preventionist
Hunterdon Medical Center
Flemington, NJ

Claudia Reed, DNP, CRNP, WHNP-BC, RNC-OB, SANE
Nurse Practitioner
OB-GYN Evaluation Center
University of South Alabama
Children's and Women's Hospital
Mobile, AL

Linda A. Roussel, PhD, RN, NEA-BC, CNL, FAAN
Nursing Education Consultant

Kathy Roye-Horn, RN, CIC
Director of Infection Prevention
Hunterdon Medical Center
Flemington, NJ

Sheri Salas, MSN, RN, CNL
Nurse Administrator and Director of Clinical Resources
USA Health
Mobile, AL

Brandy Santana, MSN, RN, CNL
Atrium Health's Carolinas Medical Center
Charlotte, NC

Laurie Sayer, MSN, RN-C, CNL
Mercy Health, Mercy Saint Mary's Grand Rapids Campus
Grand Rapids, MI

Laurie A. Schwartz, MSN, RN, CEN, CNL
Mercy Health, Mercy Saint Mary's Grand Rapids Campus
Grand Rapids, MI

Michelle Sheets, MSN, RN, CNL
Hunterdon Medical Center
Flemington, NJ

Sallie Shipman, EdD, MSN, RN, CNL
University of Alabama at Birmingham
Birmingham, AL

Libby Skaggs, RN, CCRN
Texas Health Resources
Fort Worth, TX

Janice Sills, MSN, RN, CNL
Atrium Health's Carolinas Medical Center
Charlotte, NC

Sarah Simon, MSN, RN-BC, CNL
Mercy Health, Mercy Saint Mary's Grand Rapids Campus
Grand Rapids, MI

John Sims, RN, CMSRN
Texas Health Resources HEB Hospital
Bedford, TX

Danell Stengem, MSN, RN-BC, CNL
Texas Health Resources
Fort Worth, TX

Dawn Stokley, MSN, RN, CNL
University of South Children's and Women's Hospital
Mobile, AL

Hilary Sullivan, MSN, RN, CNL, OCN
MD Anderson Cancer Center
Houston, TX

Monique Swanson, MSN, RN
Alea, HI

Maureen Tait, MSN, RN, CNL
St. Joseph Mercy Health Center, St. Joseph Mercy Hospital
Ann Arbor, MI

Amber Tarwin, MSN, RN, CNL
MD Anderson Cancer Center
Houston, TX

Vidette Todaro-Franceschi, PhD, RN, FT
Hunter-Bellevue School of Nursing
New York, NY

Jennifer H. Towery, MSN, RN, CNL
UAB Hospital
Birmingham, AL

Elizabeth Triezenberg, MSN, RN, CNL, CNRN
Mercy Health, Mercy Saint Mary's
Grand Rapids Campus
Grand Rapids, MI

Tiffany Tscherne, MSN, RN
Mobile, AL

Rebecca Valko, MSN, RN, CNL, CNRN
Mercy Health, Mercy Saint Mary's
Grand Rapids Campus
Grand Rapids, MI

Beth VanDam, MSN, RN-BC, CNL
Mercy Health, Mercy Saint Mary's
Grand Rapids Campus
Grand Rapids, MI

Teresa Vanderford, MSN, RN, CNL
Brighton, CO

Jessie Vaughn, MSN, RN, CNL, OCN
MD Anderson Cancer Center
Houston, TX

Sherry Webb, DNSc, NEA-BC, CNL
University of Tennessee, Memphis
Memphis, TN

Gabriela Whitener, MS, RN, CCRN
Texas Health Resources HEB Hospital
Bedford, TX

Elizabeth F. Williams, MSN, RN, CNL
Saucier, MS

David Wolf, RN
Texas Health Resources Plano
Plano, TX

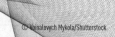

Reviewers

Helene M. Bowen Brady, DNP,
M.Ed, RN-BC, NEA-BC

Catherine M Concert, DNP, RN,
FNP-BC, AOCNP, NE-BC, CNL,
CGRN, FNAP, FNYAM
Assistant Clinical Professor
Graduate Nursing Department
College of Health Professions
Lienhard School of Nursing
Pace University
Nurse Practitioner Radiation Oncology
NYU Langone Health
New York, NY

Linda L. Cook, DNP, APRN,
NNP-BC, CNL
Program Director Clinical Nurse
  Leader Program
Clinical Associate Professor
Davis and Henley College of Nursing
Sacred Heart University
Fairfield, CT

Gordana Dermody, PhD, RN, CNL

Tonya C. Sawyer-McGee, DNP,
MBA, MSN, ACNP

Elizabeth Sloss, MSN, MBA,
RN, CNL
Department of Professional Nursing
  Practice, School of Nursing &
  Health Studies
Georgetown University
Washington, D.C.

Janice Wilcox DNP, RN, CNL
The Ohio State University College of
  Nursing
Columbus, OH

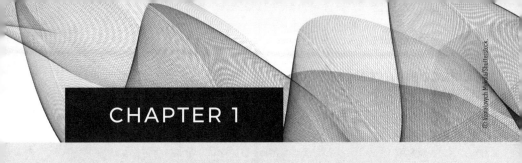

CHAPTER 1

The Clinical Nurse Leader Footprint Across the Healthcare Landscape

James L. Harris, Linda A. Roussel, and Patricia L. Thomas

LEARNING OBJECTIVES

1. Discuss how Clinical Nurse Leaders (CNLs) are transforming care in a constantly changing healthcare environment.
2. Describe the evolution of the CNL and future directions for education and practice alliances.

KEY TERMS

Communication
Education and practice alliances
Evidence-based practice
Healthcare alliances
Health equity
Lateral integration

Microsystem
Outcomes
Partnerships
Social determinants of health
Sustainability
Value

CNL ROLES

Advocate
Communicator
Coordinator
Financial steward

Leader
Lifelong learner
Risk anticipator

PROFESSIONAL VALUES

Advocacy
Collaboration

Social justice

CNL COMPETENCIES

Care coordination   Innovation
Communication   Leadership
Critical thinking

Introduction

Complexity, change, quality and safety requirements, financial viability, care fragmentation, big data challenges, and consumer demands are but a few of the issues that are commonplace in contemporary healthcare environments. Remaining
mindful of these issues, their influence, and interconnectivity challenges even the
most prepared leader and clinician. Responding to these issues requires innovative
approaches that bridge clinical demands with sustainable business approaches and
an educated workforce. Embracing a mindset of innovation and sustainability as the
linkage between improved global healthcare, lower costs, and practice/education
alliances will result in long-term solutions. Value, evidence-based solutions, and
collaborative teamwork are requisites for long-term success in healthcare as the
fourth industrial revolution evolves and is characterized by new technologies that
engage individuals rather than replace them (Edwards et al., 2020; Schwab, 2017).

For several decades, the American Association of Colleges of Nursing (AACN)
has proactively engaged in dialogue and purposeful actions in response to the demands of an evolving healthcare system. From the dialogue among a variety of
stakeholders and their subsequent actions, a preferred vision for the future of nursing and new models of nursing education have emerged. Most notable is the CNL.
Prepared at the master's-degree level, CNLs practice across populations in healthcare
settings, with a focus on quality improvement, interprofessional communication,
evidence-based practice, and care coordination at the point of care. A CNL differs
from a clinical nurse specialist (CNS) who is an expert in a specific clinical area such
as mental health nursing. CNLs and CNSs in many healthcare systems work in tandem within the same microsystem. The CNL consults with the CNS for clinical specialty intervention and then supports implementation using quality improvement
strategies that results in seamless evidence-based practices and patient outcomes.

Guiding CNL practice and education are 10 assumptions communicated by
the AACN. The assumptions guided CNL competency identification and curricula
design. These assumptions included:

1. Practice is at the microsystem level.
2. Client care outcomes are the measure of quality practice.
3. Practice guidelines are based on evidence.
4. Client-centered practice is intra- and interdisciplinary.
5. Information will maximize self-care and client decision-making.
6. Nursing assessment is the basis for theory and knowledge development.
7. Good fiscal stewardship is a condition of quality care.
8. Social justice is an essential nursing value.
9. Communication technology will facilitate the continuity and comprehensiveness of care.
10. The CNL must assume guardianship for the nursing profession (AACN, 2007).

As a leader in healthcare systems, the CNL designs, implements, and evaluates care through coordination and delegation within defined parameters. The defining aspects of CNL practice include:

- Leadership in the care of patients in and across settings
- Implementation of evidence-based practice in all healthcare settings for diverse and complex patients
- Coordination of care
- Lateral integration of care for a cohort of patients
- Clinical decision-making
- Risk anticipation, specifically evaluating anticipated risks to patient safety with the aim of quality improvement and preventing medical errors
- Participation in the identification and collection of care outcomes
- Accountability for evaluation and improvement of point-of-care outcomes
- Mass customization of care
- Interprofessional communication
- Leveraging human, environmental, and material resources
- Client and community advocacy
- Education for individuals, families, groups, and other healthcare providers
- Information management, including using information systems and technology at the point of care to improve healthcare outcomes
- Oversight of care delivery and outcomes
- Team leadership and collaboration with other professional team members (AACN, 2007)

Building on the AACN's 2007 white paper, revised expected outcomes and competencies emerged and are found in *Competencies and Curricular Expectations for Clinical Nurse Leader Education and Practice* (AACN, 2013). The revised CNL competencies build on the AACN, *The Essentials of Master's Education in Nursing* (2011), to provide a comprehensive view of expected outcomes of CNL education. The linkage of the master's essentials to the CNL competencies facilitates curriculum development. As with any expectation, outcomes, or competencies, continuous revisions of defining aspects of practice are fundamental to ongoing progress. This is evidenced by the work of a national consensus-based process to guide uniformity in curricula, student experiences, and continuous changes necessary for the CNL certification examination.

With the initiation of an AACN group tasked with revision of the Essentials, 10 domains commensurate with competencies and subcompetencies will provide a progressive link to nursing education and clinical practice. The revision provides a roadmap for achievement of competency-based outcomes that build on CNL competencies and curricular expectations. This forward approach further validates the AACN's ongoing commitment to a nursing workforce that is positioned to meet the imperatives for quality, safety, and efficiency in a global healthcare market.

CNL Footprint Past and Present

Throughout history, disruptive forces have affected organizations, individuals, and clinical practice. This is certainly evident when one considers the disruptive forces shaping healthcare's future. With health expenditures consuming more each year, one may easily question, is the future healthcare system sustainable (Cottarelli, 2010)?

CNLs are valuable assets in sustaining value-based care delivery and responding to the disruptive forces influencing healthcare. Five predominate disruptive forces are and will continue to influence healthcare beyond the present year into future decades. These forces will offer multiple opportunities for CNL interventions and collaboration. The five forces include: (1) the graying patient and provider, (2) the rise of chronic disease, (3) the information revolution, (4) the unintended consequences of technology and big data, and (5) the new healthcare consumer (Advisory Board Company, 2012). As nursing and healthcare teams respond to a global pandemic, CNLs are and will continue to be responsive to this global demand and future ones in varying microsystems.

The very nature of the CNL provides a lens for reflection and action. Specifically, Clinical (C) is the focus of healthcare—notably, access, safety, quality, care alternatives, wellness, prevention, and patient-centeredness. Nurse (N) denotes nursing actions that result in holistic care, systems-oriented thinking, relationship building, teamwork, organizational savvy, change, and increased quality. Leader (L) exemplifies leaders who work with and through others to improve and transform care (Joanne Disch, personal communication, January 16, 2016).

As Mary Wakefield stated, "This is nursing's time" (personal communication, October 17, 2015). CNL practice exemplifies Wakefield's statement, because significant impacts are evident in a variety of healthcare settings. The case for CNLs is further demonstrated because the business of care provides evidence of decreased length of stay, microsystem assessments that identify frequent causes of unexpected events, and increased quality of care. A culture of health and achievement of health equity are also essential, and CNLs will contribute to attaining this goal and its sustainability (Hassmiller & Kuehnert, 2020).

As the number of CNLs increases, outcomes and sustainable evidence-based practice will continue to be apparent. Innovation and influence by CNLs are unmistakable. However, the great need for improvement in healthcare carries with it an opportunity for priorities to be defined. Rigorous, focused inquiry that results in measurable outcomes must follow.

Priorities inform decisions for work that needs to be accomplished. CNLs will remain at the forefront of collaboratively engaging in partnerships that shape sustainable outcomes in care delivery, cost avoidance, and risk aversion. Quality improvement and patient safety are imperative clinical targets that are supported by policy, professional groups, partnerships, and patient advocacy (Kathleen Stevens, personal communication, November 21, 2015). Without CNL engagement in interprofessional partnerships, the means of gaining efficiency in care delivery may not be achieved. Likewise, rigorous inquiry that produces reliable outcome data and quantifies CNL value is imperative. Documenting the collective outcomes from interprofessional teams partnership is key in the efficacy of care delivery.

Time is a precious commodity and results must remain actionable, which are the cornerstone dating back to the first group of CNLs to enter the practice. Actionable results by CNLs continue today and create the landscape for future measurable outcomes directed at quality, safety, and value-based care across populations.

Early examples of CNL outcomes primarily focused on inpatient acute settings. While many of these outcomes were anecdotal, others were reported in professional publications and at local, regional, and national conferences. Stanley and colleagues (2008) reported care outcomes in three healthcare settings. Outcomes included improvement in the Centers for Medicare and Medicaid Services (CMS) core measures such as pain management, congestive heart failure, improved team collaboration, higher patient satisfaction, and decreased registered nurse turnover. Gabuat and colleagues (2008) described a CNL pilot initiative that resulted in decreased nursing turnover, increased patient and physician satisfaction, and improved core measures.

The Veterans Health Administration (VHA) was an early adopter of the CNL role and remains an active partner. In collaboration with the AACN, the VA Tennessee Valley Healthcare System conducted a pilot study of an evaluation tool to capture pre- and post-assignment of unit-based CNLs and was the first VHA facility to employ CNLs (Harris et al., 2006). Early findings from the pilot study were positive and included decreased length of stay for patients diagnosed with congestive heart failure (CHF), increased discharge instructions for patients with CHF, decreased falls with injuries, and decreased surgical infection rates 30 days postoperative. Additional outcome evaluations followed and were reported to include a 20% decrease in blood transfusions post-total knee arthroplasty on an inpatient surgical unit and venous thromboembolism prophylaxis protocol implementation for intubated critically ill patients and an 8% increase participation in restorative dining on a transitional care unit (Hix et al., 2009).

In keeping with the commitment of CNL that spread throughout the VHA, an evaluation and implementation section was formed. This section was charged with ensuring the ongoing expansion of the CNL initiative throughout the healthcare system, CNL transition to practice, and an avenue for disseminating impacts of the CNL within a major healthcare system. As the number of CNLs within the VHA increased, a field advisory committee was formed to advance the preceding, evaluation, and implementation section as an advisory group to advancing CNL practice throughout the healthcare system (James Harris, personal communication, January 14, 2016).

Other significant CNL reported outcomes at Maine Medical Center included an 18.2% decrease in critical care days and a 40% decrease in returns to the critical care unit. These outcomes resulted in a financial savings of $800,000 over a 14-month period after CNL-initiated interdisciplinary rounds on long-term ventilator patients. Another CNL was able to collaborate with orthopedic surgeons and blood bank personnel to eliminate retransfusion of blood cells in identified patients leading to decreased infections and a significant cost savings. As more CNLs enter the workforce and the shift from inpatient to alternative care settings occurs, numerous outcomes will be present, further demonstrating the value of embedding CNLs into existing and new models of care.

Future Implications for CNL Education and Practice

One may question, is educating CNLs and positive clinical outcomes the primary answer to care fragmentation and the multiple other issues confronting the current healthcare environment? While this is not the exclusive answer, educating nurses who function as CNLs upon graduation and become certified is one approach to a fragmented delivery system. The CNL is not a replacement for other nursing roles but rather complementary to those who work in tandem with all providers to deliver patient-centered care (Joan Stanley, personal communication, January 8, 2016). The unique education and resultant systems and leadership lens positions CNLs to contribute to care delivery that extends beyond traditional acute care boundaries. Quality improvement, project and data management, establishment of plans and projects to address resistant practice outcomes, and the impacts of mentorship to build caregiver resilience position CNLs to bring sustainable, value-added outcomes to patients and organizations alike.

The call to action for changing the ways health professionals are educated and care is delivered is now. Simulated learning experiences are increasingly available allowing care teams to learn together and share experiences that replicate real-world clinical environments. Patient care is being delivered in multiple settings. Complex procedures are delivered in ambulatory settings, home settings, and other alternative care settings. Inpatient care days will continue to decrease. Volume is no longer the goal of inpatient care. Quality is the key and will continue to be rewarded. Education must continue to embrace and include learning experiences that focus on quality, safety, and value-based care. Additionally, partnerships between education and practice are critical to making a lasting impact on care delivery. As CNLs engage in lifelong learning, opportunities to transition to doctor of nursing practice programs is encouraged and possible. This further develops the CNLs' abilities to impact care delivery at the microsystem level and beyond while responding to new reforms that secure the development of healthcare and a spirit of entrepreneurship.

From Evolution to a Peaceful Revolution

As healthcare organizations continue to integrate CNLs into care delivery models, the CNLs' impact on quality, safety, and value will be realized. During the past decade, the CNL has evolved primarily from inpatient care to a variety of care settings. The exponential growth of CNLs in practice offers opportunities to meet the challenges today and in the immediate future. Partnerships between education and practice remain pivotal in advancing CNL outcomes. A peaceful revolution of future CNL preparation will continuously result in positive outcomes and actions that complement other healthcare providers. Dissemination of information on the impacts of CNLs at national conferences must continue, and publications that highlight clinical outcomes are essential. Collaborative research is needed to identify determinants of CNL success and care models most suited for embedding CNLs into all care settings.

What started as an evolutionary process in response to fragmented care delivery has transitioned into a peaceful revolution preparing dedicated individuals to meet the healthcare challenges of today and in future decades. The time is now to adopt a culture of inclusivity where the CNL is embedded in existing and new models of care. Using experiences and CNL practice outcomes are leverage for future successes and educational directions. History repeats itself, so let us learn from the past and embrace a bright future of healthcare delivery and create alliances dedicated to greatness in the trusted profession of nursing.

It is the desire of the editors of the fourth edition of *Clinical Nurse Leaders Beyond the Microsystem: A Practical Guide* to be responsive to educating CNLs and spreading the value of CNL practice. This chapter has introduced the CNL footprint past, present, and future. The chapters that follow provide information that guide CNL education and practice. Chapter content includes:

- The CNL as a microsystem leader
- Quality and safety imperatives for CNL practice
- Managing quality data and the role of big data and analytics
- Care transitions and CNL practice
- Improvement and team sciences
- Evidence-based practice guides
- The role of CNLs in health policy, advocacy organizational influence in a global society
- Population health and management
- Mobilizing team engagement and interprofessional collaboration through microsystem leadership
- Health equity, health literacy, and attainment of social determinants of health
- Design thinking and value to CNL practice and outcomes
- Innovation
- Communication
- Community advocacy, resource mindfulness, and networking
- Selecting preceptors while readying the environment for a successful experience
- Meaningful and sustainable clinical projects
- Project management basics and tools
- Informatics and healthcare technologies
- Achieving CNL practice excellence
- Advancing the CNL initiative through certification, professional membership, and residency programs
- CNL sustainability

Summary

- The AACN was proactive in initiating dialogue and introducing the CNL in response to fragmentation of care and the demands of an evolving healthcare system.
- CNLs differ from CNSs. CNLs' work is targeted toward microsystem improvements at the point of care, whereas CNSs focus on a clinical specialty and work across healthcare systems.
- CNL practice and education is guided by 10 assumptions and expected outcomes and competencies found in *Competencies and Curricular Expectations for Clinical Nurse Leader Education and Practice* (AACN, 2007, 2013).
- CNLs are a valuable asset in sustaining value-based care delivery within microsystems and responding to disruptive forces in healthcare systems and a global society challenged with new reforms in healthcare, big data, and analytics.
- As the number of CNLs has increased during the past decade, positive outcomes and sustainable evidence-based practice have occurred.
- The CNL is not a replacement for other nursing roles but rather is complementary, working in tandem with all providers to deliver patient-centric care.

- What started as an evolutionary process in response to fragmented care delivery has transitioned into the preparation of dedicated individuals to meet the challenges of healthcare today and in future decades.

Reflection Questions

1. What value does a business case offer to support the adoption of CNLs in healthcare settings?
2. How may CNLs respond to the disruptive forces facing healthcare nationally and globally?
3. Consider the outcomes associated with CNL practice during the past decade. What strategies will prove effective in sustaining the footprint of CNLs across populations in future decades?

Learning Activities

1. Evaluate where your organization is in spreading the CNL role throughout the healthcare system. Consider the pros and cons for systemwide implementation.
2. What patient outcomes are you aware of that could benefit from the CNL role? Formulate a business plan for implementing the role within a microsystem.
3. Develop a community outreach program focusing on meeting the social determinants of health.

References

Advisory Board Company. (2012). *The five forces shaping health care's future: Determining strategy to an evolving environment.* Author.

American Association of Colleges of Nursing. (2007). *White paper on the role of the Clinical Nurse Leader* (pp. 6–11). Author. https://nursing.uiowa.edu/sites/default/files/documents/academic-programs/graduate/msn-cnl/CNL_White_Paper.pdf

American Association of Colleges of Nursing. (2011). *The essentials of master's education in nursing.* Author.

American Association of Colleges of Nursing. (2013). *Competencies and curricular expectations for clinical nurse leader education and practice* (pp. 9–22). Author.

Cottarelli, C. (2010). *Macro-fiscal implications of health care reform in advanced and emerging economies.* International Monetary Fund. https://www.imf.org/external/np/pp/eng/2010/122810.pdf

Edwards, R. L., Markaki, A., Shiley, M. R., & Patrician, P. A. (2020). A model operationalizing sustainability in global nursing. *Nursing Outlook, 68*(3), 345–354.

Gabuat, J., Hilton, N., Kinnaird, L. S., & Sherman, R. O. (2008). Implementing the clinical nurse leader role in a for-profit environment. *Journal of Nursing Administration, 38*(6), 302–307.

Harris, J. L., Walters, S. E., Quinn, C., Stanley, J., & McGuinn, K. (2006). *The Clinical Nurse Leader role: A pilot evaluation by an early adopter.* AACN. http://www.aacn.nche.edu/cnl/pdf/VAEvalSynopsis.pdf

Hassmiller, S. B., & Kuehnert, P. (2020). Building a culture of health to attain the sustainable development goals. *Nursing Outlook, 68*(2), 129–133.

Hix, C., McKeon, L., & Walters, S. E. (2009). Clinical Nurse Leader impact on clinical microsystems outcomes. *Journal of Nursing Administration, 39*(2), 71–76.

Schwab, K. (2017). *The fourth industrial revolution.* Random House.

Stanley, J. M., Cannon, J., Gabuat, J., Hartranft, S., Adams, N., Mayes, C., Shouse, G. M., Edwards, B. A., & Burch, D. (2008). The Clinical Nurse Leader: A catalyst for improving quality and patient safety. *Journal of Nursing Management, 16*(5), 614–622.

Wiggins, M. (2008, June 8). *The Clinical Nurse Leader demands in healthcare require new innovation.* Presentation made to the Joint Commission-Nursing Advisory Council.

Developing a CNL Practice Model: An Interpretive Synthesis of the Literature

Miriam Bender

Objective

The Institute of Medicine's (IOM) *Future of Nursing* report identifies the need for nurses to engage in innovative practice in order to meet higher healthcare quality standards. The purpose of this study was to clarify CNL practice components contributing to improved interprofessional collaborative patient care standards. The AACN CNL white paper defines CNL core competencies necessary for practice. The literature documents preliminary evidence of improved outcomes associated with CNL integration into clinical microsystems. However, the CNL role is not yet clearly defined in terms of the fundamental activities and responsibilities necessary to produce outcomes. Lack of practice clarity limits the ability to articulate, implement, and measure CNL-specific practice and outcomes.

Methods

An interpretive synthesis was conducted to integrate the extant CNL literature into a coherent understanding of CNL practice. A literature search was conducted in CINAHL, PubMed, Dissertations and Theses, and Google, using the search term *Clinical Nurse Leader*. Results were reviewed and included if they described any aspect of CNL practice *in action*: 30 implementation reports, 8 qualitative/mixed methods studies, 3 quantitative studies, and 244 conference abstracts were included in the final synthesis. Grounded theory methodology was utilized to reanalyze primary CNL evidence and identify domains and components of CNL practice.

Results

CNL practice encompasses five domains: preparation for CNL practice; the structure of CNL practice; the core phenomenon of CNL practice, which is continuous leadership at the point of practice; outcomes of CNL practice; and acceptance. *Preparation for CNL practice* components include a clear understanding of current care delivery deficits, strong leadership support, and an effective change management strategy. *Structure of CNL practice* components include microsystem care delivery redesign, competency-based CNL workflow, and accountability for a defined set of outcomes. *Continuous leadership at the point of practice* components include supporting staff engagement, source of constant communication/information, strengthening interprofessional relationships, team creation, and shifting focus from person to process. *Outcomes of CNL practice* components include improved care environment, improved care quality, and nursing brought to the forefront of healthcare redesign. *Acceptance* components include initial buy-in, exposure, and understanding.

Discussion

The CNL practice model proposes five domains that interact to produce the structure, function, and outcomes of CNL practice. The core phenomenon of CNL practice involves developing relationships across professions to promote and manage information exchange, shared decision making, and effective care processes. The model highlights the importance of a systematic approach to CNL development and implementation, including macro- and microsystem preparation, care delivery redesign, allowing CNLs to function to their full scope of practice, and allowing time for role acceptance. The extent to which each domain is adequately addressed influences the degree of CNL practice success.

Implications

This study advances the understanding of the relatively new CNL role by synthesizing an empirically derived model for CNL development and practice. It clarifies CNL practice components and differentiates them from existing nursing roles and practices. The model can provide a guideline to organizations wanting to implement the CNL. It can also provide a basis for future research identifying quantifiable measures of CNL practice and CNL-specific influence on outcomes.

EXEMPLAR

Transitioning into the CNL Role: One CNL, Two Perspectives

Sarah Simon

As my formal CNL education came to an end, the thought of *What's next?* ran rampant in my thinking. As most new nurses wonder what their future practice is going to look like, my CNL brain had more than enough questions. Being a Model C CNL student, I had to focus on passing my NCLEX first. Once that happened, I was embedded as a staff nurse in a fast-paced 600-bed Magnet-designated hospital. I knew I had to learn quickly and be observant of practice. After eight months as a staff nurse, I was transitioned into the CNL role. The CNL role was not only new for me but also the hospital. Three areas of focus that came to light quickly were quality, safety, and team collaboration. I experienced an interesting transition as I learned to "walk the talk" of a CNL alongside the staff I worked with. The staff were respectfully curious about what a CNL does. I must admit, it was rewarding to have them embrace me as their CNL. We quickly got started on quality and safety concerns. As a team, we went 33 days without a fall on that unit; the longest stretch prior to this was 17 days without a fall when there was no CNL. Although I was young in my nursing career, trust, dedication, and humbleness were very important in my life as a CNL.

After four months of being a CNL at that hospital, I was offered the opportunity to join a hospital that had a team of 11 very well-established CNLs. Again, I was faced with another transition, although this one was very different. Here I joined a team that knows the who, what, when, where, and why of CNL practice. That allowed me and challenged me to hit the ground running, fast and hard! I am now the CNL on a unit that I had no clinical background or expertise on. I have come to realize that this was just fine as the CNL core competencies and applications are what actually guide my daily practice. I am prepared as an advanced generalist, and by focusing to ensure quality and safety, the team's performance falls within and surpasses national standards and guidelines.

During the time I have been a CNL on this unit, the expectation to complete audits on physician and staff documentation was set. In the first month of audits, there was an average of 70.4% completion, the second month 75.4% completion, and the most recent 81.6% completion. Improvements in the completion rates can be attributed to my CNL interventions in coaching, communication, and problem-solving strategies to remove barriers that arise.

I never imagined I would be a CNL that could produce outcomes shown across the country, representing the great work that CNLs do. Although each of us will go through transitions when graduating from a CNL program, transitions from school to practice are exciting when you are able to enact what you learned in school to achieve the anticipated and expected outcomes of the CNL role.

EXEMPLAR

The Evolution of a Nurse-Driven Mobility Initiative on a Certified Stroke Unit:

Pioneering the CNL Role in a Magnet-Designated Medical Center

Gordana Dermody

Background

Stroke is the third-leading cause of death in the United States, resulting in about 137,000 deaths yearly (National Stroke Association, 2010). Approximately 795,000 individuals suffered a stroke last year, and many surviving stroke victims will face a variety of short- and long-term health consequences. Some of the adverse outcomes are directly related to immobility and may include hospital-acquired pressure ulcers, catheter-acquired urinary tract infections, aspiration pneumonia, joint stiffening, muscle atrophy, falls, and weakness from inactivity. In addition, stroke patients may experience less pain from joint stiffening and feelings of increased well-being. Rehabilitation for stroke patients should begin in the acute care setting, making it imperative to maintain and increase patient strength through nurse-driven early and frequent mobility activities as soon as deemed medically stable (National Stroke Association, 2010).

This exemplar describes one CNL student's immersion project initiated at a Magnet-designated hospital in the Midwest. The background, goals, and objectives of the mobility project Let's Move will be discussed. In conclusion, the project outcomes and future implications will be discussed.

During a CNL student practicum, a gap in care for stroke patients emerged after a microsystem and macrosystem analysis of a certified 30-bed stroke unit. A subsequent gap analysis was conducted, which revealed that the promotion of patient mobility activities by nursing assistants and nurses was not meeting clinical practice guideline (CPG) recommendations for patients with stroke or stroke-related diagnosis. Mobility activities for patients with these diagnoses include ambulation of at least 50 feet daily, active/passive range of motion (ROM) to stroke-affected joints, and promoting sitting in a chair for meals (Clinical Practice Management Resource Center, 2007).

Supporting Evidence for the Project

Studies show that early and frequent mobility activities such as ambulation, active/passive ROM, and sitting up in a chair for meals significantly improve the short- and long-term health outcomes of patients with stroke or stroke-related diagnoses (Arias & Smith, 2007; Bernardt et al., 2004; Clinical Practice Management Resource Center, 2007; Kwakkel, 2006; Ming-Hsia et al., 2010). There is agreement in the literature that therapists may have limited time at the bedside in the acute care setting. Subsequently nurses and nursing assistants need to take a proactive approach in promoting early and frequent mobility activities in stroke patients (Bernardt et al., 2004; Skarin et al., 2011).

Early, progressive mobility activities initiated within the first 24–48 hours after a stroke have shown to increase a patient's functional ability and improve health outcomes in multiple ways. Increased mobility has been shown to decrease muscle weakness and increase muscle and joint strength, allowing for more frequent ambulation and increased general well-being of the patient. A decreased rate of deep venous thrombosis is another benefit of ambulation and ROM activities. Furthermore, research shows that sitting up in a chair for meals may reduce pneumonia due to aspiration and promotes deep breathing. Last, frequent and progressive mobility activities have been shown to decrease pressure sores, urinary tract infections, and mobility-related falls and shoulder pain (Arias & Smith, 2001; Bernardt et al., 2004; Clinical Practice Management Resource Center, 2007; Kwakkel, 2006; Ming-Hsia et al., 2010). Because this healthcare organization implemented Jean Watson's relationship-centered care model to guide nursing practice, the model was used to make a case for a nurse-promoted mobility program. Watson's relationship-centered care seeks to enhance the state of wholeness for stroke patients through the alignment of body, soul, and spirit, making it necessary to provide a healing environment for patients, including nurse-driven mobility (McEwen & Wills, 2007).

Project Objectives and Timeline

The goal of this project was to promote nurse-driven mobility early, and frequent mobility in hospitalized stroke patients. The understanding that a nurse-driven mobility initiative involved many stakeholders including nurses, CNAs, physical therapists, patients, and families was imperative for project success. In addition, a strong synergistic relationship and collaboration between the CNS, CNL student, and unit manager was necessary to initiate and sustain the change processes. The literature and *Clinical Practice Guideline for Stroke* were appraised, and nurse-driven mobility protocol and guidelines were developed. In addition, education about mobility, bedside handoff, communication, gait belts and safety, and multidisciplinary collaboration was provided. The duration of the implementation of the nurse-driven mobility protocol was three months. During the last phase of the project an assessment of project outcomes was conducted.

For the purpose of planning interventions, project objectives and interventions were grouped based on the participants of the promotion of mobility including nurses, CNAs, patients, and their families. Strong collaborative relationships were formed with physical therapists that assisted in developing the mobility protocol.

Improve Documentation in the Electronic Medical Patient Record (EMR)

CNAs and nurses were instructed to document mobility activities in the musculoskeletal cells in the document flow sheets section. Ambulation documentation includes the amount of feet the patient has ambulated, sitting up in the chair for meals, and active/passive ROM. The goal was to ensure that 50% of all patients would have one or more mobility activities (ambulate, ROM, up in chair) per day documented in the EMR, under musculoskeletal interventions at the end of the project.

Increase CNA-to-CNA Communication by More Efficient Bedside Handoff

This was measured by observations that indicated that CNAs were away from the nurses' station in the rooms completing the CNA-to-CNA bedside handoff during shift change. The goal was not to observe CNAs standing at the nurses' station giving reports during shift change. Another observation included decreased call lights during shift change, compared with prior to project implementation. In addition, more patients sitting up in chairs were willing to get up at the time of the CNA handoff. Patients reported enjoying breakfast out of bed and having the opportunity to complete morning care early in the day.

Increase CNA-to-Nurse Communication

After project completion, CNAs were resurveyed regarding the communication with nurses. Due to the hectic nature of the unit, the use of the dry-erase board by CNAs and nurses to communicate ambulation goals that were met was one of the project interventions. A postimplementation survey was conducted to measure outcomes. The survey used a Likert scale with 5 = almost always, 4 = often, 3 = sometimes, 2 = rarely, 1 = never. CNAs rated the statement "I check off my patients' mobility activity on the whiteboard" as 3.8. Prior to project implementation, CNAs did not utilize the dry-erase board as a form of communicating to the nurse. In addition, CNAs were asked to report off to the nurse one hour prior to shift end. Anecdotal reports obtained through informal interviews of the unit nurses indicate that more CNAs are reporting off to individual nurses prior to shift end.

Provide Education to CNAs Regarding Safe Basic Mobility Activities for Patients

All unit CNAs received education and performed return demonstrations on how to utilize the gait belt and electronic lift equipment and safely move and mobilize patients, including performing active and passive ROM during the yearly skills lab. Preproject implementation, the unit CNAs rated their comfort with the gait belt and mobility-related assistive devices and equipment between 90–100%. However, gait-belt use on the Likert scale for the question "During the last 30 days I used the gait belt" was rated between "never" and "rarely" (1.43). The postproject survey rating of gait-belt use in the last 30 days is rated between "sometimes" and "often" with 3.5.

Patients and Family

Improve patients and family understanding that participation in rehabilitative activities will enhance functional ability. Provide education to patients and family regarding mobility activities, gait-belt use, and assistive devices. Patient education was provided by the CNL student during daily rounding and working together with the nursing staff to provide the same education to patients. In addition, a patient-friendly brochure was developed and provided, which described the necessity for early and frequent mobility and its benefits. Previous satisfaction surveys indicated that patients felt like they were not involved in their care. In addition, patients and families reported that not enough physical activity was provided for the patient who had suffered from stroke on a certified stroke unit. To help patients understand the importance of mobility, patients received a pictorial handout with active ROM exercises that patients could practice on their own. An informational handout regarding gait-belt use was provided, and patient families received training on how to utilize the gait belt to help their loved one at home prior to discharge. Anecdotal reports from family and patients suggested that the education was helpful and indicated the beginning of rehabilitation for stroke patients while in the acute care setting.

While improving the hospital consumer assessment of healthcare providers and systems (HCAHPS) scores was not a specific goal, unexpectedly an improvement of the HCAHPS ratings related to patients feeling that they are involved in their care and being listened to was found. The unit manager has reported a significant upward trend in patients' rating of the HCAHPS for the three months of project intervention implementation. Prior to project implementation the HCAHPS rating had been reported as being below the 50th percentile, which steadily increased to the 75th percentile concerning items such as "Nurses treat you with courtesy and respect" and "Nurses listen carefully to you."

Nurses

Increase utilization of the patient dry-erase board to improve goal setting with patients, increase patient and family communication, and interdisciplinary collaboration. Set mutually agreed on mobility goal with patients during bedside handoff by inviting patients to be involved in their care. Educate nurses to assess a patient's mobility status and perform basic mobility activities. Prior to the project only 6% (n = 65) of all unit patients had a measurable mobility goal on the whiteboard. The goal was for at least 50% of all patients on the unit to have a specific and measurable mobility goal on the whiteboard. For the purpose of continuity of care for nonstroke patients, and due to low numbers of stroke patients, the interventions were applied to all patients. Prior to the project implementation, nurse-to-nurse patient handoff occurred outside of the patient room, and patients had little opportunity to be involved in the planning of their mobility. Patients' families had expressed feeling disconnected from the progress their loved one was making.

Outcomes

A new bedside handoff tool was created for a new bedside handoff initiative, which was imperative to set mutually agreed on mobility goals with the patients. During the handoff nurses were at the bedside talking with patients and setting mutually agreed on mobility goals with the patients. Nurses then wrote the specific and measurable mobility goal on the dry-erase board and drew simple check-off boxes. For example, "walk in hall ×3, 25 feet." The dry-erase board was a cost- and time-effective method for communicating with CNAs, physical therapists, and physicians. In addition, as patients completed the goals, check-off marks later informed the family members coming to visit about the progress their loved one had made. Nurses' use of the whiteboard to set mutually agreed on mobility goals with patients were measured with biweekly observation of each patient's whiteboard. A steady increase of mobility goals on the board was evident: Week two 48% ($n = 23$); week four 46% ($n = 46$); week six 75% ($n = 28$); week eight 77% ($n = 27$). During week 10 of project implementation 94% ($n = 24$) of all unit patients had at least one specific measurable mobility goal on the whiteboard. Nurse documentation of mobility improved and patients were observed being mobilized significantly more often (**Table 1-1**). The distance of ambulation in feet improved significantly (**Table 1-2**). Anecdotal reports revealed that the presence of physical therapists on the unit increased, and collaborative relationships were being strengthened.

Nurses were surveyed at the end of the project. Nurses rated "I set specific, measurable mobility goals with my patients" between "often" and "almost always" (4.5)

Table 1-1 Documentation of Mobility in EPIC

	Preintervention $n = 19$	Postintervention $n = 36$
ROM	16.1%	17.5%
Ambulation	3.6%	43.7%
Chair	5.4%	37.1%
Positioning	48.2%	64.9%
p < .05 p < .01		

Table 1-2 Distance of Ambulation

Ambulation in Feet	Preintervention ($n = 19$)	Postintervention ($n = 36$)
	no documentation	47% Mean = 247.29 ft Median = 150 ft

on the postmobility project survey. Prior to the project this was rated as "sometimes" (3.2). The statement "I write specific, measurable mobility goals on the whiteboard" was rated "often" (4.1), and prior to project implementation, this was rated as "sometimes" (3.4). Nurses who reported feeling confident in using the gait belt increased from 63% (n = 20) to 79% (n = 19) after project conclusion.

Sustainability and Project Impact on the Organization

The mobility project impacted the organization in multiple ways. First, the organization had the opportunity to experience the CNL role in the microsystem. The organization, a Magnet-designated facility, valued innovative patient care approaches to improve patient outcomes while increasing efficiency. The utilization of existing nursing staff to mobilize patients was a cost-effective approach and was made possible by changing the handoff and rounding process, which resulted in more efficient nursing staff workflow. Furthermore, in light of the limited therapist time at the bedside, utilizing the nursing staff to provide the needed mobility activities helped to increase mobility in stroke patients without requiring a budget increase for more full-time equivalents (FTEs).

In addition, as HCAHPS scores for patient satisfaction significantly increased during the short time of project intervention implementation, the organization has noted the possibility of increased financial benefits due to the CNL role practicum. This has resulted in the creation of a CNL position. This development affected the sustainability of the project in several ways. First, the chief nursing officer has expressed a desire to spread the project to other units, eventually spreading throughout the entire organization. Second, the continued presence of the CNL role and beneficial outcomes of the mobility and other such projects could result in employing CNLs in the future (Harris & Roussel, 2010).

One barrier to the nursing staff that emerged during the project was that the gait belt to safely ambulate patients was frequently lost or was inconveniently located when needed most. In addition, nursing staff expressed concerns about using gait belts in the isolation rooms, fearing cross-contamination. There was no process in place to launder the gait belts. With the CNL student leading the effort, the organization investigated the use of single patient-use gait belts as a dispensable and chargeable patient item. The utilization of single-patient use gait belts was thought to reduce cross-contamination, increase use of gait belts, and improve the safety for patients. To obtain stakeholder buy-in, the physical therapy department was approached to trial single-patient use gait belts in collaboration with nurses from this unit. The cost to patients for this gait belt was minimal ($4), effectively contained the cost of frequently lost unit gait belts, and may help to reduce the severity of injury if a patient has to be lowered to the floor. Through the collaborative work of the CNL student, single-patient use gait belts were adopted systemwide one year later.

In conclusion, it has been said that US healthcare is riddled with costs spiraling out of control, rapid change and growth in biomedical technology, professional shortages, and high turnover, as well as ever-increasing demands for cost containment coupled with better health outcomes for patients (Harris & Roussel, 2010). To bridge the fragmentation of healthcare in the United States, a call for action to impact the current healthcare delivery has been issued (Berwick, 2002; Harris &

Roussel, 2010; IOM, 2011). CNLs across the nation are embarking on responding to the call to improve healthcare delivery. This CNL student project was an example of how the CNL role brings value to healthcare organizations by improving patient outcomes in efficient and cost-effective ways.

References

Arias, M., & Smith, L. N. (2007). Early mobilization of acute stroke patients. *Journal of Clinical Nursing, 16,* 282–288.

Bernardt, J., Dewey, H., & Donnan, G. (2004). Inactive and alone: Physical activity within the first 14 days of acute stroke unit care. *Stroke, 35,* 1005–1009.

Berwick, D. M. (2002). A user's manual for the IOM's "Quality Chasm" report. *Health Affairs, 1*(3), 80–90.

Clinical Practice Management Resource Center. (2007). *Clinical practice guideline: Stroke/transient ischemic attack (TIA).* OSF St. Anthony Medical Center. http://www.osfhealthcare.org

Harris, J. L., & Roussel, L. (2010). *Initiating and sustaining the clinical nurse leader role.* Jones & Bartlett Publishers.

Harris, J. L., Roussel, L., Walters, S. E., & Dearman, C. (2011). *Project planning and management: A guide for CNLs, DNPs, and nurse executives.* Jones & Bartlett Learning.

Institute of Medicine. (2011). *The future of nursing: Leading change, advancing health.* National Academies Press.

Kwakkel, G. (2006). Impact of intensity of practice after stroke: Issues for consideration. *Disability and Rehabilitation, 28*(13), 823–830.

McEwen, M., & Willis, E. M. (2007). *Theoretical basis for nursing* (3rd ed.). Lippincott Williams & Wilkins.

Ming-Hsia, H., Shu-Shyuan, H., Ping-Keung, Y., Jiann-Shing, J., & Yen-Ho, W. (2010). Early and intensive rehabilitation predicts good functional outcomes in patients admitted to the stroke intensive care unit. *Disability and Rehabilitation, 32*(15), 1251–1259.

National Stroke Association. (2010). *Stroke 101* [Fact sheet]. http:///www.stroke.org

Skarin, M., Bernardt, J., Sjoholm, A., Nilsson, M., & Linden, T. (2011). "Better wear out sheets than shoes": A survey of 202 stroke professionals' early mobilization practices and concerns. *International Journal of Stroke, 6,* 10–15.

CHAPTER 2

Clinical Nurse Leaders in the Global Community

Gordana Dermody and Patricia L. Thomas

LEARNING OBJECTIVES

1. Explore the CNL role and competencies and the ways they can contribute to global health outcomes.
2. Discuss the unique interaction among environmental and sociocultural and political context, healthcare settings, and implementation of best practice.
3. Discuss models and frameworks that can be used to facilitate CNL praxis in the global community.
4. Describe how CNL competencies can make valuable contributions to address health inequities, disparities, and outcomes aligned with international goals.

KEY TERMS

Collaboration
Systems thinking
Evidence-based practice
Cultural sensitivity
Health equity
Macrosystem
Mesosystem
Microsystem

Lateral integration
Outcomes
Praxis
Partnerships
Health disparities
Sustainable development goals
Social determinants of health
Sustainability

CNL ROLES

Advocate
Communicator
Coordinator
Financial steward

Leader
Lifelong learner
Risk anticipator

IAL VALUES

Social justice

CNL COM. ETENCIES

Care coordination   Innovation
Communication   Leadership
Critical thinking

Introduction

Healthcare has joined other industries in becoming globalized in recent years. With the rise in medical tourism, appreciation about global shortages of healthcare professionals, and the consequences of social determinants of health on outcomes, efforts to engage nurses in interprofessional solutions have grown exponentially (Drennan & Ross, 2019). Nurses have a long and rich history of engaging in international or global work since Florence Nightingale; however, deliberate and focused interest has expanded since the 2015 UN Sustainability and Sustainable Development Goals were endorsed (United Nations Sustainable Goals, n.d.). Represented by 17 universal goals, the purpose of this work is to engage various sectors that include governments, businesses, health, institutions of higher education, and local nongovernmental organizations to improve the lives of people globally (Bleich & Thomas, 2021; Dossey et al., 2019). The Sustainable Development Goals (SDGs) are a call to action globally to end poverty and improve lives. Nurses are positioned to address 9 of the 17 goals directly by virtue of the universal values, and expectations of nursing practice and health disciplines have identified 16 of the 17 described issues residing in the delivery of health services (Dossey et al., 2019; Figueroa et al., 2019; United Nations Sustainable Development Goals, n.d.; WHO, 2020). Over 1,000 indicators have been established to address poverty, education, health literacy, erasing hunger, promoting health and well-being, and improving clean water and sanitation among others. These are areas that CNLs can contribute to through collaboration, understanding process and quality improvement, risk anticipation, and outcome management within the unique contexts where care is delivered. This chapter posits CNLs as one vehicle to accomplish this work given the unique knowledge, skills, and competencies CNLs possess.

CNL competencies were developed initially in response to calls to overcoming fragmentations and errors in healthcare that required a clinician with unique competencies and skills (AACN, 2007, 2013). The central goals of this new master's-prepared RN were safety, quality, and cost-effective care in any practice setting. Enactment of the role centered on advanced skills and knowledge of care coordination, team building, risk anticipation, lateral integration, leadership at the point of care, quality and process improvement and outcomes management. Expectations for professional practice included patient and professional advocacy and serving as a change agent, educator, information manager, and team leader (AACN, 2007, 2013; Harris et al., 2018). There were 10 assumptions for preparing CNLs:

1. Practice is at the microsystems level.
2. Client care outcomes are the measure of quality practice.
3. Practice guidelines are based on evidence.
4. Client-centered practice is intra- and interdisciplinary.
5. Information will maximize self-care and client decision-making.
6. Nursing assessment is the basis for theory and knowledge development.
7. Good fiscal stewardship is a condition of quality care.
8. Social justice is an essential nursing value.
9. Communication technology will facilitate the continuity and comprehensiveness of care.
10. The CNL must assume guardianship for the nursing profession (AACN, 2007).

Subsequently CNLs were branded as *generalists* who primarily work in the microsystem, which is also known as the place where patient care is provided (AACN, 2013; Bender et al., 2013; Harris et al., 2018; Huber et al., 2003; Rankin et al., 2018). Notably, microsystems were defined as small, interdependent groups of people who work together regularly to provide care to specific groups of patients (Institute for Healthcare Improvement [IHI], 2020). It is important to recognize this definition does not include "on a particular nursing unit or clinic" and supports CNL practice outside acute care settings. Likewise, it supports the notion that patient populations can be considered a microsystem when their needs are similar irrespective of the location where care is provided. While many healthcare leaders and systems view CNLs as unit-based or department-based clinicians, this stifles opportunities to engage CNLs in meeting needs outside the traditional confines of health systems. When this definition is viewed with a wide lens, the work of CNLs expands to include groups of patients and multisector team members who would come together to discuss concerns not readily addressed in traditional delivery models. It opens the door to global CNL practice by leveraging the 10 assumptions of CNL practice to address disparities in healthcare delivery. The unique context of care defined by location, resources, culture, and values would shape leadership and interventions.

Ongoing work of nurse scientists to develop theory and practice models useful for CNL transitions into healthcare systems is promising (Kaack et al., 2018). Conceptual frameworks that depict the logical progression of CNL education (Maag et al., 2006), in addition to conceptualization of CNL practice, are critical for the continued progression for CNL integration and replication of CNL practice across healthcare systems (Bender, 2016; Bender et al., 2012; Harris et al., 2018).

After the conception of the generalist-microsystem expert, which quickly became known as the *CNL role*, clinicians who had been trained to function as CNLs started to make impressive headway in overcoming what we may call *wicked* healthcare problems (Bender et al., 2012; Clingerman & Thomas, 2020; Donnelly, 2006) by transforming care at the point of care. Soon, the realization of the potential implications the CNL role may have in a global sphere emerged in the literature. As early as 2010, the idea to consider the CNL role in a global context with the goal of improving the quality of healthcare delivery systems came to the forefront (Baernholdt & Cottingham, 2011). Late adopters to this idea may have argued that it was too early to tell if the CNL was sustainable locally or nationally because there were difficulties with the integration of the role into existing healthcare systems. However, over a decade later the competencies and skills of the CNL have become desirable by other nations around the world (Dermody et al., 2016; Figueroa et al., 2019; Katsumata et al., 2016; Pavlic et al., 2019; Thomas & Dermody, 2020), and with good reason as health crises abound and countries are endeavoring to stem the tide of health disparities and inequities.

The Challenges of Using Best Practice in the Global Community

Evidence-based practice is only as good as the supply chain and the person delivering the clinical service. During the ongoing COVID-19 crisis, hospital leaders and politicians in every nation became acutely aware that they needed both a supply chain to deliver a steady flow of supplies such as personal protective equipment (PPE) and clinicians who were trained in donning and doffing without contaminating themselves. As the crisis unfolded, supply chains were fragmented, with reports that nurses had to wear their face mask for several consecutive shifts (Burki, 2020; Cohen & Rodgers, 2020). Ventilators were also in short supply initially, causing hospitals to enter crisis mode to meet patient needs. While these scenarios represent significant challenges in the United States, broken supply chains and a lack of trained clinicians to overcome healthcare challenges is a common occurrence in developing countries, and nations that have experienced environmental or man-made challenges such as conflict and wars, which may have resulted in humanitarian disasters. During the last decade, CNLs have become more globally minded, which is critical for the time we live in (Baernholdt & Cottingham, 2011).

Humanitarian and Health Crisis

Humanitarian and health crises usually occur in tandem. Humanitarian crises include: (1) man-made disasters, including armed conflict, forced displacement, and refugee crises; (2) natural disasters, such as floods, hurricanes, earthquakes, and droughts; and (3) major infectious disease outbreaks (Kohrt et al., 2019, p. 1). Man-made disasters such as terrorist attacks and disease outbreaks such as the current COVID-19 pandemic, the Ebola outbreak, and the Zika virus outbreak have received wide exposure in the media. A humanitarian crisis will transpire into a health crisis, with acute and long-term health impacts that affect hundreds of millions of people globally every year. Low- and middle-income countries are often more affected compared to higher income countries because they already have weak or developing healthcare systems and supply-chain problems (United Nations Office for the Coordination of Humanitarian Affairs, 2018). Major disease outbreaks in a particular country can quickly become an international crisis as we have seen with Ebola and now also with COVID-19, leading to potential displacement and socio-economic displacement (Kohrt et al., 2019).

"If one looks at climate change, population growth, urbanization, many times chaotic urbanization, food insecurity, water scarcity, massive movements of people—all of these trends are becoming also more and

more interlinked . . . generating dramatic humanitarian situations." António Guterres, UN Secretary-General, 2017 (United Nations Office for the Coordination of Humanitarian Affairs, 2018, p. 4)

Vulnerable populations such as undocumented migrants, young children, mothers, the elderly, people with mental health issues and those with preexisting disease and chronic conditions are at risk for health inequities. In 2017, over 95 million people were affected by natural disasters alone, and 65.8 million people were forcibly displaced by violence and conflict (United Nations Office for the Coordination of Humanitarian Affairs, 2018). Thinking back to the Ebola crisis, healthcare leaders did not seem to take too much notice, until the first case of Ebola was discovered in the United States. While delayed (and slow) responses to global disease outbreaks are unfortunate, healthcare systems quickly scramble to develop protocols and procedures to meet population health needs (Hoffman & Silverberg, 2018).

This shows that while healthcare systems can be slow to learn, they are complex organisms continually evolving to adapt to demographic, epidemiological, sociopolitical, and environmental needs (Figueroa et al., 2019). Further, persistent gaps in translation of evidence into practice continue to be problematic for countries known as first nations, for example the United States, Canada, and England, and developing nations (Bussières et al., 2016).

CNL competencies and skills are optimally situated to meet the healthcare challenges of the global population. Therefore, CNLs are a critical commodity in these uncertain times in the global sphere (Dermody & Van Son, 2016) and they have opportunities to evolve and adapt their CNL practice with the challenges that will change the way care is delivered nationally, and in a global context (Dermody et al., 2016; Gerard & Hughes, 2020).

Models and Frameworks to Facilitate CNL Praxis in the Global Community

There is a unique interplay between the context and setting of care delivery—the type of intervention or change that is desired and whether it is to be implemented in the microsystem, the mesosystem, or the macrosystem, and the processes that will be used to make the impossible possible. While the "evidence" may be based on research, implementing the evidence into an environment with supply chain issues can make "evidence-based practice"—which has come to be the expected standard in wealthy nations—improbable. CNLs must consider many factors that impact the implementation of best practice into healthcare systems in the global community including geographic, epidemiological, socioeconomic, political, ethical, and legal polices, and processes (Pfadenhauer et al., 2017). For example, frequent handwashing before and after patient contact is standard procedure, with ample industry-grade antibacterial soap and plenty of paper towels and waste removal being the norm. However, clinical practice in the African bush may see several limitations due to shortages of running water and soap. The vast differences of what is available in different countries requires CNLs to be flexible and pragmatic problem solvers, readily able to adapt to what is available to them in the clinical setting to practice as close to evidence as possible. The development of conceptual models for CNL praxis in the global community would be helpful to provide an overarching guide for CNLs who may be practicing in a variety of global settings.

Leveraging Digital Health to Overcome Global Health Problems

Although knowledge about healthcare technologies is an expected competency in CNL practice, very little is known about how CNLs make use of innovative technologies to address healthcare challenges. Using digital technologies in developing countries can be useful to overcome healthcare challenges such as COVID-19. For example, there is a potential for digital health technologies to facilitate healthcare delivery remotely, using computing devices and client-facing AI-powered apps. Developing nations are very creative in developing innovative solutions to overcome healthcare challenges. For example, lessons from African countries include the development of geospatial technologies, for example, dashboards for detection of infections in communities, and a tracing mobile phone app (COVID-19 Tracker), which is GPS fitted to track movement. In Ghana and Nigeria, drones are used for disinfecting public places and the rapid transport of critical items like PPEs and samples for testing (Prah & Sibiri, 2020; Sarfo & Karuppannan, 2020). Telemedicine kits and mobile health units are other examples of what CNLs may be working with when they are practicing in another country. For example, mobile health units are usually powered and have Wi-Fi and help remotely located clinicians have access to experts for quick diagnosis and triage. In addition, mobile health units can also include mobile virus testing labs, and they can provide remote training for medical staff. CNLs are optimally positioned to develop and implement innovative technologies to overcome healthcare challenges located in the global sphere.

CNL Praxis in Global Communities

The concept of *praxis* has been defined as "the coming together of theory and practice" (Rolfe, 1993, p. 173). While the CNL competencies and skills are practical, they are grounded in nursing and social science theories because CNLs are nurses. To accelerate the translation of evidence into practice in the global setting, CNLs need to be able to identify the system level of implementation (macro, meso, or micro) and begin a dialogue and synergistic collaboration with both academic and clinical stakeholders to determine the most efficacious implementation plan (Rolfe, 1993). There are several evidence-based practices and translational frameworks that are useful to implement evidence into the clinical setting. However, for CNLs who may be working in the global community, either formally, as a consultant, or as a medical volunteer, it is important to include an assessment of the environmental, geographic, and sociopolitical climate of the setting as a foundation to guide the implementation process (Figueroa et al., 2019; Pfadenhauer et al., 2017).

To maximize this synergistic collaboration between stakeholders to translate evidence into practice in the global setting, we propose this CNL global praxis model (**Figure 2-1**). This model may be useful to advance global population health because it conceptualizes the praxis of CNLs in a global context, not only as a

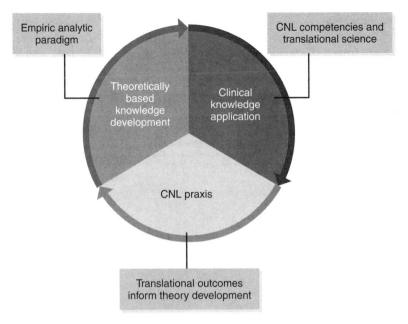

Figure 2-1 CNL global praxis model

microsystem expert. Working in a developing nation may require CNLs to move among micro-, meso-, and macrosystems as the hierarchies may be flatter, experts may be lacking, and cultural and ethnic factors require an adaptive approach to obtaining stakeholder engagement. Therefore, this initial praxis model could be useful to develop educational programs that can guide CNLs and students who desire to use their CNL competencies and skills in the global community. Educational programs should create translational science courses where praxis among global health, translational science, and CNL competencies and skills can be fostered through didactic and practical application.

Global health and translational science concepts should be a foundation for CNL programs with the aim of decreasing the knowledge-practice gap and improving healthcare quality and patient outcomes in global communities. CNL students should gain experience collaborating synergistically with stakeholders in the global community during activities specially designed to translate evidence into practice. Examples of application are offered in exemplars at the conclusion of this chapter.

Application of CNL Competencies in the Global Community

The fundamental aspects of CNL practice are well suited to translate into the global healthcare context. Further, the curriculum framework for client-centered healthcare span nursing leadership, clinical outcomes management, and clinical environment management aspects. While all educational aspects are critical for CNL practice, several are important to practice in the global setting including: global healthcare, human diversity, social justice, healthcare policy, and finance including

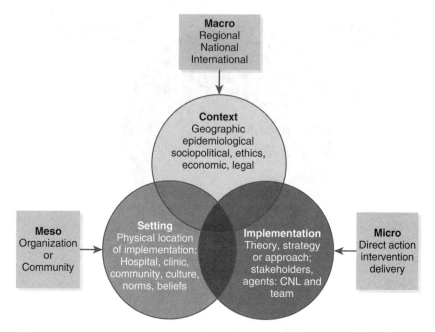

Figure 2-2 Application of the CNL lens to the global practice

Data from Pfadenhauer, L. M., Gerhardus, A., Mozygemba, K., Lysdahl, K. B., Booth, A., Hofmann, B., Wahlster, P., Polus, S., Burns, J., Brereton, L., & Rehfuess, E. (2017). Making sense of complexity in context and implementation: The Context and Implementation of Complex Interventions (CICI) framework. *Implementation Science, 12*(1), 21. https://doi.org/10.1186/s13012-017-0552-5

resource allocation and biostatistics. **Figure 2-2** shows the CNL leader's system lens in relation to the global setting. The microsystem continues to be the place where direct action is implemented. The mesosystem includes aspects of the setting and the community within which the setting is located. These aspects include the physical location of best-practice implementation such as hospital, clinic, community, and the culture, norms, and beliefs of the people living there. The macrosystem refers to the regional, national, or international context including geographic, epidemiological, sociopolitical, ethics, economic, and legal aspects of a country.

Table 2-1 displays how the fundamental aspects of CNL practice as described by the American Association of Colleges of Nursing (AACN) Competencies and Curricular Expectation for Clinical Nurse Leader Education and Practice (2013) are related to the domains suggested by the Context and Implementation of Complex Interventions (CICI) framework. Because most translational frameworks emphasize organizational assessment, the CICI framework was developed to facilitate a complex assessment of the healthcare setting context including macrolevel aspects such as geographic location, sociopolitical, cultural, and epidemiologic and other factors (Pfadenhauer et al., 2017). The implementation of evidence into a global setting will be a complex endeavor. Accordingly, it is important for CNLs to be able to conduct robust and comprehensive assessments beyond the traditional organization and health specialty settings. Table 2-1 describes the dynamic interacting dimensions of the CICI framework including context, implementation, setting, and intervention. Future work should involve adapting CNL tools such as micro-, meso-, and macrosystem assessment and analysis, and implementation frameworks so that they can be used in the global context.

Table 2-1 CNL Global Community Praxis

Fundamental Aspects of CNL Practice		Global Domains
■ Team leadership, management, and collaboration with other health professional team members ■ Information management or the use of information systems and technologies to improve healthcare outcomes ■ Stewardship and leveraging of human, environmental, and material resources ■ Assessment of systems	Context	■ Geographic location: Landscapes, resource infrastructure (water, electricity, finances, delivery systems), level of isolation ■ Epidemiology: Demographics, disease burdens, life expectancies, health needs ■ Sociocultural: Ways of living including language, spiritual beliefs, historically derived ways of living, symbols, artifacts, local customs ■ Socioeconomic: Types of social and economic resources and access to these resources, and differences in different subpopulations ■ Ethical: Norms, implicit and explicit rules (legal), and standards for behavior ■ Political: Leadership and governance, distribution of power, organizational political and power structures ■ Legal: Legislative rules and regulations that can be legally enforced
■ Design and implementation of evidence-based practice(s)	Implementation	■ Process of implementing change (i.e., best practice intervention) ■ Strategies used to implement the change
■ Practice across all settings ■ Advocacy for patients, communities, and the healthcare professional team	Setting	■ Physical setting in which the best evidence will be implemented (i.e., clinic, hospital, community, legislative, educational)

(continues)

Table 2-1 CNL Global Community Praxis   *(continued)*

Fundamental Aspects of CNL Practice		Global Domains
■ Clinical leadership for patient-care practices and delivery, including the design, coordination, and evaluation of care for individuals, families, groups, and populations ■ Participation in identification and collection of care outcomes ■ Accountability for evaluation and improvement of point-of-care outcomes, including the synthesis of data and other evidence to evaluate and achieve optimal outcomes ■ Risk anticipation for individuals and cohorts of patients ■ Lateral integration of care for individuals and cohorts of patients	Intervention Levels	■ Macrosystem: National, regional, or international (i.e., policies or regulation for a particular country) ■ Mesosystem: Community or organization (i.e., clinical practice guidelines for a hospital system) ■ Microsystem: Direct patient care setting (i.e., palliative care, medical surgical)

Data from American Association of Colleges of Nursing. (2013). Competencies and curricular expectations for clinical nurse leader practice and education. https://www.aacnnursing.org/Portals/42/News/White-Papers/CNL-Competencies-October-2013.pdf; Pfadenhauer, L. M., Gerhardus, A., Mozygemba, K., Lysdahl, K. B., Booth, A., Hofmann, B., Wahlster, P., Polus, S., Burns, J., Brereton, L., & Rehfuess, E. (2017). Making sense of complexity in context and implementation: The Context and Implementation of Complex Interventions (CICI) framework. *Implementation Science, 12*(1), 21. https://doi.org/10.1186/s13012-017-0552-5

Conclusion

The influence and impact of CNLs are demonstrated at local, national, and global levels through the leverage of the unique competencies and skills established through their education. While extending CNL practice into global communities adds to the complexity in understanding macro-, meso-, and microsystem functioning, it is the awareness of practice context including culture, resources, and multisector team members with shared goals and purpose that will bring improvement in the area of health disparities. Team building, empowerment, collaboration, and leadership are cornerstones of CNL practice that enable care redesign with sustainable outcomes. The CNL lens, grounded in systems thinking and horizontal leadership, not bound to the traditional delivery model, offers significant opportunity for CNLs to address complex and recalcitrant disparities in healthcare and health outcomes.

Summary

- Healthcare, and therefore nursing practice, is now recognized as a global industry.
- The World Health Organization (WHO) and the United Nations have embraced universal goals to address health inequities across the globe.
- CNL competencies and education have applications to global health delivery.
- CNLs are well positioned to adapt to unique clinical practice experiences expressed in countries beyond the United States and are accustomed to building multisector teams and coalitions to address complex issues.
- Context and praxis models will assist CNLs in implementing their roles globally.

Reflection Questions

1. Review the United Nations SDGs. Select one goal that is interesting to you and identify three ways a CNL could develop projects that would impact outcomes.
2. Identify a country you would like to visit. What questions would you ask nurses and nurse leaders to gain perspective on the healthcare delivery process and practice of nursing in that country?
3. Examine **Figure 2-2** and create a list of CNL activities that align with the macro-, meso-, and microsystem components. Compare and contrast how this list might be influenced if viewed from the perspective of the United States and another country of your choice.

References

American Association of Colleges of Nursing. (2007). *White paper on the role of the Clinical Nurse Leader.* Author. https://nursing.uiowa.edu/sites/default/files/documents/academic-programs/graduate/msn-cnl/CNL_White_Paper.pdf

American Association of Colleges of Nursing. (2013). *Competencies and curricular expectations for Clinical Nurse Leader practice and education* [White paper]. https://www.aacnnursing.org/Portals/42/News/White-Papers/CNL-Competencies-October-2013.pdf

Baernholdt, M., & Cottingham, S. (2011). The Clinical Nurse Leader—new nursing role with global implications. *International Nursing Review, 58*(1), 74–78.

Bender, M. (2014). The current evidence base for the Clinical Nurse Leader: A narrative review of the literature. *Journal of Professional Nursing, 30*(2), 110–123. https://doi.org/10.1016/j.profnurs.2013.08.006

Bender, M. (2016). Conceptualizing Clinical Nurse Leader practice: An interpretive synthesis. *Journal of Nursing Management, 24*(1), E23–E31. https://doi.org/10.1111/jonm.12285

Bender, M., Connelly, C., & Brown, C. (2013). Interdisciplinary collaboration: The role of the Clinical Nurse Leader. *Journal of nursing management, 21*(1), 165–174. https://doi.org/10.1111/j.1365-2834.2012.01385.x

Bender, M., Connelly, C. D., Glaser, D., & Brown, C. (2012). Clinical Nurse Leader impact on microsystem care quality. *Nursing Research, 61*(5), 326–332. https://doi.org/10.1097/NNR.0b013e318265a5b6.

Bleich, M., & Thomas, P. (2021). Data as an Influencer of Policy and Regulation. In P. Thomas, J. Harris, & B. Collins (Eds.), *Data-Driven Quality Improvement and Sustainability in Health Care*, (pp. 117–130). New York, NY: Springer Publishing.

Burki, T. (2020). Global shortage of personal protective equipment. *The Lancet, 20*(7), 785–786. https://doi.org/10.1016/S1473-3099(20)30501-6

Bussières, A. E., Al Zoubi, F., Stuber, K., French, S. D., Boruff, J., Corrigan, J., & Thomas, A. (2016). Evidence-based practice, research utilization, and knowledge translation in chiropractic: A scoping review. *BMC Complementary and Alternative Medicine, 16*, 216.

Clingerman, E., & Thomas, P. (2020). Polarity thinking: A lens for embracing wicked problems, conflict, and resistance in healthcare. In L. Roussel, P. Thomas, & J. Harris (Eds.), *Management and leadership for nurse administrators* (8th ed.). Jones & Bartlett Publishers.

Cohen, J., & Rodgers, Y. (2020). Contributing factors to personal protective equipment shortages during the COVID-19 pandemic. *Preventive Medicine, 141*, 106263. https://doi.org/10.1016/j.ypmed.2020.106263

Dermody, G., Katsumata, A., & Lizer, S. (2016). *Fostering the integration of the Clinical Nurse Leader role in Japan through a multidisciplinary clinical immersion program in the United States.* Sigma Theta Tau International Repository. https://sigma.nursingrepository.org/handle/10755/602947

Dermody, G., & Van Son, C. (2016). Evidence-based practice in the global community: Building bridges. In H. R. Hall, & L. A. Roussel (Eds.), *Evidence-based practice: An integrative approach to research, administration and practice* (2nd ed., pp. 357–371). Jones & Bartlett Publishers.

Donnelly, G. (2006). The transformation of healthcare: A wicked problem. *Holistic Nursing Practice, 20*(5), 215–216.

Dossey, B., Rosa, W., & Beck, D. (2019). Nursing and the Sustainable Development Goals: From Nightingale to now. *American Journal Nursing, 119*(5), 44–49. https://doi.org/10.1097/01.NAJ.0000557912.35398.8f

Drennan, V., & Ross, F. (2019). Global nurse shortages—the facts, the impact and action for change. *British Medical Bulletin, 130*(1), 25–37. https://doi.org/10.1093/bmb/ldz014

Figueroa, C. A., Harrison, R., Chauhan, A., & Meyer, L. (2019). Priorities and challenges for health leadership and workforce management globally: A rapid review. *BMC Health Services Research, 19*(1), 239. https://bmchealthservres.biomedcentral.com/articles/10.1186/s12913-019-4080-7

Gerard, S., & Hughes, D. (2020). Clinical Nurse Leaders address a call to action on human trafficking. *Journal of Nursing Care Quality, 35*(3), 195–198.

Harris, J., Roussel, L., & Thomas, P. (2018). *Initiating and sustaining the Clinical Nurse Leader role: A practical guide* (3rd ed.). Jones & Bartlett Publishers.

Institute for Healthcare Improvement. (2020). *Clinical microsystem assessment tool.* http://www.ihi.org/resources/Pages/Tools/ClinicalMicrosystemAssessmentTool.aspx#:~:text=Background,embedded%20in%20a%20larger%20organization

Hoffman, S., & Silverberg, S. (2018). Delays in global disease outbreak responses: Lessons from H1N1, Ebola, and Zika. *American Journal of Public Health, 108*(3), 329–333.

Huber, T., Godfrey, M., Nelson, E., Mohr, J., Campbell, C., & Batalden, P. (2003). Microsystems in health care: Part 8. Developing people and improving work life: What front-line staff told us. *Joint Commission on Quality and Safety, 29*(10), 512–522. https://clinicalmicrosystem.org/uploads/documents/JQIPart8.pdf

Kaack, L., Bender, M., Finch, M., Borns, L., Grasham, K., Avolio, A., Clausen, S., Terese, N. A., Johnstone, D., & Williams, M. (2018). A Clinical Nurse Leader (CNL) practice development model to support integration of the CNL role into microsystem care delivery. *Journal of Professional Nursing, 34*(1), 65–71. https://doi.org/10.1016/j.profnurs.2017.06.007

Katsumata, A., Lizer, S., & Dermody, G. (2016). *Implementing the Clinical Nurse Leader (CNL) role in Japan.* Sigma Repository. https://sigma.nursingrepository.org/handle/10755/602800

Kohrt, B., Mistry, A., Anand, N., Beecroft, B., & Nuwayhid, I. (2019). Health research in humanitarian crises: An urgent global imperative. *BMJ Global Health, 4*(6), e001870. https://doi.org/10.1136/bmjgh-2019-001870

Maag, M., Buccheri, R., Capella, E., & Jennings, D. (2006). A conceptual framework for a Clinical Nurse Leader program. *Journal of Professional Nursing, 22*(6), 367–372. https://doi.org/10.1016/j.profnurs.2005.11.002

Pavlic, D., Burnsa, H., Wonga, A., Lehmera, J., & Baek, H. (2019). An immersion program for Clinical Nurse Leader students: Comparing health care systems in South Korea and the United States. *Journal of Professional Nursing, 36*(2), 83–95. https://doi.org/10.1016/j.profnurs.2019.07.006

Pfadenhauer, L. M., Gerhardus, A., Mozygemba, K., Lysdahl, K. B., Booth, A., Hofmann, B., Wahlster, P., Polus, S., Burns, J., Brereton, L., & Rehfuess, E. (2017). Making sense of complexity in context and implementation: The Context and Implementation of Complex Interventions (CICI) framework. *Implementation Science, 12*(1), 21. https://doi.org/10.1186/s13012-017-0552-5

Prah, D., & Sibiri, H. (2020). The resilience of African migrant entrepreneurs in China under COVID-19. *Journal of Entrepreneurship in Emerging Economies.* https://www.emerald.com/insight/content/doi/10.1108/JEEE-05-2020-0111/full/html

Rankin, V., Ralyea, T., & Sotomahor, G. (2018). Clinical Nurse Leaders forging the path of population health, *Journal of Professional Nursing, 34*(4), 269–272. https://doi.org/10.1016/j.profnurs.2017.10.008

Rolfe, G. (1993). Closing the theory-practice gap: A model of nursing praxis. *Journal of Clinical Nursing, 2*(3), 173–177. https://doi.org/10.1111/j.1365-2702.1993.tb00157.x

Sarfo, A., & Karuppannan, S. (2020). Application of geospatial technologies in the COVID-19 fight of Ghana. *Transactions of the Indian National Academy of Engineering, 5,* 1–12. https://doi.org/10.1007/s41403-020-00145-3

Thomas, P., & Dermody, G. (2020). *CNLs going global,* CNL Summit. https://www.aacnnursing.org/Professional-Development/Conferences/Presentations-and-CEs/Presentations/2020/CNL-Summit

United Nations Office for the Coordination of Humanitarian Affairs. (2018). *World humanitarian data and trends 2018.* Author. https://www.unocha.org/sites/unocha/files/WHDT2018_web_final_spread.pdf

United Nations. (n.d.). Sustainable Development Goals-About. https://www.un.org/sustainabledevelopment/development-agenda/

World Health Organization. (2020). Health topics: Sustainable Development Goals. https://www.who.int/health-topics/sustainable-development-goals#tab=tab_1

EXEMPLAR

Creating Clinical Immersion Experiences in the United States for Japanese Nurses

Shannon Lizer, Minami Kakuta, Brandie Messer, and Patricia Thomas

The relationship between Japanese nursing colleges and universities and Saint Anthony College of Nursing (SACN) in Rockford, Illinois, has been well established. Initially, this relationship began with two annual visits to Japan by nursing faculty and the graduate dean. At the onset, the purpose of these visits was to share concepts of US nursing with Japanese nurses, hospital leaders, and academicians. Concepts shared included the role of the advanced practice registered nurse (APRN), ANCC Magnet designation, shared governance, professional communication, evidence-based practice, and curricular structure in undergraduate and graduate nursing programs.

As experienced APRNs, we noted that throughout many interactions it was quite apparent that the APRN role did not fit well within the structure of Japanese healthcare, which is very traditional and clearly physician driven. As time progressed, there was a growing mutual awareness, by both US and Japanese nurses, that the Japanese culture was ideally suited to the role of the CNL. This was clearly identified through a careful assessment of cultural norms.

Japanese healthcare supports teamwork, a focus on patient outcomes, and a systems approach to problem solving. Aligning the CNL role with the meso/microsystem of the specific health system and hospital, specific attributes of the CNL role, such as team management, clinical leadership, lateral integration, and data-driven methods of decision-making and change could be easily assimilated into the leadership style and hierarchy of Japanese healthcare in general, and to nursing practice specifically.

Japan has a government-driven healthcare model (macrosystem) with very large mesosystems (for example the Japanese Red Cross [JRC] Society Health System), which is perfectly aligned with microsystems in the individual JRC hospitals throughout Japan. Three partnerships emerged—the JRC Kyushu International College of Nursing, University of Tsukuba, and Kyoto University—and demonstrated potential to drive change through CNL leadership. The alignment of US nursing and Japanese nursing through shared professional values, congruent organizational priorities, and similar academic obligations created a springboard to leverage the CNL role as defined by the AACN white paper on the role and curricular expectations for collaboration (2007). As nurse leaders in practice and academe explored the CNL role together and evaluated the gaps in practice that could be addressed throughout Japan, the recognition of the potential of the CNL became more apparent.

Academic nurse leaders from Kyoto University, JRC Kyushu International College of Nursing, JRC College of Nursing, and University of Tsukuba joined forces to present seminars with CNL content to nurses from multiple organizations across Japan. This work was sponsored through a grant provided by the JRC Society. Participants in the CNL seminars included Japanese nurse leaders from health systems across Japan, including Kyoto City Hospital, Kyoto University Hospital, and many of the JRC hospitals. These seminars were aimed to provide immersive learning about the education and practice of CNLs and support of CNL content delivery in Japan. This experience was developed to include weeks-long didactic learning by professors, deans, faculty, hospital directors, chief nursing officers, and graduate students followed by a CNL immersion experience in the United States.

Consequently, annual visits of SACN and other faculty to Japan focused on didactic sessions about CNL role, competencies, and metrics. This content was brought to life in the clinical immersions in three US hospitals and health systems annually. Nurse academic leaders, operational leaders, faculty, and students were partnered with colleagues in clinical immersions that brought the focus of real CNL work to Japanese nurses who were then able to plan and operationalize their new knowledge and skills in their home Japanese institution.

EXEMPLAR

Recognizing Microsystem-Macrosystem Interfaces with International Partners: Using Dialogue, the CNL Lens, Cultural Awareness, and Shared Values to Address Needs

Patricia Thomas

As part of an international research team comprised of nurse leaders from practice and academe in eight countries, the microsystem-macrosystem assessment components provided a framework to explore and evaluate the construct of caring and its influence on job satisfaction and clinical care outcomes. Participants representing the United States, Canada, Scotland, Brazil, Slovenia, China, and Turkey have engaged in ongoing collaboration and dialogue about how nurses are educationally prepared, the structures and models of care delivery in each country, the distinctions in health provider roles and titles in respective countries, and the influence of health policy and governance and cultural norms that impact individual and organizational decision-making. The research team members are part of an international consortium that was established to promote collaboration, dissemination, and uptake of empiric research findings to build an international community of practitioner-scholars.

In 2016 nurse leaders in the eight countries received institutional review board (IRB) approval in their respective organizations to launch a research study to examine principles of caring theory and sociotechnical theory and the impacts on nurse job satisfaction. Aligned with the thesis of the quadruple aim, each country committed to launch the Healthcare Environment Job Satisfaction Survey (HES) every other year and use the unit and organizational results to establish deliberate and focused interventions to improve results. This group of leaders met face-to-face once a year in one of the members' countries to discuss the status of each study, progress to date, and results. Additionally, they explored and consulted with one another regarding unit- and organizational-level interventions described in the literature to address results in their respective organizations.

In 2017 the consortium research team members met in Slovenia and in 2018 they met in Turkey. During these visits the team members also provided formal presentations on topics identified by the host country. Topics represented current trends and issues in nursing practice and were aimed to share knowledge and best evidence to inspire translation and uptake of best evidence. Experts from the group presented to academic and operational nurse leaders, staff nurses, students, and community members. Follow-up conference calls were held throughout the year to report progress and support one another through consultation and sharing best evidence and lessons learned.

One of the premises underlying the work was that unit-level data aggregated to the organizational level provided general information, but unit-specific information needed to drive focused intervention if improvements were to be sustained. Each country was at a different phase in the research process, and all had committed to resurveying nurses every two years. While visiting Turkey, it became apparent that the microsystem-macrosystem interface was the critical foci of work serving as the vehicle or engine to improve and sustain outcomes.

A critical first step in entering work with international partners is conducting organizational and microsystem assessments centered on cultural context to build awareness and common language. Identifying the shared values of the nursing profession served as the starting point. From there, building awareness of the social, political, cultural, and economic influences that include resource distribution, decision-making, health policy, and leadership actions in an inclusive and a nonjudgmental manner were foundations for our collaboration. Using published literature, shared academic knowledge, and showcasing experts on different topics of interest from each country framed the collaboration and agendas. Formal presentations with health system operational nurse leaders, academic nurse leaders, and students provided a venue for dialogue that all were accustomed to.

During visits to each country, at least two full days were dedicated to sightseeing and learning the history and culture of the sponsor country. This provided a rich experience for the participants to explore history and culture while getting to know one another personally.

What we have learned from this work is how the shared values and desired outcomes of nurses across the globe establish a shared and common foundation for dialogue and collaboration. Language and time barriers are overcome by the transcendent commitment to excellence in nursing practice irrespective of our country of origin. Each participant in the collaborative brought forward individual strengths and abilities to build a network of capability that could not have been accomplished by a single individual. Using a systems lens coupled with a commitment to shared understanding, cultural respect and awareness, and disciplined organizational and microsystem assessments frame dialogue to advance nursing science, practice, and in turn nurse job satisfaction and nurse leader development. The translation of empiric research outcomes coupled with the implementation of best evidence and consultations positively impact health systems and academic institutions globally.

EXEMPLAR

Monthly CNL Certification Preparation Study Sessions Promote Collaboration and Success of Japanese Nurse Leaders in Academe and Practice

Minami Kakuta, Shannon K. Lizer, and Patricia Thomas

For the past four years, SACN graduate faculty have partnered with nursing faculty from Tsukuba University and Kyoto University in Japan to host monthly virtual study sessions aimed to promote successful CNL certification of Japanese nurses. These study sessions were initiated to address the areas of focus Japanese nurses identified as stumbling points when taking the CNL certification examination. Differences between US and Japanese health delivery systems, health policies, leadership development, and academic norms were identified as distinct content areas that undermined successful completion of the board certification process. Japanese nurse leaders, nurse educators, and staff nurses across Japan were invited participants. Parallel participants in the United States serve as facilitators of the sessions.

A team of graduate faculty who teach CNL curriculum prepare study session content framed by the AACN CNL white paper and AACN CNL role and curricular expectations. Specific areas of focus include nursing theory, leadership development, points of contrast between US and Japanese healthcare policy, process and quality improvement strategies, microsystem assessment, and evidence-based data-driven nurse-led improvement projects. Exercises and assignments are developed that mirror the Commission on Nurse Certification (CNC) CNL board certification requirements.

All study sessions are delivered in the Japanese language to promote assimilation of the content. The study groups align participants in a unique fashion, dissimilar to the typical Japanese nursing structures. The participants developed a standardized template for session assignments including: title, page, name of submitter, translated content, content interpretation, and related resources. All information is shared in a cloud-based application accessible by all team members. Subsequently, all participants review the assigned content prior to the session and are prepared to actively engage in the discussion. Faculty facilitators also take notes and post them in the cloud.

Sessions are planned during nighttime hours in the United States to promote participation of Japanese nurses. In true team fashion, participants take turns as the leader in organizing the upcoming session. The participant leaders organize the schedule, plan content to be covered, and create individual assignments for completion. The participant leader facilitates discussion. Prior to each session, participants translate assigned readings published in the CNL textbook, CNL board preparation text, or assigned journal articles that are published in English and translated into Japanese, so they are prepared for the study session in their native language.

The session process is relatively consistent. At the beginning of each session, participants take turns sharing what they have learned from the current readings. Further, session participants summarize and post their analysis in a Word document for all to use as a future reference. These summaries also inform the group faculty about individual progress and perspective.

During each session, participants share how they will incorporate the particular CNL topic into their respective practice as nurses within their respective organizations. An example of this is a discussion of root cause analysis—focusing on the process, not on "who did something wrong." This represents a huge cultural shift for Japanese nurses. When an error occurs, the typical focus in Japan is not on the process but rather on who made a mistake. This change in perspective offers the opportunity to put emphasis on the importance of systems thinking, a shift away from blame, and application of the CNL role.

The role of faculty facilitators is to clarify content that is not understood, expand on the discussion based on their knowledge and experience, and promote an active dialogue. The role of the team participant leader has truly engaged the group, and this systematic organizational role has led to the success of the group. While the focus of this group was originally intended to simply provide support for participants to successfully pass the CNL certification exam, it has truly become a coalition of Japanese nurses who want to learn together and share knowledge to improve academic and practice outcomes.

Culturally, nurses in Japan typically stay in the same organization, and it is not common to discuss nursing practice and nursing issues beyond their home organization or outside of their job position. These study sessions provide Japanese nurses a safe environment to share their issues or questions and exchange and learn other nurses' perspectives outside typical organizational boundaries and titles such as chief nursing officer (CNO), staff nurse, and educator. As a result, these study sessions promote informal academic and clinical partnerships. To date, over 45 Japanese nurses, educators, and leaders have participated in these sessions. This coalition has been particularly important during the current COVID-19 pandemic in sharing emerging practice guidelines, strategies to implement rapid system-wide uptake of evidence, and situational awareness to build resilience as they share experiences in managing the COVID-related issues in clinical and academic settings.

Engaging with International Partners

Linda A. Roussel

The author had a wonderful opportunity to engage international partners in Turkey and Saudi Arabia on executive and clinical leadership. While partners were familiar with executive leadership and management (which was my first connection), the concept of the CNL was a new role that they were curious about. The primary participants during the international work were the nurse leaders and managers in service lines and unit levels. While nurse leaders were familiar with care coordination and interprofessional collaboration, *lateral integration* was a new term. As a lateral integrator, the CNL, as a process expert, coordinates various functions to expedite efficiency and effectiveness. This is particularly important with healthcare reform and the mandate for reducing costs with the CNL providing important services required for effective care transitions. CNLs directly care for individuals and populations and require this important role function to provide oversight and ensure that the clinical care meets high-quality standards and affords seamless continuity of care for patients. The author further emphasized CNLs' skill set and knowledge base including systems thinking, political savvy, teamwork and team building, positive interpersonal skills, and a high degree of clinical expertise. Through a series of interactive exercises, the nurse managers and directors were able to align their role in the management area as both roles necessitated authentic leadership skills. The nurse managers were particularly interested in clinical leadership at the microsystem's level from the patients' and frontline workers' perspectives.

CHAPTER 3

The Prominence of CNL Microsystem Leadership for High-Reliability and Value-Added Outcomes

Patricia L. Thomas

LEARNING OBJECTIVES

1. Describe attributes of high reliability in organizations and ways CNLs support establishment and sustainability.
2. Explore value aligned with clinical and financial outcomes in CNL practice.
3. Examine the impact of healthcare economics and risk mitigation as key concepts for CNL practice.
4. Discuss ways CNLs ready the practice environment for improvement and excellence.
5. Examine the triple aim and movement toward the quadruple aim enhanced by CNL leadership.
6. Discuss the CNL role in value-driven, high-performing microsystems through process excellence and communication of results.

KEY TERMS

Economic value
Enterprise risk management
Evidence-based practice
Risk management

Root cause analysis (RCA)
Safety
Value
Value-driven care

CNL ROLES

Advocate
Catalyst
Integrator

Member of a profession
Risk averter

CNL PROFESSIONAL VALUES

Accountability
Integrity
Financial stewardship
Interprofessional teamwork

Outcomes management
Quality improvement
Social justice

CNL CORE COMPETENCIES

Assessment
Communication
Critical thinking
Data analysis
Design/Manage/Coordinate care

Ethical decision-making
Information and healthcare
   technologies
Resource management

Introduction

The *triple aim*, as defined by the IHI, calls for "improving the individual experience of care; improving the health of populations; and reducing the per capita costs of care for populations" (Berwick et al., 2008, p. 759; IHI, 2020). The only means by which this can be accomplished is through improving existing care delivery systems across the continuum of care. Although multiple care providers should be involved in these efforts, in multidisciplinary teams, CNLs are uniquely positioned by their organizational skills, leadership abilities, and advanced clinical and quality improvement education to be key players.

Recently, the triple aim has been expanded to a quadruple aim whereby attention to the well-being of care providers and care team members is viewed as a foundation to improve healthcare delivery. In addition to cost, quality, and populations, the quadruple aim emphasizes the provider of care and the meaning and joy they find in their work as central to the patient experience. Recognizing the experiences of healthcare providers across disciplines, the quadruple aim highlights the need for physical and psychological safety and attention to the work environment for success in healthcare transformation. Exacting the meaning and joy healthcare providers find in work with the impact it has on the experience of care is the addition of the quadruple aim, endorsed by organizations, providers, and policy makers but not the IHI. The point of divergence resides in the patient focus of the triple aim wherein the quadruple aim adds the satisfaction of care providers (Feeley, 2017). For organizations implementing a quadruple strategy, measurement will be quantified through workplace safety and engagement surveys noting not only accomplishments in safety but also attending to burnout and its mitigation as a means to accomplish the quadruple aim. Recent attention has centered on building resilience and self-care skills to help distill the joy in work and support care redesign that benefits patients and providers alike (Bachynsky, 2020; Bowles et al., 2019; Sikka et al., 2015).

A triad of organizational constructs contributes to the environment in which the CNL functions; those concepts involving high-reliability, evidence-based practice, and process excellence derived from quality improvement principles of reducing waste and developing consistency in practice to provide a sound performance framework from which to function. High-reliability organizations (HROs) focus on mindfulness and perfection, according to the June 2012 report from The Joint Commission. Evidence-based practice (EBP) has been defined as integrating clinical expertise with the best available clinical evidence from systematic reviews to influence and achieve patient management (Sackett et al., 2000, p. 3). This has been extended to include the values and beliefs of individuals as they influence how we engage in decision-making and choices related to health practices. Process excellence entails continuous improvement through the elimination of waste and the reduction of variation recognizing standardization and consistency in care delivery is key to repeated positive outcomes. As the CNL embraces and employs the constructs of HRO, EBP, and process excellence, the capacity for enhancing the value of the organization improves.

Each of these focal points underscores the need to lead in new, transformative, and responsive ways. With extensive leadership literature to support the concepts of transformation, high reliability, evidence-based intervention, and expected excellence, a distinctive role for CNLs emerges. Not only are CNLs academically and experientially prepared to accomplish this work, but they are also uniquely positioned at the point of care as generalists to work in complex adaptive systems. This distinction provides breadth (rather than specialization), and is an expectation of distilling the most salient focal points within and across microsystems to achieve desired outcomes. Given the national concerns about access to care, cost, health literacy, and social justice, this is a clarion call to action for every CNL.

The CNL's Role

The CNL's role is that of a leader in the delivery of care to patients, in sickness and in wellness, across the continuum of care. In this assigned leadership position, the CNL is responsible for myriad accountabilities that are inclusive of care design and delivery, risk anticipation and management, quality monitoring and improvement, collaboration and team management, education, and advocacy (AACN, 2007, 2013).

To optimally fulfill the role, the CNL must be prepared to meet the assigned responsibilities. The AACN (2007, pp. 6–10, 2013) lists the following 10 assumptions for preparing the CNL:

1. Practice is at the microsystems level.
2. Client care outcomes are the measure of quality practice.
3. Practice guidelines are based on evidence.
4. Client-centered practice is intra- and interdisciplinary.
5. Information will maximize self-care and client decision-making.

6. Nursing assessment is the basis for theory and knowledge development.
7. Good fiscal stewardship is a condition of quality care.
8. Social justice is an essential nursing value.
9. Communication technology will facilitate the continuity and comprehensiveness of care.
10. The CNL must assume guardianship for the nursing profession.

The assumptions for CNL role preparation are important to note, as they reflect the relationship of EBP and the desire to embed process excellence training into the CNL curriculum to facilitate a best practice foundation to high reliability, outcomes management, and risk mitigation.

Through leading interdisciplinary teams, guiding actions by enacting horizontal leadership, and the application of an EBP model, CNLs function as role models in change leadership. Guided by system thinking, and the alignment of principles in high reliability and process excellence, the CNL provides care to individuals, groups, and the community using a disciplined and systematic approach to process and quality improvements in microsystems. The CNL is intentional with regard to the identification of performance metrics and outcome monitoring, and as a team leader, CNLs model interdisciplinary collaboration. The CNL influences the team and provides stewardship of resources—human, material, and financial. Having an appreciation for the interrelated functions of multiple microsystems, the CNLs' unique knowledge to lead and manage changes positions this leader to exact improvement rather than unintended harm in other microsystems in the organization. Information management and technology are tools CNLs use to perform their work that has expanded with telehealth, interoperable EMRs, and app technology (Harris & Thomas, 2021; Thomas & Harris, 2021). In total, the CNL is responsible and highly qualified to integrate principles of high-reliability process excellence and EBP at the point of care.

High-Reliability Organizations

The constructs of high reliability, EBP, and process excellence, when present in an organization and utilized by the CNL, contribute to making the organization value driven. Each of the constructs contributes distinctive elements to the environment; the constructs are interdependent and synergistic. For the CNL to be successful in the pursuit of delivering value, the organization must support these constructs, and the CNL must be diligent in the application.

HROs, as discussed earlier, need to focus on mindfulness and perfection. These foci are outcomes of several core principles that move organizations toward the ultimate goal of high reliability—consistent quality results, in every location, every time. When enacted and embedded in the organization's culture, there is transformation. Multiple industries possess characteristics that challenge their ability to deliver such consistency. From the aviation industry to correctional services, the constructs of high reliability exist. In healthcare, HROs deliver an outcome of "exceptionally safe, consistently high-quality care" (Agency for Healthcare Research and Quality [AHRQ], 2008, p. 6, 2015). An exploration of the characteristics and principles of high reliability showcases how the CNL skill set of advanced clinical and quality knowledge, leadership, and outcomes management generates performance that creates a value-driven HRO through interacting microsystems.

Organizations face myriad challenges that contribute to their ability to perform consistently. Healthcare organizations are not unique in that they demonstrate many, if not all, of these challenges, including the following identified by AHRQ:

- *Hypercomplexity:* multiteam systems that must coordinate processes and performance to provide consistent results.
- *Tight coupling:* closely aligned teams whose members are dependent on one another for the completion of tasks contributing to overall performance.
- *Extreme hierarchical differentiation:* well-defined roles requiring extensive coordination; those team members considered "expert," regardless of rank, assume the position of "decision maker" during times of crisis.
- *Multiple decision makers in a complex communication network:* many positions that make decisions that are interdependent and interconnected.
- *High degree of accountability:* high level of responsibility and liability when errors occur.
- *Need for frequent, immediate feedback:* continuous need for communication and feedback, presenting ongoing opportunities to make adjustments.
- *Compressed time constraints:* processes, systems, people, and culture to identify when time is needed to consistently perform as desired (AHRQ, 2008, 2015; Chassin & Loeb, 2013).

Healthcare is replete with these challenges. The CNL, as the leader of the microsystem, is immersed within them and must be well prepared, both with awareness of the challenges and with strategies to mitigate them. Respecting the following five core principles can assist in addressing the challenges that most complex organizations face on the journey to becoming highly reliable:

1. *Sensitivity to operations:* HROs continuously monitor processes and systems to identify and eliminate errors. Developing associates with "situational awareness" and a sensitivity to operations facilitates an environment that promotes consistent performance. CNLs in their microsystems are well positioned for early identification of defects to address upstream impacts. By engaging his or her team members in process and quality improvements, the CNL uses knowledge of systems, quality improvement, and measurement to lead interdisciplinary teams that address concerns leading to errors.
2. *Reluctance to simplify:* HROs understand that work is complex and recognize one-dimensional systems will not suffice to resolve the challenges. Associates in HROs recognize that processes and systems evolve and can fail in new and unimaginable ways. With the recognition of complexity and the acceptance that many of the systems cannot be simplified, healthcare associates in HROs remain vigilant and simplify those processes that they can, using multidisciplinary teams trained in systems design. CNLs consider this when examining and streamlining processes.
3. *Preoccupation with failure:* HROs continually consider the prospect that systems may fail and errors may occur. Healthcare organizations anticipate that these errors will put patients at risk and therefore when the errors or "near misses" occur, investigations follow, and systems are redesigned to mitigate future errors. CNLs use this knowledge when engaging in process redesign.
4. *Deference to expertise:* HROs respect knowledge and reinforce a culture where the associates with the greatest knowledge take the lead in resolving issues. In such a culture, the leadership defers to those with the best understanding. In

this culture, it is also the responsibility of those with the knowledge to share information. In creating teams to address practice and process concerns, CNLs use this strategy to engage all the parties that touch a process, recognizing that clinicians, support staff, and ancillary department team members influence outcomes and need to be involved in process design and improvements.

5. *Resilience:* HROs strive to develop a capacity to respond quickly to errors. HROs are dependent on the result of honoring expertise and a relentless attention to process. CNLs, possessing nursing expertise and a foundational knowledge of process excellence, are integral stakeholders in the creation and sustainability of high reliability in organizations.

Process Excellence

Just as healthcare HROs are synergistic with EBP, the same is true with process excellence. Process excellence can be appreciated as the vehicle for enhancing HROs and EBP, through a continuous improvement cycle using proven methodologies that span all industries. Process excellence represents the embodiment of all types of process, quality, or performance improvement: Lean, Six Sigma, and total quality management (TQM). Process excellence is distinguished from quality improvement as a framework that embraces principles of Lean and Six Sigma to reduce waste and variation while enhancing standardization (Martin & Osterling, 2014). Process improvement practitioners have long understood that the persons who are most effective in leading quality initiatives are those who understand the principles of improvement and are closest to the work that requires improvement. As such, there is an acknowledgment of the people, the process, the leadership, and the commitment to replicable outcomes. The CNL, enhanced with process excellence skills, becomes that effective person who leads quality initiatives when working within microsystems. Prepared with advanced knowledge, team-building skills supported by collaborative interprofessional relationships, and an understanding of measurement and value, CNLs' leadership, mentorship, and modeling behaviors bring process excellence and systems thinking into daily practice.

A microsystem is defined as the smallest unit on the front line of healthcare delivery systems. The clinical microsystem provides direct care to patients and families, establishing the essential building blocks of the organization. It is within this microsystem that the quality of care is defined, and the reputation of the organization is created (Dartmouth Institute for Health Policy and Clinical Practice, 2015; Nelson et al., 2007). To prepare CNLs to become process excellence practitioners for microsystems, an understanding of improvement methodology within the construct of microsystems and integration of improvement methodology into the CNL curriculum is essential. The creation of HROs in healthcare depends on EBP and a culture that embraces continuous improvement through process excellence. The CNL, as a practitioner of EBM and process excellence, is seen as a leader of the movement toward high reliability.

Evidence-Based Practice

A significant factor that shapes the CNL's environment is EBP, earlier defined as an integration of "individual clinical expertise with the best available external clinical evidence from systematic research"; initially this concept was termed "evidence-based medicine" (EBM; Sackett et al., 1996, p. 71). Additional components of EBP are patients who have individual expectations for care and the value to be derived from the encounter. A contributing factor in the creation of an HRO, EBP places emphasis on knowledge and expertise. The CNL is in a key position to play an active role in each of the HRO and EBP environments.

Sackett and colleagues (2000) identified five essential steps in the EBM/EBP process that facilitate the integration of internal practice, external practice, and the expectations of the patient:

1. *Assess the patient:* Start with the patient—the clinical problem or question arises from the patient.
2. *Ask the question:* Construct a well-built clinical question derived from the case.
3. *Acquire the evidence:* Select the appropriate resource(s) and conduct a search.
4. *Appraise the evidence:* Appraise the evidence for its validity (closeness to the truth) and applicability (usefulness in clinical practice).
5. *Apply:* Talk with the patient. Return to the patient—integrate that evidence with clinical expertise and patient preference and apply it to practice.

The outlined process embeds a discipline and standardization that impels high reliability. The CNL, through education and practice, develops the expertise to accurately assess the patient and ask appropriate questions. Through the acquisition of evidence and appraisal, the CNL, proficient in the microsystem, determines the degree of usefulness. The CNL, through the relationship established with the patient, integrates the determined evidence with the patient's preference to deliver EBP. Additionally, CNLs observe patterns in microsystems and populations to leverage evidence and principles of high reliability to bring systematic quality and process improvements.

Process Excellence Training

The AACN, in collaboration with nurse executives, health systems, and educators, proposed the CNL as a nursing solution to address gaps in healthcare quality by addressing patient needs, safety, and quality improvement through a systematic and deliberate approach to implementing EBP, quality management, and clinical leadership at the point of care. CNLs are prepared as advanced generalists accountable for identifying outcomes of practice at points of care. This can be accomplished by participating in a range of quality improvement projects aimed at collecting and creating evidence, leading multidisciplinary teams, and incorporating interventions with the greatest likelihood of producing high-quality care outcomes (AACN, 2007, 2013).

For the CNL to function in this manner—to lead through quality and process improvement—foundational knowledge is needed. Microsystems, as the smallest unit of the frontline healthcare delivery system, can also be considered the smallest unit of a value stream. In process excellence terms, a value stream is defined as all the activities required to bring a specific product, whether it be goods or a service, to the customer; in healthcare, the product is often a combination of goods and services. This is a key distinguishing point in process excellence; awareness of interacting systems and a commitment to ensuring negative impacts from an improvement activity are minimized throughout the value stream. Critical tasks for managing the value stream are problem solving, information management, and transformation.

Problem solving entails following an idea from detailed design to the launch. Information management includes order taking, scheduling, and creating detailed documentation. Transformation entails the movement from raw materials to delivery of the completed product to the customer (Nelson et al., 2011; Womack & Jones, 2003, p. 19). Individual value streams may be composed of multiple microsystems, all of which contribute to the products or services of the whole system. It is important to note that products and services may also be produced at the microsystem level.

In process excellence terms, items are identified as adding value when the customers' needs are met. Often this entails meeting the following three challenges:

1. *Identifying the customer:* Customers in healthcare are the patient, families, healthcare providers, the community, and payers. The challenge, in light of reform, is to redefine the true value of the service to be delivered to each customer.
2. *Defining value in terms of the whole product or service:* The delivery of a product or service occurs across a continuum. The Affordable Care Act challenge is to improve care across the care continuum, providing it to an increased percentage of the population.
3. *Achieving target cost:* When the target cost is identified, the key stakeholders across the continuum work collaboratively to maintain or lower the target (Nelson et al., 2011; Womack & Jones, 2003, pp. 31–36).

The concept of value is important in today's healthcare landscape, as the economic model transforms from a focus on volume (quantity) to a focus on activities that contribute to high-value outcomes (quality). Value-based purchasing connects performance to reimbursement by rewarding and incentivizing excellence in care measured by clinical care processes and the patient experience (CMS, 2013). Demonstrating higher quality at lower costs becomes a driver for transformation (Aroh et al., 2015). The CNL has the capability and capacity to greatly impact value-based purchasing, which is defined as the unification of "information on the quality of health care, including patient outcomes and health status, with data on the dollar outlays going toward health. It focuses on managing the use of the healthcare system to reduce inappropriate care and to identify and reward the best-performing providers" (Aroh et al., 2015; CMS, 2013; Meyer et al., 1997, p. 1).

Heightened attention to pay for performance, new bundled payment reimbursement strategies, and focused risk contracting for value and quality have accelerated organizational responsiveness to high-reliability, performance excellence, and evidence-based practices to achieve consistent and replicable outcomes. The CNL's role in creating a value-driven approach to care in an HRO is dependent on the optimized environment of high reliability, the incorporation of EBP concepts, and the CNL's ability to help create those two constructs. The CNL's role in creating value is further enhanced when the principles of process excellence are applied. This chapter explores how each of the constructs of the environment contributes to value and the role that the CNL plays in the formation of both.

Healthcare Economics

More than at any other time in history, the cost of healthcare has become a common household conversation. As health reform and the implementation of the Affordable

Care Act have progressed, the cost of care in the United States has come into question. Compared to other civilized countries, the United States lags in clinical care outcomes but nevertheless has the distinction of being the costliest system in the world. The IOM conducted a workshop series, "Healthcare Imperative: Lowering Costs and Improving Outcomes," which found that "[t]he United States spends far more on health care than any other nation. In 2018, healthcare costs reached $3.6 trillion—or $11,172 per person representing 17.57% of the GDP. Total healthcare spending is anticipated to reach $6.2 trillion in 2028 meaning it will represent 20% of the GDP or one-fifth of the US economy" (CMS, 2018). Despite this spending, health outcomes in the United States fall below the performance in other countries, notably below Australia, Canada, France, Germany, the Netherlands, New Zealand, Norway, Sweden, Switzerland, and the United Kingdom (IOM, 2011; Mahon, 2014; Tikkanen & Abrams, 2020).

Relative to this data, the relationship between process, structure, and outcomes assumes greater importance, especially as organizations strive to reduce errors, bring greater consistency to care delivery, and develop process improvements to decrease waste. Likewise, as one considers principles of high reliability and value, the need for evidence-based interventions and desired replicable outcomes are significant. Elements of pay for performance are based on the assumption that consistent EBP is the most cost-effective care, building the line of sight among high reliability, cost, error prevention, risk reduction, and showcasing the role of the CNL. Bundled payment, accountable care organizations, integrated clinical networks, and population health management initiatives are driving change and innovation across the care continuum. CNLs as advanced generalists, with a system lens and advanced knowledge in quality and process improvements, are well positioned to develop, lead, and implement this phase of healthcare reform.

Risk Management

The definition of high reliability implies a parallel path of assessment of risk and risk management in managing microsystems. Once it is recognized that clinical operations need interdependent microsystems to deliver safe, appropriate, and consistent care, risks can be managed through a lens of preoccupation with error. Traditionally, risk assessment and risk management have been retrospectively viewed in clinical situations that did not produce a desired outcome. Risk mitigation has entered the vernacular based on the recognition that preoccupation with error highlights the many variables that contribute to harm.

The landscape of healthcare delivery today is focused on quality and safety and is dedicated to understanding systems and processes that result in outcomes. Commitment to value, rather than volume, and strategic initiatives aligned for reliability, consistency, and safety are gaining attention as organizations strive for seamless, efficient, error-free care. With the development of the CNL role, organizations have embraced those closest to the patient (in a microsystem) who have unique and desirable insights about where gaps exist in our current processes, which are ripe for contributing to errors. As CNLs have demonstrated sustainable change and improved outcomes in responsive quality and process improvement activities, CNL knowledge, skill set, and contribution to organizational effectiveness have been established.

In designing the CNL role, the AACN (2007, 2013) established risk anticipation, or the ability to critically evaluate and anticipate risks to client safety, was determined to be a critical component of the role. At the system level (risk to any client) and the individual level (by review of patient history and comorbidities), CNLs anticipate risk when new technology, equipment, treatment regimens, or medication therapies are introduced (AACN, 2007, 2011, 2013). Tools for risk analysis, for example, failure mode evaluation analysis, root cause analysis, and quality improvement methodologies, are the levers and tools consistently employed by CNLs. Because CNLs are embedded in a microsystem, their knowledge of systems, leadership, quality improvement, and measurement uniquely qualify them to scan the clinical environment to identify potential risk.

Conclusion

The era of high-reliable care that is effective, efficient, seamless, and cost-effective is the CNL's playground! Positioned as a clinical leader in microsystems that span the continuum of care, the CNL has the opportunity to emerge as a leader in creating HROs. CNL education has focused on quality improvement, risk anticipation, measurement, monitoring, and assessing care practices. What is needed now are deliberate tactics and strategies to showcase how the unique attributes of CNL education place them in a ready position to replicate accomplishments as a leader in complex adaptive systems. With the expanded definition of microsystems that extend beyond a traditional unit or service line, CNLs are transforming care and care outcomes. CNLs function as mentors and team leaders in pursuit of improvements in the patient care experience and have the opportunity to optimize the care environment through high-reliability principles and integration of EBP to create value when the principles of process excellence are applied.

Summary

- The principles of high reliability, EBP, and process excellence are integrated into the CNL role and serve as the foundational elements to improve quality and patient safety.
- Continuous systematic assessment of the clinical environment is essential for situational awareness in HROs.
- Hypercomplexity is a characteristic of healthcare, and respect of this complexity is essential for meaningful quality improvement.

Reflection Questions

1. If you were having lunch with a nurse on your unit and were asked to define high reliability, how would you answer?
2. Think about a recent experience on your unit where an error occurred. Can you identify elements of high reliability that were enacted? Are there elements of high reliability that might have prevented the error?

3. Consider a "near miss" that you or a coworker has experienced. What process was undertaken to review the incident? Were any tools used to document it? What recommendations would you make based on the principles of high reliability and risk anticipation?

Learning Activities

1. Consider your most recent work shift. Identify a process that would benefit from a process excellence value stream review.
2. Obtain a copy of a policy or procedure that is commonly used on your work unit. Is there an evidence base that supports the steps in the policy or procedure? Were the references from literature published less than five years ago? Who was involved in the development of the policy or procedure?
3. Keep a journal for one week of occurrences in your workday that do not achieve the desired outcomes despite multiple attempts at improvement. Using a system lens and drawing from improvement and high-reliability principles, what would you recommend to the unit leaders or clinical practice council as part of the microsystem assessment?

References

Agency for Healthcare Research and Quality. (2008). *Becoming a high reliability organization: Operational advice for hospital leaders*. https://archive.ahrq.gov/professionals/quality-patient-safety/quality-resources/tools/hroadvice/hroadvice.pdf

Agency for Healthcare Research and Quality. (2015). *High reliability*. https://psnet .ahrq.gov/primers/primer/31/high-reliability

American Association of Colleges of Nursing. (2007). *White paper on the role of the Clinical Nurse Leader.* Author. https://nursing.uiowa.edu/sites/default/files/documents/academic-programs/graduate/msn-cnl/CNL_White_Paper.pdf

American Association of Colleges of Nursing. (2011). *CNL job analysis study*. http://www.aacn.nche .edu/cnl/publications-resources/job-analysis-study

American Association of Colleges of Nursing. (2013). *Competencies and curricular expectations for clinical nurse leader education and practice*. http://www.aacn.nche.edu/publications/white-papers/cnl

Aroh, D., Colella, J. Douglas, C., & Eddings, A. (2015). An example of translating value-based purchasing into value-based care. *Urologic Nursing, 35*(2), 61–74.

Bachynsky, N. (2020). Implications for policy: The triple aim, quadruple aim, and interprofessional collaboration. *Nursing Forum, 55,* 54–64. https://doi.org/10.1111/nuf.12382

Berwick, D., Nolan, T., & Whittington, J. (2008). The triple aim: Care, health, and cost. *Health Affairs, 27*(3), 759–769.

Bowles, J., Batcheller, J., Adams, J., Zimmermann, D., & Pappas, S. (2019). Nursing's leadership role in advancing professional practice/work environments as part of the quadruple aim. *Nursing Administration Quarterly, 43*(2), 157–163. https://doi.org/10.1097/NAQ.0000000000000342

Centers for Medicare and Medicaid Services. (2013). *Expanded coverage under the Affordable Care Act: Information for health care professionals*. http://www.cms.gov/outreach-and-education/medicare-learning-network-mln/mln products/downloads/acamarketplacefactsheet-icn908826.pdf

Centers for Medicare and Medicaid Services. (2015). *National health expenditure data: Historical*. https://www.cms.gov/research-statistics-data-and-systems/statistics-trends-and-reports/nationalhealthexpenddata/nationalhealthaccountshistorical.html

Centers for Medicare and Medicaid Services. (2018). *National health expenditure data*. https://www.cms.gov/Research-Statistics-Data-and-Systems/Statistics-Trends-and-Reports/National HealthExpendData/NHE-Fact-Sheet

Chassin, M., & Loeb, J. (2013). High-reliability health care: Getting there from here. *Milbank Quarterly, 91,* 459–490.

Dartmouth Institute for Health Policy and Clinical Practice. (2015). *Clinical microsystems*. https://clinicalmicrosystem.org/

Feeley, D. (2017). *The triple aim or the quadruple aim? Four points to help set your strategy*. http://www.ihi.org /communities/blogs/the-triple-aim-or-the-quadruple-aim-four-points-to-help-set-your-strategy

Harris, J., & Thomas, P. (2021). Data as the centerpiece of administrative and clinical decisions. In P. Thomas, J. Harris, & B. Collins (Eds.), *Data-driven quality improvement and sustainability in healthcare*. Springer Publishing.

Institute of Healthcare Improvement. (2020). *Initiatives: The triple aim*. http://www.ihi.org/Engage /Initiatives/TripleAim/Pages/default.aspx

Institute of Medicine. (2011). *The healthcare imperative: Lowering costs and improving outcomes*. http://www.iom.edu/Reports/2011/The-Healthcare-Imperative-Lowering-Costs-and-Improving -Outcomes.aspx

Mahon, M. (2014). US health system ranks last among eleven countries on measures of access, equity, quality, efficiency, and healthy lives: Investment in primary care is essential to improving access and care coordination as Affordable Care Act expands coverage. *The Commonwealth Fund*. http://www.commonwealthfund.org/publications/press-releases/2014/jun/us-health -system-ranks-last

Martin, K., & Osterling, M. (2014). *Value stream mapping: How to visualize work and align leadership for organizational transformation*. McGraw-Hill.

Meyer, J., Rybowski, L., & Eichler, R. (1997). *Theory and reality of value-based purchasing: Lessons from the pioneers*. Agency for Health Care Policy and Research. Publication No. 98-0004.

Nelson, E., Batalden, P., & Godfrey, M. (2007). *Quality by design: A clinical microsystems approach*. Jossey-Bass.

Nelson, E., Batalden, P., & Goldfrey, M. (2011). *Value by design: Developing clinical microsystems to achieve organizational excellence*. Jossey-Bass.

Sackett, D., Rosenberg, W., Muir-Gray, J. Haynes, R., & Richardson, S. (1996). Evidence based medicine: What it is and what it isn't. *BMJ, 312,* 71–72.

Sackett, D., Straus, S., Richardson, S., Rosenberg, W., & Haynes, R. (2000). *Evidence-based medicine: How to practice and teach EBM* (2nd ed.). Churchill Livingston.

Sikka, R., Morath, J., & Leape, L. (2015). The quadruple aim: Care, health, cost and meaning in work. *BMJ Quality & Safety, 24*(10), 608–610.

Thomas, P., & Harris, J. (2021). Application of data science in healthcare. In P. Thomas, J. Harris, & B. Collins (Eds.), *Data-driven quality improvement and sustainability in healthcare* (pp. 87–100). Springer Publishing.

Tikkanen, R., & Abrams, M. (2020). US health care from a global perspective, 2019: Higher spending, worse outcomes? *The Commonwealth Fund*. https://www.commonwealthfund.org /publications/issue-briefs/2020/jan/us-health-care-global-perspective-2019

Tomey, A. (2010). *Guide to nursing management and leadership* (8th ed.). Mosby-Elsevier.

Womack, J. P., & Jones, D. T. (2003). *Lean thinking*. Free Press/Simon & Schuster.

EXEMPLAR ·

Resource Management in the Intensive Care Unit

Elizabeth F. Williams

The Patient Protection and Affordable Care Act instituted value-based purchasing to healthcare organizations resulting in a dramatic change in the ways these organizations receive reimbursement from the government. The focus is now on quality and satisfaction of care rather than quantity. Healthcare organizations are now required to meet 18 core measures and 17 HCAHPS metrics. Failure to do so could potentially result in a reduction of 1% of total payments (Johnson et al., 2012). These new requirements are one source for the relentless budget crunches that many health-care organizations experience. Budget cuts are now more important than ever. The CNL has an important role in aiding to identify areas for savings in the microsystem. This exemplar will focus on how the intensive care unit (ICU) CNL can exhibit fiscal stewardship by actively participating in resource management of clinical supplies in the microsystem.

Resource Management's Relation to the Delivery of Quality of Care

Healthcare delivery costs are multifaceted. Resource leveling entails ensuring the necessary clinical supplies are available to providers to deliver care while also curtailing any surplus or deficiency of essential supplies. If a change in supplies is identified, costs must be taken into consideration. However, those involved in the supply change must be cognizant that costs are not solely monetary. The people involved in the decision must also question the expense of not carrying out the supply change (J. Harris, personal communication, August 25, 2015). If the supply is causing harm to patients by way of increased infection rates or pressure ulcers, then the costs of not replacing the item with a more suitable item would have a negative impact on the quality of care for the patient. This illustration shows why resource management has a direct impact on quality of care. Appropriate supplies must be available for providers to deliver quality care.

Resource Management/Clinical Supplies in the ICU

Experts predict that 30% of hospital costs come from the ICU. The culture of critical care nurses has the expectation that supplies management should never allow them to run out of a product and should not refute supplies for low par volumes. But there is often faulty communication between nursing and supply management (Barlow, 2005). To have successful resource management in regard to clinical supplies, nursing and those in charge of supply management must have an open line of communication where compromise is present equally. It is vital for supply management to include clinical input in product decisions to avoid disparate supplies being replaced in inventory.

Individual materials distribution (IMD) houses and distributes supplies to the clinical areas at the facility. The clinical areas consist of the hospital (10-bed ICU/20-bed medical-surgical unit/emergency department/surgical suites), specialty and primary care clinics, long-term care, and inpatient mental health. The ICU is a 10-bed unit with a ratio of two patients per one nurse. No clinical area has a specific budget for supplies; rather, there is one global shared budget for all clinical areas: $4.1 million per fiscal year. The ICU has used $89,353.28, of the clinical budget, in supplies between fiscal year to date (FYTD) October 2014–August 2015. The corporate office determines what specific products are purchased for inventory. If problems are noted with a certain product, employees are encouraged to report the concern with a complaint form available on the intranet. Unlike most healthcare facilities, the patients at the facility do not get charged for medical supplies.

Consequently, nurses are not aware of the cost or accountability of products resulting in avertible waste.

The following supplies were identified by polling registered nurses in the ICU as the most frequently used supplies. The individual costs of the supplies are included as well as the total dollar amount used this FYTD, October 2014–August 2015.

Supply	Unit $	FYTD $
1. Purple Wipes	1.72	2,053.85
2. Oxygen sensors	11.67	1,633.37
3. Tegaderms	0.27	247.27
4. IV start kits	7.55	4,059.00
5. 20G PIVs	1.96	1,098.00
6. 19G needles	0.23	454.69
7. 12cc syringes	0.08	185.26
8. 2 × 2 sterile gauze	0.05	107.22
9. Lab tubes (average cost for most used tubes)	0.36	1,248.65
10. Primary IV tubing	6.00	3,771.01

CNL Role in Supply Management

Value-based purchasing is the culmination of evidence on the quality of healthcare with regard to patient outcomes, level of health, and dollar expenditures applied toward healthcare (Meyer et al., 1997). The CNL has the competence necessary to positively influence value-based purchasing through resource management. The CNL's presence in the microsystem positions them to be able to directly observe the product flow in the unit (Archbold & Thomas, 2014). The CNL should be mindful and observant of product waste, product par level overages/shortages, and product needs. Additionally, it is essential that the CNL ensure the staff are educated regarding supply expenditures as well as engage them in opportunities for improvement in the reduction of supply cost (Johnson et al., 2012). The identification of supply issues should be brought to the attention of those in charge of ordering supplies in the unit by the CNL. It is the role of the CNL to not only recognize these issues but to develop potential solutions and present them appropriately. In the ICU, the nurse manager is in charge of ordering the supplies and deciding what supplies will be kept in the supply room.

Conclusion

The current paradigm of performance-based payment necessitates healthcare providers to emphasize ways to reduce healthcare costs. CNLs are perfectly positioned to aid in resource management and improvement initiatives in their microsystem.

CNLs have the potential to prove their value to organizations by way of resource management, particularly in supply management.

References

Archbold, L., & Thomas, P. (2014). Creating a value-driven approach to care in a high-reliability organization. In J. Harris, L. Roussel, & P. Thomas (Eds.), *Initiating and sustaining the clinical nurse leader role: A practical guide* (2nd ed., pp. 197–209). Jones & Bartlett Learning.

Barlow, R. (2005). Critical conditioning: Supply strategies for ICU demand. *Healthcare Purchasing News, 29*(5), 10–12.

Johnson, D., Bell, B., Elgendy, J., Mcdonald, E., West, F., Wenzel, L., & Distefano, M. (2012). Don't waste green! Launching a budget awareness campaign. *Nursing Management, 43*(8), 51–54. https://doi.org/10.1097/01.NUMA.0000416412.14098.79

Meyer, J., Rybowski, L., & Eichler, R. (1997). *Theory and reality of value-based purchasing: Lessons from the pioneers.* Agency for Health Care Policy and Research. Publication No. 98-0004.

EXEMPLAR

Improving Patient Handoffs: Standardizing Workflows Using Lean Methodology and a Collaborative Team Approach

Melanie Hamilton

The application of Lean principles to existing workflow processes is a practical approach to improving value and efficiency in healthcare. A comprehensive microsystem assessment, completed on a 34-bed respiratory acute care unit at a large, urban pediatric hospital, revealed inefficiencies in the patient handoff process during shift changes. The patient handoff process lacked standardization; frequent interruptions, inconsistent practices, and fragmented workflows contributed to negative patient outcomes and staff dissatisfaction. In collaboration with unit leadership, the CNL student implemented a process improvement project to standardize the unit workflow during shift changes to limit interruptions and improve patient outcomes.

To promote a partnership approach to improvement efforts, an interdisciplinary project team was formed, and included registered nurses (RNs), patient care technicians (PCTs), unit secretaries (US), leadership, the CNL, and a clinical educator. Through the use of Lean methodology principles, the team identified inefficiencies and gaps in the current workflow processes during shift changes. Approaching the unit workflow as a complex system, the team separated and analyzed each workflow according to role (nurse, charge nurse, PCT, and US). Team members for each role served as workflow experts, providing expert knowledge on role-specific processes. Current state analysis identified process gaps and nonessential tasks that could be eliminated from each workflow; new process flow improvements were identified and developed for each role and included a set of standardized improvement interventions to be integrated into future state workflows. Each improvement idea was assigned a lead and a completion date. Staff-led education and training were developed and provided to all unit staff, promoting ownership and commitment of the workflow improvements.

Through effective integration of Lean methodology and facilitation of teams, the CNL successfully utilized the expert knowledge of each team member in waste identification to improve efficiency and standardize unit workflows during shift changes.

Patient Handoff: Imperatives for Quality, Safety, and Satisfaction Outcomes

Jessica R. Driscoll

At an emergency department (ED) in Southern Florida, nursing handoff was typically communicated by phone from ED to ICU nurses. After completing a needs assessment, it was determined handoff communication was an area of opportunity in the ED to improve nursing satisfaction, improve patient safety, increase patient-centered care, and improve the overall quality of care patients received. Patient handoff is a critical point in patient care where mistakes or miscommunication can easily occur. For example, The Joint Commission (2012) states that an estimated 80% of medical errors occur due to miscommunication during patient handoff. Therefore, the implementation of bedside handoff can improve communication, nursing satisfaction, and patient satisfaction.

Surveys were distributed to nurses before and after implementation to determine needs and outcomes. A total of 45 nurses completed the survey before implementation and 55 completed the survey one month after implementation. The bar

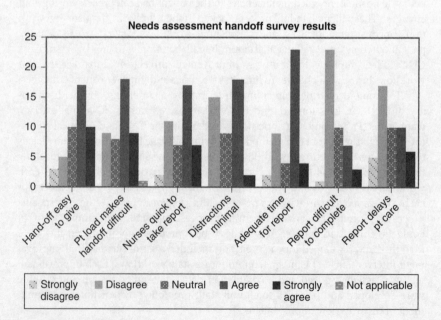

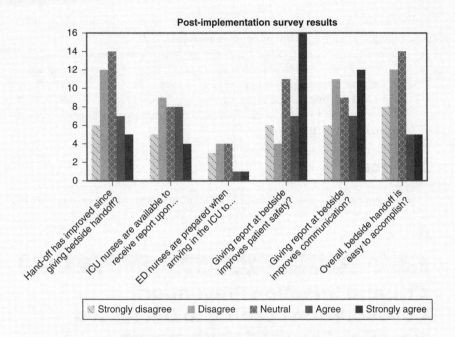

graphs display findings from the survey followed by various staff comments. Staff members stated they were content with the process; however, areas of improvement could prove beneficial. Staff indicated bedside handoff improves patient safety and communication. However, the process implemented was still in need of improvements to be the most valuable to patients. Bedside handoff is thought to be significant in patient safety. However, nurses believe the process was taking too long and not as efficient as possible.

Nursing Comments Regarding Bedside Handoff

- "Giving bedside report encourages teamwork among units. It facilitates rapport between team members more efficiently than over the phone."
- "Assisting in situating the patient on the bed and monitor as a team also improves bedside report and builds rapport and trust among units."
- "Getting a handoff tool with what the ICU expects from the ED may be helpful."
- "I believe bedside report helps nurses and patients understand their care and what is going on, but still a work in progress."
- "ED nurses care about specifics that are not as important to ICU nurses and vice versa."
- "The handoff is much better. I get to see the nurse who cares for the patient face to face. They can also answer why the patient has a new procedure/tube inserted at the bedside."
- "I prefer to give report while in ER because having patients charts in front of me helps to remember details that may be missed or forgotten."

- "It is taking too long to give report. We are off the floor for an average of 20 minutes, leaving our other patients unattended."
- "Difficulty writing stuff down, because of getting patient situation."
- "ICU nurses not available. Report takes longer. ED nurses do not have computers available to pass information from. ICU nurses seem rushed when taking report and less information is shared."
- "ED nurses tend to rush during report at bedside, making it difficult to collect important information."

Reference

The Joint Commission. (2012). Transitions of care: The need for a more effective approach to continuing patient care. *Hot Topics in Healthcare, 1*(8). http://www.jointcommission.org/assets/1/18/hot_topics_transitions_of_care.pdf

---

EXEMPLAR

CNL and Infection Prevention Collaboration Leading to Decreased Hospital-Acquired Vancomycin-Resistant Enterococcus on a Medical Specialty Unit

Jennifer Kareivis, Barbara Bonnah, Michelle Sheets, Kathy Roye-Horn, and Lisa Rasimowicz

Background

At Hunterdon Medical Center (HMC), the efficacy of the CNL is based on measurable indicators unique to each unit's population, as formulated by the chief nursing officer. Health care–acquired infections are one of the indicators. A 48-bed medical specialty unit, 3 West, screens all patients on admission for methicillin-resistant *Staphylococcus aureus* (MRSA) and vancomycin-resistant *Enterococcus* (VRE) to identify community-acquired cases.

Aim

To illustrate the correlation between the collaboration of CNLs and the infection prevention (IP) department and the decrease in hospital-acquired (HA) VRE at HMC.

Methods

In February 2010, an increase in the rate of HA VRE was noted. The CNLs collaborated with the IP department to decrease infection rates on the unit. A committee was formed to improve the rates of HA VRE. Staff nurses, housekeeping, patient care assistants, the IP department, unit management, and the CNLs on 3 West were included on the team. Observations were conducted to evaluate compliance with hand hygiene, use and cleaning of equipment, and wearing of PPE in isolation rooms. If a patient was positive for HA VRE, a review of his or her record was conducted. The CNL and IP department assessed if there was proximity to a patient with a known positive VRE, if the patient was on telemetry, or if the patient was utilizing a commode during his or her stay. An educational program was developed for the nursing staff, informing them of the increased rate of HA VRE and data from observations. The education focused on hand hygiene before/after patient contact and wiping of equipment before/after patient use.

Results/Conclusion

The overall rate of HA VRE decreased on the 3 West medical specialty unit from February 2010 to September 2010. The CNL cannot effect changes, such as decreasing HA VRE, without collaboration with other departments such as the IP department.

EXEMPLAR

Predictive Assessment Tool: Prevention of Return to ICU Post Transfer to Lower Level of Care

Sheri Salas and Lisa Mestas

Patients who are discharged from the ICU to medical surgical floors before they are stable are at risk for deterioration and readmission to the ICU. Early discharge from the ICU can increase the likelihood of ICU readmission and postdischarge unanticipated death if patients are discharged before they are stable (Badawi & Breslow, 2012). There are many negative implications related to readmission to the ICU. Readmission to the ICU is associated with worse outcomes and increased cost.

A postsurgical/trauma floor had 60 rapid response (RR) events from March–August 2012. Thirty-five percent (21) of those RR took place within 24 hours of transfer from the surgical trauma intensive care unit (STICU), and 13 of those patients had to transfer back to STICU (bounce backs). Sixty-two percent of patients that had an RR event within 24 hours of transfer out of the ICU bounced back.

RR events showed that patients were being transferred to the floor with high acuity levels at risk for adverse events on the medical surgical unit. No standard assessment tool is in place to ensure patients are stable to transfer to the floor. RR events take floor nurses away from the bedside of other patients while the ICU is interrupted with a declining patient when an RR results in a bounce-back transfer. Continuity of care is compromised in these events and length of stay is increased when a patient has complications after an RR event. An RR event raises the cost of the hospital stay by adding ICU days due to ICU readmission.

Data from six months of RR events that occurred in patients recently transferred from STICU to the floor was analyzed. Indicators that led to the events were utilized to create a predictive risk tool with a scoring system that would categorize patients as high, medium, or low risk to have an RR event within 24 hours of transfer to the floor when assessed in STICU prior to discharge from the unit. Data was shared with the surgical trauma team who agreed to participate in a pilot of the tool. The staff of both the ICU and floor were educated on the utilization of the tool. Staff were also educated on guidelines for patients that score within a high-risk category on the tool, which included consulting provider regarding patient status/readiness for transfer to a lower level of care based on indicators.

The pilot was initiated in March 2012 with a baseline annualized readmission rate within 24 hours (bounce back) from the floor to STICU of 70%. The tool was adopted and has been sustained for three years with bounce-back rates of 13% for 2014 and 2015. The rate for 2016 decreased to 10%. The total cost avoidance since initiation in 2012, based on average length of stay of return to ICU, is $472,038.

Since the tool has proven to be successful in this patient population, it will be integrated into the new electronic medical record system. The method for developing the tool is being utilized to develop similar evaluation screening mechanisms for other care areas.

Reference

Badawi, O., & Breslow, M. J. (2012). Readmissions and death after ICU discharge: Development and validation of two predictive models. *PLoS ONE, 7*, e48758. https://doi.org/10.1371/journal .pone.0048758

EXEMPLAR

Sustaining Heart Success Education Compliance

Noel Mendez and Myrna Martinez

In a 600-bed National Cancer Institute (NCI) designated hospital, a Heart Success program was implemented to ensure patients with heart failure (HF) or patients receiving cardiotoxic drugs are promptly screened and evaluated for HF. CMS requires hospitals to report CORE measures in patients who have HF and that they receive appropriate management and education about HF, including postdischarge follow-up to prevent readmission within 30 days related to HF symptoms.

The CNLs were instrumental in staff education, compliance monitoring, and sustainability efforts in this program. The CNLs used PowerPoint and case presentations to prepare the nurses on how to identify at-risk patients, collaborate with the primary team, and educate patients with HF. The process includes identifying patients with possible HF diagnosis based on set criteria including physical assessment, symptoms, history, and review of current medications. After which, the nurses collaborate with the primary team to confirm the HF diagnosis and start patient education comprised of a video, booklet, and teach-back session to ensure comprehension and provide opportunities for questions and clarification.

The CNLs use daily team briefs in identifying patients and providing appropriate resources to the nursing staff. The CNLs also identified unit champions by involving the charge nurses and unit secretaries to help with monitoring compliance with the Heart Success program. Compliance rate is audited every month based on the completion of interdisciplinary patient education records and discharge instructions. In the two years since the implementation of the program, the compliance rate has consistently been 90% to 100%.

EXEMPLAR

Understanding Nursing Workflow in Relation to Medication Administration Errors

Bethel Guk-Ong

The British Journal of Clinical Pharmacology defined medication error as a "failure in the treatment process that leads to or has the potential to cause patient harm" (Aronson, 2009). Medication administration errors are reported to the Safety Intelligence (SI) database. The unit's two CNLs collaborate with a nurse manager, an associate director, and charge nurses to prevent, monitor, investigate, trend, and formulate action plans for medication administration errors.

The estimated cost of medication errors that lead to an adverse event is $5.6 million per year (Walker, 2016). A process improvement initiative spearheaded by a CNL to decrease medication errors was implemented. It was identified that the error occurs during preparation and administration. Medication error and medication-related errors have been the highest SI events reported in fiscal year (FY) 2015.

As a means of engaging the frontline staff, their feedback was solicited during a monthly meeting. The action plan was the feedback of the staff that focused on the five rights of medication administration. The associate director's support was valuable in leading a cohesive work group. Leadership observations and on-the-spot coaching provided a second line of defense in preventing medication errors.

The lack of compliance with the use of the medication administration record (MAR) to verify medications during preparation and administration was related to MAR unavailability. The unit practice of clustering three to four patient MARs in one binder was the indirect start of medication errors. Before implementation of our electronic medical record, the unit workflow became a competition between RNs and patient service coordinators (PSCs) of who is holding the binder. The unavailable binder with three to four patient MARs causes a disruption in the workflow. The staff offered a suggestion to separate the MARs and place them in individual binders. The new process made the MAR available for the unit staff like PSC and RN.

The medication error data were made available on a unit board that includes the plan-do-study-act (PDSA) format, run chart, fishbone chart, and a table for prioritizing causes. This initiative was submitted to the institution's Celebrate Improvement department. There was a significant drop in medication errors in the unit after two months. From the identification of a unit opportunity to implementation, the reported medication error has steadily dropped from 13 to 1 after seven months.

While the institution was undergoing an electronic medical record implementation, medication errors were still the focus for the unit to monitor. There was only one medication error reported after the go-live of the electronic medical record, and it was non-nursing related.

References

Aronson, J. K. (2009). Medication errors: Definitions and classifications. *British Journal of Clinical Pharmacology, 67*(6), 599–604.
Walker, E. E. (2016). Medication errors. *Imperial Journal of Interdisciplinary Research, 2*(5).

Visible Teamwork: Primary Team Nursing and the Influence of a Newly Formed Leadership Team and Its "Going for the Gold Campaign"—The P7 Beacon Journey at MD Anderson Cancer Center

Christine Rudzinski Raby and Lyzanne Mason

The University of Texas MD Anderson Cancer Center (MDACC) is a 656–licensed bed NCI designated comprehensive cancer center located in the Texas Medical Center in Houston, Texas. MDACC is the number one cancer hospital in the nation and has achieved Magnet recognition for nursing excellence since 2002. The AACN confers a Beacon award for excellence to nursing units for a period of three years with a gold, silver, or bronze designation for meeting national criteria consistent with Magnet Recognition, the Malcolm Baldrige National Quality Award, and the National Healthcare Award (AACN, personal communication, July 2015).

The setting for our Beacon journey takes place on P7, a 32-bed progressive care unit. Our team specializes in providing care for patients undergoing thoracic/cardiovascular surgery and surgical oncology patients requiring postsurgical cardiac monitoring and complex care. Our unit is comprised of two 16-bed circular pods, with cardiac monitoring capabilities in every room. Additionally, 4 of the 32 rooms are equipped with arterial line monitoring.

In 2012, P7 achieved a Silver Beacon Award for Excellence. It was a great honor for the entire staff and an extraordinary achievement. This marked a major milestone not only for our unit but for our institution as P7 became the first unit to receive a Beacon Award for Excellence! As with Magnet redesignation, the Beacon redesignation journey was our unit's commitment to exceptional patient care, dedication to our team, and upheld our core values of caring, integrity, and discovery. Would this journey be possible and realistic given the fact that we had a newly formed leadership team and new nursing care model?

In June 2013, the CNL role was established on P7 along with primary team nursing (PTN). This created a new leadership structure for the unit and in turn resulted in the loss of three long-standing members of its team. The unit was in a state of transition for a lengthy period of time and expressed ongoing fear, anxiety, and concern with the new nursing model. Over time, the staff began to understand and appreciate the CNL's role as vital to the quality and safety of our patients. The CNLs had such a positive influence on our teams; they encouraged staff participation in unit committee meetings, promoted certification, and completed case presentations and a monthly educational series geared toward topics such as failure to rescue, safety events, civility, and care coordination. The staff changed their mindset from one that was focused on, "What else is going to happen to us?" to that of, "Let's make things happen for the patients!"

At the time of our Beacon redesignation, the P7 Leadership team was comprised of a new associate director (AD), two CNLs, one nurse manager (NM), and one educator. The skill mix of the P7 staff included 62 bachelor's-prepared RNs, 5 master's-prepared RNs, 10 certified nursing assistants, and 8 PSCs. The staff questioned the possibility of redesignation with the new leadership team because we only had six months to complete the application. However, with the support and encouragement from the leadership team, the staff was determined to "Go for the Gold!"

The P7 leadership team worked diligently with all staff members on both shifts to review the feedback report from our 2012 Silver Beacon application. The feedback report attributed to many visible improvements and practice changes that occurred on our unit since the inception of our new leadership team and PTN. Although the current leadership team was not part of the staff for the first application, they were able to articulate how important the redesignation was for both the unit and the institution. How did we rejuvenate the enthusiasm and passion within our team?

The CNLs distributed questions from the Beacon application to appropriate P7 committee team members, clinical charge nurses, members of the leadership team, and other staff who volunteered their responses. Weekly Beacon meetings were hosted by the CNLs and our AD and occurred weekly from July 2014 to November 2014 until all the questions on the application were answered. We used these sessions to brainstorm and provide feedback to staff as a team; we truly wanted the voice of staff to be heard throughout the application. Our 48-page Beacon application was submitted to the AACN in December 2014 after many collaborative editing sessions with the CNLs and AD. As soon as our application was finalized and submitted, an announcement was made to staff, and we waited anxiously for news about the status of our redesignation.

After a well-deserved wait, we received an email on July 6, 2015, from the AACN Beacon team stating, "Congratulations to the P7 Thoracic/Cardiovascular Surgery at U of TX MD Anderson Cancer Center on successfully achieving a SILVER-level AACN Beacon Award for Excellence. Your unit's accomplishment represents one of many significant milestones on the path to optimal outcomes and exceptional patient care" (AACN, personal communication, July 2015). Even though our team was striving for the gold, the Silver Beacon Award was gold to them. Moving forward, staff members now make it a point to collect exemplars of extraordinary care practices for our next Beacon redesignation in 2018. We all agree: This will be gold!

The honor of achieving the redesignation of the Silver Beacon Award is best stated by a P7 clinical charge nurse, "The Beacon Award is such an honor for our team. It reflects and validates our unit's commitment to exceptional patient care and continued learning while showcasing MD Anderson's core values: Caring, Integrity and Discovery. I am proud to work with such an accomplished group of healthcare providers" (K. Berg, personal communication, April 2016).

Contrasting the CNL Versus the Advanced Practice Provider: Evidence for a Different but Valuable Role

Sarah Price and Janice Sills

The role of the CNL as an advanced master's-prepared generalist is easily misinterpreted or minimized when compared to the role of Advanced Practice Providers (APP). Without diagnostic responsibilities or prescriptive rights, for example, how does the CNL clinically practice beyond the scope of other nurses and healthcare providers? The answer lies within their unique position of expertise and presence. Many graduate-level nursing positions arguably decrease nurse-to-patient face time, however, the CNL is uniquely immersed in their population regardless of whether this is at the micro-, macro-, or mesosystem level. This frontline presence in addition to advanced clinical education empowers the CNL to foster collaborative relationships and improve outcomes. Consider the following example:

> A patient was admitted for an elective lumbar fusion. While participating in nurse-provider rounds over postoperative days (POD) 1 and 2, the CNL noted marked pancytopenia. The provider justified these abnormalities to be a result of surgical blood loss and hemodilution and gave orders to trend labs. The CNL continued to investigate. The patient's history provided no diagnosis to support such findings. Surgical blood loss was minimal and postoperative IV fluid therapy was routine. Upon interaction with the patient, she did not display the typical signs and symptoms of volume depletion such as low blood pressure, light-headedness, or dizziness. Additionally, the CNL continued to coach the bedside nurse regarding the abnormal findings and persistently advocated to the provider the need to work up the pancytopenia of unknown etiology. Finally, on POD 4, a hematology consult was initiated, which triggered an urgent bone marrow biopsy, transfer to the oncology unit, and probable diagnosis of acute myeloid leukemia.

This example highlights the CNL's role as an advanced generalist trained to contribute to the plan of care in a different but much needed way, offering expertise beyond that of the bedside nurse and a frontline presence beyond that of the provider. Another differentiating aspect of the CNL's role is that the CNL's work is not complete nor fully satisfied with one clinical save such as the one outlined previously. Alternately, findings such as this trigger other CNL core roles such as risk anticipator, advocate, catalyst, and outcomes manager to lead change, maintain patient safety, and improve outcomes. The CNL is called not only to care for individual patients during one shift but for populations throughout the care continuum as well. Thus, the CNL recognizes that each clinical save reveals an opportunity for process improvement with the ability to spread positive change from one bedside to the microsystem and beyond. For example, the CNL has used the knowledge gained from this clinical save combined with other evidence to make a case for initiating structured interdisciplinary rounding as a standard of care on the unit. In this way, the CNL truly maximizes the value of the role to improve outcomes by filling gaps that otherwise might allow patients to fall through the proverbial cracks. So, while CNLs are not APPs, their work provides positive results that should be valued as such.

Geriatric CNL Ensuring Geriatric-Friendly Care Provision Beyond the Microsystem

Tru Byrnes

Background

Since the implementation of the CNL role at Carolinas Medical Center (CMC) about 10 years ago, the CNLs had always been focused on the care of diverse patient populations within their 12-bed microsystem. In 2019, the Chief Nurse Executive (CNE) of CMC changed the CNL practice model for over 30 practicing CNLs and CNL students from a 12-bed microsystem focus to a population-based focus—meaning the CNLs concentrate on improving the care for a specific population. They would follow their patients throughout the care continuum from admission to discharge. This change allowed the CNLs to hone their clinical expertise, which provides a better opportunity to develop process improvement and standardize care to impact patient outcomes. In 2020, the first geriatric CNL role at CMC was implemented. The geriatric CNL oversees at least 24 inpatient adults across two hospitals. These units admitted more than 20,000 older adults annually. Her focus was geared toward ensuring safe care provision of high-risk patients aged 65 and older.

Bridging the Gap of Geriatric Care

To improve the geriatric population outcomes, the geriatric CNL would need a team to help create and implement processes. She then formed and led the Nurses Improving Care for Health System Elders (NICHE) Steering Committee. This committee consisted of multidisciplinary team members, including geriatric providers, a pharmacist, an occupational therapist, a nurse leader, a nurse educator, clinical nurse leaders, an informatics specialist, and clinical nurse specialists. When reviewing 2019 delirium data, it showed that older adults who had delirium had at least seven extra hospital stays, costing additional billions of dollars annually in healthcare costs. The patients with delirium were more likely to be discharged to a skilled nursing facility instead of home. Thus, the first task that the NICHE committee focused on was the delirium prevention initiative in hospitalized older adults by creating a nursing education program, which provided education to more than 700 nurses across two hospitals, developed delirium patient education, and integrated the education into the interactive patient care system (IPCS). Further, the NICHE committee developed a delirium risk stratification strategy to predict high-risk patients, created a nursing nonpharmacological delirium protocol, and incorporated the delirium management treatment guidelines into the electronic medical record.

The geriatric CNL performs daily rounds on high-risk patients and patients with delirium on the unit. During these rounds, she provides family education, ensures that staff implements the delirium prevention protocol, and discusses in real time the possibility of removing harmful treatments and high-risk medications with the physician. In the future, the hope is to have the delirium risk stratification tool implemented in the electronic health record to capture more patients and at the point of hospital entry for early identification.

Outcomes

As a result of this extensive work, the geriatric CNL has already identified a reduction in length of stay and cost savings. On a medical-surgical unit, 40% of delirium incidence reduction was achieved with a potential cost avoidance of $187,000 to $704,000. While performing chart audits, she found many high-risk medications based on the BEER criteria were used (American Geriatrics Society, 2015), particularly medicines that could induce delirium. Within two months, she found 79 out of 179 (45%) older adults age 65 and older had one or more high-risk medications on the MAR. When the geriatric CNL discovered something, she would contact the provider to have those medications removed. For example, she noticed Lorazepam was prescribed for an 82-year-old patient for agitation. She recommended discontinuing it due to the risk of delirium and falls. Later that day, she discovered 20 mg of Zyprexa was ordered for this patient. She immediately contacted the physician and suggested a safe starting dose of 2.5 mg for an older adult. Even though it is challenging to attach the cost savings to these events, we know from the literature that potential inappropriate medications can increase healthcare costs (Hyttinen et al., 2016).

Conclusion

In less than a year of implementing this role, the geriatric CNL has impacted older adults' outcomes in many ways. In addition to the previous examples, she has served as a geriatric clinical expert for healthcare team members, including a CNL colleague, nurses, providers, and even a nurse executive consulted for advice regarding complex geriatric care. When fully supported by the nursing leader, this role demonstrates the extensive bandwidth of the CNL's role. It also displays the extraordinary power the role can have on patient outcomes.

References

American Geriatrics Society. (2015). American Geriatrics Society 2015 updated BEERs criteria for potentially inappropriate medication use in older adults. *Journal of the American Geriatrics Society, 63*(11), 2227–2246.

Hyttine, V., Jyrkka, J., & Valtonen, H. (2016). A systematic review of the impact of potentially inappropriate medication on health care utlization and costs among older adults. *Medical Care, 54*(10), 950–964. https://doi.org/10.1097/MLR.0000000000000587

CHAPTER 4

CNLs Creating a Culture of Quality, Safety, and Value

James L. Harris and Patricia L. Thomas

LEARNING OBJECTIVES

1. Provide a case for quality, safety, value, and risk aversion/management.
2. Analyze how a culture of quality improvement and evidence-based practice improves CNL practice and value across healthcare settings.
3. Discuss how CNLs contribute to the attainment of core measures, identified performance standards, and markers of success.
4. Discuss the link to quality, safety, and value in clinical immersions, including failure modes and effect analysis (FMEA) and root-cause analysis (RCA).
5. Identify how to use data sets for assessing need and project management success.
6. Identify how the clinical value compass can improve quality care.
7. Identify crucial measurement systems that quantify quality and safety processes and project sustainability.
8. Discuss how using the logic model and other improvement models with accompanying metrics, including summative and formative evaluation, result in sustainable project outcomes.

KEY TERMS

Organizational learning
Culture of safety
Quality improvement
Planning
Quality patient care and safety
Cyclical review

Needs assessment
Metrics and measurement
Microsystems
Evidence-based practice
Risk aversion
Value

CNL ROLES

Member of a profession

Outcomes manager

Team manager

Information manager

Systems analyst/risk anticipator

Coordinator of care

PROFESSIONAL VALUES

Accountability

Outcome measurement

Quality improvement

Interprofessional teams

Integrity

Financial stewardship

Microsystems management

Evidence-based practice

Social justice

Quality patient care and safety

CNL COMPETENCIES

Critical thinking

Ethical decision-making

Communication

Team leader

Assessment

Information and healthcare
   technologies

Healthcare systems and policy
   designer/manager/coordinator
   of care

Assessment environment of care
   manager

Nursing technology and resource
   management

Introduction

The AACN's role expectations for the CNL place an emphasis on the need to redesign care delivery for improved patient safety, effectiveness, and efficiency (AACN, 2007). In 2013, the AACN stipulated in the *Competencies and Curricular Expectations for Clinical Nurse Leader Education and Practice* white paper that "the CNL assumes accountability for patient-care outcomes through the assimilation and application of evidence-based information to design, implement, and evaluate patient-care processes and models of care delivery" (p. 4). Highlighting alignment between the AACN's *The Essentials of Master's Education in Nursing* (2011) and the CNL competencies and accountability for quality, safety, and value, the expectations for CNL practice and action were apparent. Integral to the care delivery redesign process are interprofessional team members committed to excellence and quality improvement quantified through metrics and measurement (National Quality Forum, 2017). By acknowledging the need to decrease fragmentation of care in the delivery system, processes underlying care delays, redundancy or gaps in service, and dissatisfaction within provider, patient, and stakeholder groups, a quality improvement framework offers methods to support changes in interrelated systems aimed toward better clinical and financial outcomes.

Several landmark studies have influenced the trends in quality improvement to address real and pressing concerns in the US health system. In 1999 the IOM published *To Err Is Human: Building a Safer Health System*, which stated that between 44,000 and 98,000 Americans die each year as a result of medical errors; this exceeds the annual loss of lives from car accidents, breast cancer, and AIDS. Additionally, the cost of preventable errors resulting in injury was reported between $17 and

$29 billion. The fragmentation of the healthcare delivery system was identified as a major contributor to these errors. In response to these findings, building a safer, outcomes-driven care delivery system relying on quality improvement tools to increase efficiency, cost effectiveness, and high performance became a focus (AACN, 2007; The Joint Commission, 2008).

A second IOM report, *Crossing the Quality Chasm: A New Health Care System for the 21st Century* (2001), made an urgent call for change that emphasized safety, effectiveness, patient-centeredness, and care that is timely, efficient, and equitable. This landmark study stressed the environment of care and systems issues as pivot points that negatively impact safety and effectiveness, noting that the care patients receive in today's healthcare delivery system has become increasingly complex, with nurses simultaneously interacting with multiple systems, processes, and technologies (Healthcare Information and Management Systems Society, 2015; Kelly et al., 2014; Nelson et al., 2007). In a follow-up report, *Health Professions Education: A Bridge to Quality*, the IOM (2003) recommended that health professionals be educated to deliver patient-centered care as members of an interdisciplinary team, emphasizing implementation of evidence-based practices, quality improvement practices, and informatics (AACN, 2007). In 2015, *Measuring the Impact of Interprofessional Education (IPE) on Collaborative Practice and Patient Outcomes* emphasized interprofessional collaboration, team-based healthcare delivery, and enhanced personal and population health. This report acknowledged definitive evidence linking IPE to outcomes does not yet exist. The gap in evidence and the challenges present to close this gap warrant attention and will need to include strategies to overcome barriers that limit a clear connection between IPE and health and system outcomes (p. 8).

In 2008, The Joint Commission published a report, *Health Care at the Crossroads: Guiding Principles for the Development of the Hospital of the Future*, which emphasized the increasing complexity of care delivery and the pace of change and innovations that make it difficult for clinicians to keep up. Recognizing that hospitalized patients have higher acuity, more comorbid conditions in need of management, and shortened hospital stays, The Joint Commission report stated that the average length of stay has decreased 25% since the 1980s. At the same time, the Food and Drug Administration approved more than 500,000 new medical devices. Advances in pharmaceuticals and genomic developments have exploded onto the health delivery landscape during this time period as well. Although advances in technology help improve patient outcomes, the volume of technology and the requisite knowledge to manage new technology have made care delivery more complex, with unforeseen opportunities for error. This multifaceted complexity weighs heavily on conscientious clinicians. To respond to these demands, The Joint Commission identified the CNL as the clinician best suited to manage the "real-time" care of patients within the microsystem to ensure the use of evidence-based practices and quality improvement principles, measurement, and evaluation to improve patient care outcomes.

The CNL role creates an opportunity for new care models and team configurations in every delivery setting. Regulatory and accreditation pressures to increase safety and reduce costs are mounting as health outcomes are examined. Similarly, access to timely and cost-effective care for underserved populations is central to meeting the social determinants of health in a safe and cost-effective manner (Chang et al., 2018). Unprecedented attention to cost, dwindling human and financial resources, and acknowledgment of increasing complexity underpin the desire to systematically address historical practices that present threats to patient safety (Bender, 2016; Bender et al., 2012; The Joint Commission, 2008; Newhouse, 2006; Rusch & Bakewell-Sachs, 2007).

The assumptions underpinning the CNL role competencies are translated into daily operational performance in a microsystem where the CNL interacts at the point of care across the care continuum. Cost evaluation, return on investment, and cost-benefit analyses will be essential to validate the CNL's impact on cost reductions in an environment where pay for performance and the expectation of reducing errors and improving safety and efficiency are paramount to future organizational success (Bender, 2016; Crema & Verbano, 2013; Stavrianopoulos, 2012; Williams & Bender, 2015). Anticipating risks that influence safety and care outcomes, the CNL is positioned to scan the practice environment to identify system issues that could result in error, harm, or added costs based on the underlying processes embedded in care delivery. CNLs are uniquely qualified by their education in advanced clinical knowledge, understanding of systems, attention to measurement and outcomes, and firm grounding in quality improvement principles to lead teams of clinical professionals through risk identification, assessment, and planning to improve patient safety (AACN, 2013). CNLs target interventions that are specific to identified needs and populations based on assessments that ensure accountability across disciplines.

Background

The AACN, in collaboration with nurse executives, health systems, and educators, proposed the CNL as a nursing solution to address gaps in healthcare quality by addressing patient needs, safety, and quality improvement through a systematic and deliberate approach to implementing evidence-based practice, quality management, and clinical leadership at the point of care. CNLs are educationally prepared as advanced generalists accountable for identifying outcomes of practice on assigned patient care areas. CNLs can accomplish their goals by participating in a range of quality improvement projects aimed to collect and create evidence, by leading multidisciplinary teams, and by incorporating interventions with the greatest likelihood to produce high-quality care outcomes (AACN, 2007, 2013; Bender, 2016).

In 2008, Berwick, Nolan, and Whittington articulated the "triple aim" for health care: "improving the experience of care, improving the health of populations, and reducing per capita costs of health care" (p. 579). The preconditions include enrollment of an identified population, a commitment to universality for members, and the existence of an organization (an "integrator") that accepts responsibility for all three aims for that population. The organization's responsibilities highlight partnerships with patients and families, redesign of primary care, population health management, fiscal responsibility, and macrosystem integration. The CNL is positioned to address the triple aim and support organizational integration through meticulous application of quality and risk management principles and processes in microsystems to support the macrosystem integration.

Recently, the triple aim has been expanded to the quadruple aim, adding well-being of the care team members in the equation of better care experiences, care of populations, and efficient lower cost care. Recognizing care providers' engagement and resilience are central to quality and safety, attention to the team members who care for patients is emphasized. In addition to reasonable workloads and practices that support engagement, satisfaction, and meaning in work, the quadruple aim also focuses on recognition of burnout and issues in the environment to enhance work life. Examples of ways to incorporate this into work include team documentation, use of protocols for health preventative interventions by nurses and medical assistants, close proximity to team members, use of preappointment testing to expedite care at laboratories, standardized prescriptions and refills, training and orientation of staff coupled with redesign of work to eliminate unnecessary elements (Bodenheimer & Sinsky, 2014).

Supporting a Culture of Safety

Developing a culture of safety and supporting the basic tenents are critical to improving quality, safe care, and value-based operations (Weaver et al., 2013). Given the general agreement that patient safety needs improvement, it is important for healthcare providers to have a consistent, clear, and concise definition of what quality encompasses. Lohr (1990) defined quality as "the degree to which health services for individuals and populations increase the likelihood of desired health outcomes and are consistent with current professional knowledge" (p. 4). Systematic, deliberate, and defined methods will be needed to measure, understand, improve, and communicate internal progress at the unit and organization level. Regulatory agencies and groups external to the organization (including professional organizations, payers, and policy makers) will also need this information to make policy decisions based on clear measurements, shared goals, and systematic approaches toward improvement (Strome, 2013; Williams & Bender, 2015).

Wilson (2013) emphasized that most studies related to the perceptions of patient safety culture were associated with professional characteristics like role, rank, and practice settings or work design and workforce deployment. Wilson contends that the organizational contextual factors such as teamwork, communication openness, manager support, organizational learning, feedback about errors, error reporting, and nonpunitive responses to errors influence perceptions of safety and a culture of safety. The collective safety organizing behaviors heightened team awareness of safety and provide the psychological safety for reporting errors and recovering from mistakes. In this study, collective safety organizing behaviors were associated with more positive perceptions of a patient culture of safety.

CNLs are situated to mentor, coach, and guide teams to enact the paradigm shift necessary to sustain a culture of safety found in the application of evidence-based practices and actionable quality improvement that is supported by data. In addition to advanced clinical knowledge, CNLs examine the care delivery system from the perspective of individual patients or a microsystem population framework, recognizing the interrelated functions of process, information management, and outcomes (AACN, 2007, 2013; Bender, 2016; Nelson et al., 2007). As such, CNLs have the opportunity to influence safety culture through microsystem leadership, safety awareness, leading teams, and relationship building aimed toward organizational learning.

Risk Anticipation, Risk Assessment, and Risk Management

For many clinicians, discussion of "risk" conjures up visions of litigation, malpractice, and blame. Risk management historically focused on reducing liability, but in recent years, risk management has been closely aligned to quality improvement through the identification of processes to reduce errors, increase communication, and develop standardization in processes to establish consistency in care. The American Society for Healthcare Risk Management (ASHRM), affiliated with the American Hospital Association, provides the following definition of risk management: "Enterprise risk management in healthcare promotes a comprehensive framework for making risk management decisions which maximize value protection and creation by managing risk and uncertainty and their connections to total value" (ASHRM, 2014, p. 5). This process involves risk identification, analysis, treatment, and evaluation inclusive of monitoring, identification, and prevention of situations that could result in injury, financial loss, or regulatory noncompliance (ASHRM, 2014). Common elements of risk management programs include review of policies, procedures, and protocols; incident reporting; claims management; review of standards of care; and awareness of regulatory and accreditation requirements.

"Enterprise risk management," as defined by Carroll (2009), is a structured analytical organizational process that focuses on risk exposures that are both proactive and reactive. It includes identifying and eliminating the financial impact and volatility of a portfolio of risks rather than on risk avoidance alone. Essential to this approach is an understanding that risk can be managed to gain competitive advantage. Risk anticipation becomes part of a systematic process review found in process redesign or process flow diagramming in quality improvement projects.

Enterprise risk management (ERM) uses a process or framework to complete a comprehensive assessment and measurement of risk throughout an organization. It relies on stratification of risk into domains, looking for interrelatedness or interdependencies that allow the development of strategies to manage each risk. The domains include clinical operations, finance, human, strategic, legal/regulatory, and technological risks (ASHRM, 2014).

Two principles guide ERM: the recognition that risk represents capital or potential for loss, and the belief that holistic or comprehensive approaches are critical to manage diverse risks. This framework requires awareness that risks are not isolated; although organizations are often structured in operational silos, the risks do not occur in isolation. Traditional healthcare risk management takes a clinically focused approach and examines risks individually. The ERM model defines risks in terms of the probability that adverse events will occur and result in financial losses. Risk management focuses on protecting the organization's assets. Instead of handling risk in functional silos where measurements of success are variable, an enterprise-wide risk management approach employs common metrics across risk domains to determine the effectiveness of risk management strategies that focus on both opportunity and risk (ASHRM, 2014).

Risk assessment is often undertaken as a vehicle to improve safety. Recent initiatives to reduce hospital infections and falls, to improve and increase effective communication between healthcare team members, and to reduce errors have been showcased in regulatory requirements, reimbursement policies, and patient satisfaction results. Improvement activities highlight the ways organizations leverage opportunity in replicating successes achieved in different parts of an organization or microsystems, stressing that quality, safety, and cost can all improve when a risk is addressed and avoiding legal action germane to improving care outcomes. Value-based care, bundled payments, and pay-for-performance have shifted the financial risk for payers to providers. A broader range of risk management and aversion is therefore required (New England Journal of Medicine Catalyst, 2018).

Many clinicians view the mitigation of risk in the context of quality improvement activities for good reason. Many of the tools used in quality improvement work, like root-cause analyses, fishbone diagrams, FMEAs, and monitoring of outcome metrics, are common to risk management. Regulatory bodies also advocate risk anticipation and management through expectations of high reliability in healthcare organizations.

CNLs have an opportunity to identify high-risk processes in their assessment of the microsystem and guide improvement work to mitigate risk. Because CNLs have knowledge of process streams in the clinical environment, awareness of inputs and outputs, or gaps in care, they are positioned to lead interprofessional efforts to improve outcomes using evidence-based practices to manage risk. Likewise, as risks are identified, the CNL can support unit-level practice and process changes by mentoring and coaching team members through the change. As CNLs expand practice to include additional microsystem settings, a broader lens is available to view risk. This has opened new opportunities for CNLs to proactively engage in legal, political, and risk mitigation efforts.

Recent focus on CMS and The Joint Commission core measures have provided CNLs opportunities to improve outcomes and sustain change by affording common definitions of expected outcomes. At the microsystem level, care for patients with acute myocardial infarction, heart failure, pneumonia, stroke, surgical care, and vaccination rates have been identified as a priority for organizations recognizing interventions at the point of care that are timely, consistently executed, and effective lead to exemplary practices and results. Nursing sensitive indicators related to falls, catheter-associated urinary tract infections, central line infections, ventilator-associated pneumonia, patient satisfaction, and hospital associated pressure ulcers are common focal points for CNLs given their embeddedness on the unit and awareness of gaps or barriers that impede performance (Bender, 2016; Bender et al., 2012; Ott et al., 2009; Stavrianopoulos, 2012; Wilson et al., 2013).

Quality Improvement, Evidence-Based Practice, and the CNL Role

Quality improvement is known by many names but holds in common the real-life experiences and data within an organization to rapidly cycle through a defined process to evaluate outcomes (McLaughlin & Kaluzny, 2005; Strome, 2013; White et al., 2016). The terms *continuous quality improvement*, *total quality management*, *performance improvement*, and *process improvement* are often used interchangeably to describe efforts geared toward data-driven, process-oriented, outcome-focused activities. These efforts were originally established in the business world and have recently been applied in the healthcare industry. Often, quality improvement is offered as a framework to examine long-standing clinical and systems issues in a different way (McLaughlin & Kaluzny, 2005; Nelson et al., 2007; Strome, 2013; White et al., 2016).

The key feature of quality improvement is the cyclical nature of the process, which is designed to evaluate workflow and processes built from value-added actions that are performed by work teams in a system (McLaughlin & Kaluzny, 2005; Newhouse, 2006; Strome, 2013; White et al., 2016). Quality improvement processes do not meet the standards of rigor found in scientific research and have neither theoretical underpinnings nor an aim to generate new knowledge. Rather, quality improvement aims to bring individuals who work together into a venue where systematic review and evaluation of work processes can be examined in a cyclical fashion as a means to evaluate and improve established practices and outcomes (Newhouse, 2007; White et al., 2016).

Philosophical Elements of Quality Improvement

Continuous quality improvement has several characteristics that are evident in organizations. According to McLaughlin and Kaluzny (2005), they include the following:

1. Strategic focus drawing on the mission and values of the organization
2. A customer focus directed toward patients, providers, and stakeholders
3. A systems perspective, revealing emphasis on the interdependence of interacting processes that influence outcomes
4. Data-driven analysis emphasizing the gathering of objective data to influence decision-making
5. Team involvement inclusive of representatives that implement current work processes and those who will implement the resulting workflow change
6. Multiple causations requiring identification of root causes
7. Sets of solutions identified to enhance system functions and outcomes
8. Process optimization supported by alignment of tools and structures to evaluate interventions
9. Continuous improvement supported by ongoing analysis of outcomes directed toward ongoing modification of processes to enhance system performance
10. Organizational learning so the capacity to generate future improvements is enhanced (White et al., 2016)

Several quality improvement methodologies reside in health systems, identified as Lean, Six Sigma, or TQM structures. Irrespective of the quality improvement methodology selected by an organization, there are eight common steps in quality improvement:

1. A clear and defined aim or purpose
2. A review of the literature
3. Examination of current resources to facilitate quality improvement
4. Mapping the current processes

5. Root-cause analysis (RCA)
6. Selecting appropriate tools for process analysis
7. Selecting measures and metrics (baseline and outcome)
8. Rapid cyclical review of the plan, data, interventions, and outcomes (McLaughlin & Kaluzny, 2005; White et al., 2016).

Defined Aim or Purpose

Having a clear purpose or aim in any project seems logical, but this is a part of quality improvement that can lead to frustration when project teams engage in work. Because the team is composed of individuals from varied disciplines, many assumptions are made that define how clinical issues are individually viewed. Additionally, because processes are complex and interrelated, it is easy for a team to lose focus or expand the project scope if the aim or purpose is not clearly and explicitly defined.

When creating an aim or purpose for a quality improvement team, answering the "who, what, when, where, and how" of a project is key. *Who* refers to the people affected by the concern; *what* refers to the problem identified; *when* refers to the timing of the issue; *where* refers to the specific unit or location of the concern; and *how* refers to the measures, metrics, or standards that alert the team to an issue. Once the team can establish these parameters, elevator discussions or concise yet informative language suitable to a conversation that lasts through the duration of an elevator ride can be crafted. Additionally, when the team starts to drift into processes or topics that do not relate specifically and directly to the purpose or aim of the team, these issues for the "parking lot" can be documented for future discussion or communication to other project teams.

Review of the Literature

EBP has been defined as a problem-solving approach to clinical decision-making that ingrates the best available scientific evidence with the best available experiential evidence from patients and practitioners; it incorporates the organization's culture, internal and external influences on practice, and critical thinking that supports judicious application of the evidence to the care of an individual, a population of patients, or the system. EBP and research inform quality improvement through review of the literature. By providing interventions with a great likelihood of success, both research and EBPs inform quality improvement (DiCenso et al., 2005; Hall & Roussel, 2014; White et al., 2016).

Central to the CNL role is the expectation that clinical practice and interventions will be evidence-based. Driven from past experiences in not achieving consistent and sustainable improvements and increasing regulatory demands to demonstrate the inclusion of evidence in processes, protocols, and policies, EBPs are gaining attention (Hall & Roussel, 2014). National patient safety goals based on The Joint Commission's requirements and supported by the National Quality Forum set the overarching goal for establishing EBP as the norm in clinical care (Department of Health and Human Services, 2011; The Joint Commission, 2008).

Resources to Facilitate Improvement

When undertaking a quality improvement initiative, it is important to explore, examine, and establish both internal and external resources for support. Internal resources can include individuals from quality management departments, finance, information services, libraries, and education departments. Books, websites, and discussions with members of the interdisciplinary team who have experience with quality improvement activities can provide important resources to support a team's efforts. External resources include professional organizations, internet resources, quality improvement organizations, and members of other industries with knowledge of quality management or RCA.

Mapping Current Processes

Several methods for mapping current processes exist. When initiating the mapping process, CNLs will engage members of the interdisciplinary team in exercises to identify, define, and document process steps, decision points, and inputs from other departments or disciplines that lead to the current outcomes (McLaughlin & Kaluzny, 2005; White et al., 2016). This stage involves a detail-specific discussion between members of the team to capture the complexity of the process intended for improvement.

Design Thinking

As CNLs engage with teams to map processes and select tools for improvement, design thinking is a useful process to approach unresolved complex issues. Design thinking is a solution-based process that provides a different perspective centered on empathy where stakeholder experiences and needs are highlighted and problems are framed in human-centric terms, ideas evolve, prototypes/interventions are created and tested/implemented (Dam & Siang, 2019). Hasso, Meinel, and Weinberg (2009) identified six stages of design thinking to include the following.

1. *Understanding* through a process of empathizing with individuals to gain perspectives on experiences and motivations.
2. *Observing* the physical environment of individuals within the context of experiences and motivations.
3. *Identifying* a point of view that culminates in defining a problem in human-centric terms.
4. *Ideating* offers individuals and teams to view problems in an alternative manner.
5. *Prototyping* is the opportunity where the product/intervention is tested, approved, or rejected based on individual and team perspectives.
6. *Testing* is the final stage where opportunities exist to make final refinements toward solving the identified problem, as it is ready for implementation. This stage also provides opportunities for individuals to gain an understanding of the uniqueness of the solution toward solving the problem.

Through this nonlinear process, individuals and improvement teams empathize, define problems, generate alternative solutions to a problem, develop and test solutions to a product and/or intervention. This process engages interprofessional teams and individual providers to generate quality, safe solutions whereby new techniques are generated.

Root-Cause Analysis

The Joint Commission established expectations for organizations to proactively identify high-risk processes that are likely to contribute to errors. Within this process is the realization that systems and processes contribute to adverse events and errors. Because quality improvement initiatives are focused on addressing processes, it is important to use systematic approaches to guide teams in identifying the root cause or process that breaks down and leads to an undesired result. Once a process flow is completed, further analysis of each process is required to identify the underlying cause or step in a process that sets into motion a cause and effect that drives an occurrence or problem. Drilling down on process steps to identify a root cause can be accomplished using different tools, but cause and effect or fishbone diagrams are most common. Fishbone diagrams delineate the causes of a situation centered on predefined categories of people, materials, methods, machinery, and policy (McLaughlin & Kaluzny, 2005; Strome, 2013).

Selecting Appropriate Tools

Several tools are used to represent data collected before, during, and after quality improvement efforts are undertaken. Each tool has a distinct purpose and provides a fact-based approach to identify concerns, propose solutions, and monitor outcomes of the process changes. The most common tools include brainstorming, cause and effect diagrams, Pareto charts, control charts, process flow diagrams, fishbone diagrams, surveys, pie charts, histograms, and run charts (McLaughlin & Kaluzny, 2005; Strome, 2013).

Selecting Measures and Metrics

Measurement and metrics are the foundation of quality improvement, as they are the basis for evaluating the impact of quality improvement activities. Defining the metrics at baseline is the starting point for quality activities, as these measures typically inform and define how a problem was recognized. Equally important are the primary and secondary metrics the quality improvement team selects as they modify processes to achieve the team's goals and purpose. Metrics can include clinical indicators of care and process or business metrics (McLaughlin & Kaluzny, 2005; Nelson et al., 2007; Strome, 2013).

Technology, and therefore electronic medical records and informatics, has been infused into the care arena at a rapid pace during the last decade. Clinicians are often bombarded with more data than could possibly be analyzed and reviewed. With this in mind, it is important for the CNL to consider how information is gathered, where it is stored, and what tools, methods, and resources are available to access data. When reviewing data stored in data warehouses, repositories, and databases, it is important to clarify terms and data definitions to ensure consistency and understanding of how data will be used in the quality improvement process (Strome, 2013).

Nurses are generally comfortable assessing clinical outcomes and indicators of care, but it is also important for CNLs to incorporate business metrics and measurements when planning quality improvement projects. These measures are important to the administrators and regulators of care accustomed to quantifying and articulating value at a systems level (Bender, 2016; Williams & Bender, 2015). Quantifying the return on investment, impacts on costs of care, and articulating system improvements could establish the value of the CNL's role in organizations. With rising pressures regarding pay for performance, trended outcomes of care in public reporting, and rising interest from accreditation and consumer groups, selection of business indicators aimed at cost-effectiveness and efficiency is essential.

Rapid Cycle Review

A cornerstone and distinguishing characteristic of quality improvement is a rapid cycle review that encourages continuous and ongoing efforts to improve outcomes. The plan-do-check-act (PDCA) cycle is frequently referenced in quality improvement methodologies. Discussed by Deming (and attributed to Shewhart's work at Bell Laboratories), the PDCA cycle of improvement offers a cyclical process to structure tests of change identified by team members as being most likely to improve outcomes in a disciplined and rapid manner (McLaughlin & Kaluzny, 2005; Strome, 2013). *Plan* involves the definition of the problem, examination of the processes that contribute to it, and devising a plan to address the problem. *Do* involves identifying the steps in a plan and carrying them out. *Check* involves analyzing the data collected to summarize what was learned. *Act* involves examining outcomes with an eye toward further modifications so that the cycle can be initiated again to refine and bring further improvements (McLaughlin & Kaluzny, 2005; Nelson et al., 2007; Strome, 2013).

Relevance of the Microsystem

Microsystems are defined as the smallest functional unit on the front line of healthcare delivery systems. The clinical microsystem provides direct care to patients and families, establishing the essential building blocks of the organization. It is within this microsystem that the quality of care is defined and the reputation of an organization is created (Bender, 2016; Nelson et al., 2007; White et al., 2016).

Microsystems include members of the interdisciplinary team in various roles who work together on a regular basis to provide care to discrete subpopulations of patients. A microsystem has business and clinical aims, linked processes, and a shared information environment that produces performance outcomes (Bender, 2016; Nelson et al., 2007; White et al., 2016). Microsystems are represented in all practice settings and specialties and evolve over time, but they always have a patient at the center. Microsystems vary widely in terms of quality, safety, and costs because they are embedded in a context where providers, support staff, information, and processes converge to support individuals who provide care to meet the unique and individual health needs of patients and families. Microsystems are loosely or tightly connected to one another and are the functional, interdependent systems that create an organization or macrosystem (Bender, 2016; Nelson et al., 2007; White et al., 2016).

Tornabeni, Stanhope, and Wiggins (2008) noted that "the CNL role focuses on understanding the interdependency of all disciplines providing care and the need to tap into the expertise of the team, rather than individual providers" (p. 107). By understanding the roles of the interdisciplinary team, the CNL laterally integrates the team to provide patient-centered care. CNLs use their interpersonal communication skills, clinical leadership skills, and knowledge of group dynamics to facilitate care, leveraging their knowledge of internal and external resources to provide lateral integration (Bender, 2016).

Assessment of the Microsystem for Selection of Quality Improvement Projects

Many tools have been created to support CNLs in the assessment of their microsystems. Irrespective of the tool selected, a thorough and systematic assessment is needed before embarking on a quality improvement project. The microsystem assessment elements to be examined include: unit descriptors; skills, composition, and competence of team members; presence of formal and informal leaders; interdisciplinary team relationships and communication; accountability and control over practice; support for education; experience with quality improvement processes and resources; and readiness for change.

The 5 Ps framework offers a deliberate framework for clinicians to assess microsystems in a systematic manner. The 5 Ps are purpose, patients, professionals, processes, and patterns. Each *P* has a definition associated with it, and these categories set a framework to inform the selection of improvement themes and aims. To be most effective, the exploration of the 5 Ps should include all the members of a clinical microsystem. Nelson and colleagues (2007, p. 265) offer a series of questions and exercises to lead interdisciplinary teams through the microsystem assessment to establish the *health* of the microsystem, making obvious the areas that require attention (diagnosis) and solutions (treatment) to be evaluated by the team (follow-up).

Systematic and Purposeful Identification of Quality Improvement Initiatives

When considering initiatives to improve quality and safety, project selection in an organization is of paramount importance. By using a gap analysis or microsystem assessment, CNLs can align quality improvement efforts in the microsystem to strategic initiatives and organizational goals while simultaneously focusing attention on the front lines to impact change. The CNL is in a unique position to manage change, apply quality improvement methods, and incorporate team learning by leading interdisciplinary members through a disciplined, systematic approach of problem identification, process analysis, measurement, and evaluation that is meaningful in daily operations.

A potential pitfall for CNLs is the identification of quality improvement projects that extends beyond the microsystem. Scoping a project through a defined aim or purpose at the onset of quality improvement activities is essential to success. Because there are many priorities that overlap at the organizational level, concentrating on improvements at the microsystem level is key. Problem identification through brainstorming with members of the microsystem team is a mechanism to support unit-level activities that will be meaningful and appropriate for CNL intervention (Bender, 2016; Rusch & Bakewell-Sachs, 2007).

Structure for Monitoring Quality Improvement Projects

Many organizations have quality departments that distribute quality reports monthly, quarterly, and annually as a part of a quality dashboard, benchmarking, or quality report card process. In addition to these contributions, many quality departments distribute reports for quality improvement initiatives and regulatory obligations. There is a wealth of knowledge contained in these departments, and before engaging in a quality improvement project, the CNL team leader should explore what tools, report development, and distribution supports are available.

Team Leader Tools for Success

Once the philosophy of quality improvement has been embraced and the tenets of quality improvement have been articulated, the progress toward improvement needs to be monitored and evaluated. Irrespective of the methodology selected to guide the organizational quality improvements, team member roles, responsibilities, and ground rules need to be discussed and documented. This step is commonly avoided or driven by assumptions, but failing to explicitly address it is a critical mistake. If CNLs are going to embrace quality improvement, setting team expectations and responsibilities from the onset of the group's work is essential. The documents created during this phase of the team's interactions will be referenced throughout the quality improvement process as the agreed on guiding principles, rules, and accountabilities each team member holds.

Several forms or documents can be found to document the team's expectations. At a minimum, the team will want to identify the team leader, the secretary (responsible for documenting and distributing meeting minutes and agendas), and the responsibilities of each team member based on expertise. Attendance requirements, frequency of meetings, length of meetings, and commitment to completing work between meetings are the focal points of discussion among the team members.

Searching the internet for sample team charters provides a wealth of templates or formats for teams to consider if the organization does not have a preferred or approved template. A charter is a written agreement defining what a team is going to accomplish and how success will be measured. The charter focuses the team's efforts and documents the expectations that team members have of one another. By using a team charter, discussion between multidisciplinary team members can be guided to include key focal points in team dynamics and important issues can be agreed on before the team engages in change. A signed charter indicates the formal beginning of a project and an equitable commitment for completion.

Most professionals hold common beliefs about group process and goal attainment, but ground rules provide the boundaries for how team members will interact. Many organizations have established ground rules for team interactions based on their mission and shared values. Although these ground rules provide basic tenets for group interactions, it is important to offer team members the chance to modify rules to reflect what they believe the guiding principles should be. Common content for ground rules includes valuing each person and their input; anticipating unique contributions from all team members; courteous, honest, and respectful communication; and the agreement that each member will represent the work of the team in a positive manner.

CNLs are positioned to monitor the improvement activities from the team leader position as a coordinator and manager of care through teaching, guidance, mentoring, and leveraging the language of the improvement process. Effective use of team tools can set expectations and provide elements that document activities and progress that lead to the attainment of project goals.

Linking Quality Improvement to the Clinical Immersion Experience and the Daily Life of a CNL

Embedded in the CNL role are expectations of accountability for patient-centered, cost-effective care across practice settings and measurable outcomes that demonstrate improved safety, quality, and EBP. The CNL curriculum supports the development of clinical leaders who can manage change by leading members of the interdisciplinary team in complex care environments (AACN, 2007, 2011, 2013).

All CNLs are required to complete 400 clinical hours throughout their educational experience, with 300 to 400 hours devoted to a clinical immersion experience. During the clinical immersion experience, the student enacts the CNL's role and competencies in an organization (AACN, 2007, 2013). Quality improvement may be offered as a separate course in the curriculum or threaded throughout the educational experience in several courses, but the culmination of the CNL clinical immersion experience is grounded in principles demonstrated through quality improvement projects. As members of the nursing profession, CNLs will be expected to identify areas for improvement within the care delivery system, assess and plan meaningful change at the microsystem level, and measure clinical and financial outcomes to demonstrate improved outcomes that align with strategic organizational goals aimed at improving cost, quality, and safety.

As clinical leaders and members of the nursing profession, CNLs are also expected to participate in self-evaluation and reflective thinking (AACN, 2007, 2013). This includes examining individually held assumptions, values, and beliefs with an open mind, supported by the use of critical-thinking skills to explore different perspectives, solutions, and options offered by members of the interdisciplinary team or the literature. The clinical immersion experience offers CNL students a venue to share the outcomes of quality improvement activities, as well as the reflective practice, learning, and insights gained related to leading teams, evaluating practice and implementing EBPs, and guiding or mentoring others in quality improvement processes aimed at patient safety and improved care delivery. Documents assembled during the quality improvement process can then become a part of the students' clinical immersion portfolios.

After completion of the clinical immersion experience in their formal education, CNLs are expected to replicate elements of the clinical immersion in daily practice. Often, organizations rely on the CNL to bring quality improvement strategies into a microsystem to support organizational change and performance. This means working within the microsystem culture to implement change without the educational process as a guide. The scope and anticipated duration of an improvement project may be more or less than the 15-week semester, but the elements of the clinical immersion experience can be replicated to map the process steps required when leading a microsystem quality improvement. The discipline of documenting process steps, gaining consensus around the problem, establishing ground rules, engaging interdisciplinary team members, and using quality and sustainability tools is unchanged. A common pitfall experienced by graduate CNLs is the omission of different steps in the process (believed to be academic exercises) that leads to frustration and delays in achieving desired results.

The Spectrum of Value Related to Quality Immersion Projects

The spectrum of value is not inherently evident across healthcare settings. Different meanings of value are attributed from its meaning across settings that are dependent on the situation or a strategic initiative. Rather, value stems from its meaning.

Value is a key component of any CNL immersion project and fundamental to continuous and sustained improvement. Fundamental to immersion projects is shifting from volume to value that is centralized within a microsystem patient-centric needs assessment (Marzorati & Pravettoni, 2017). As immersion projects are developed, a consistent question must be answered: Will the change of project activities link to one another to create and sustain value beyond completion? Porter's value chain concept is an applicable framework to answer this question (Porter, 1985). Applying this concept provides a framework to answer the question and assess if the activities will create, deliver, and capture value at each step throughout the process for the spread across any microsystem.

While value has different meaning across healthcare settings, CNLs remain a valuable resource necessary to engage teams that embrace opportunities associated with value and sustainable improvement. Ultimate outcomes will consistently be measured as quality and safe care is evident in empirical terms.

Conclusion

With increasing national demands from regulators, payers, and consumers to support effectiveness of interventions to improve patient safety, quality of care, and value, change efforts formed by quality improvement initiatives provide a systematic, disciplined, and reliable process to support decision-making and measurement aimed to improve patient care quality in the healthcare delivery system. Developing a data-driven, outcomes-oriented structure grounded in role accountability will be essential. The CNL is well positioned to lead interdisciplinary teams in their efforts to implement quality improvement, safety, and value at the microsystem level regardless of the setting.

Summary

- As a coordinator of care with a system focus, the CNL has a responsibility to lead interprofessional teams in quality improvement, safety, and value-driven initiatives.
- Quality frameworks and various tools are used in an organization; quality improvement relies on a systematic and disciplined approach to understanding care processes.
- Disciplined use of quality improvement tools and evidence are foundational to outcomes management.
- Understanding stakeholder expectations coupled with interprofessional collaboration generate meaningful quality improvement initiatives that are sustainable.
- Scanning the environment for individual and system risks is an important responsibility of CNLs.

Reflection Questions

1. What part of the quality improvement process do you think that you are most prepared to complete? What part are you least least prepared to accomplish?
2. What resources are available in an organization to assist you with quality improvement?
3. How do your see the CNL interacting with other members of the clinical team to advance quality improvement, risk anticipation, evidence-based practices, and value-based outcomes?
4. Identify a process in a microsystem that could benefit from an interprofessional team effort. Talk to members of the team to create an action plan.
5. Identify how design thinking is an avenue to change practice at the microsystem and healthcare setting level.

Learning Activities

1. Interview a member of an organization's quality improvement department. Identify the quality methods, tools, and measurement techniques used in the organization.
2. Meet with a member of a risk management team. Explore the tools and reports they create for members of the senior leadership team. Explain the CNL role and inquire about the risks this person believes a CNL could address in a microsystem.
3. Locate the quality reports and metrics that are distributed to leaders throughout the organization. Identify three metrics that you believe the CNL could impact.
4. Outline the steps you would take if tasked to develop a quality improvement plan to address a metric CNLs could impact.

References

American Association of Colleges of Nursing. (2007). *White paper on the role of the Clinical Nurse Leader*. Author. https://nursing.uiowa.edu/sites/default/files/documents/academic-programs/graduate /msn-cnl/CNL_White_Paper.pdf

American Association of Colleges of Nursing. (2011). *The essentials of master's education in nursing*. http://www.aacn.nche.edu/education-resources/MastersEssentials11.pdf

American Association of Colleges of Nursing. (2013). *Competencies and curricular expectations for clinical nurse leader education and practice* [White paper]. https://www.aacnnursing.org/Portals /42/News/White-Papers/CNL-Competencies-October-2013.pdf

American Society for Healthcare Risk Management. (2014). *Enterprise risk management: A framework for success* [White paper]. http://www.ashrm.org/pubs/files/white_papers/ERM-White-Paper 8-29-14-FINAL.pdf

Bender, M. (2016). Conceptualizing clinical nurse leader practice: an interpretive synthesis. *Journal of Nursing Management, 24,* E23–E31.

Bender, M., Connelly, C., Glaser, D., & Brown, C. (2012). Clinical Nurse Leader impact on microsystem care quality. *Nursing Research, 61*(5), 326–332.

Berwick, D., Nolan, T., & Whittington, J. (2008). The triple aim: Care, health, and cost. *Health Affairs, 27*(3), 759–769.

Bodenheimer, T., & Sinsky, C. (2014). From triple to quadruple aim: Care of the patient requires care of the provider. *Annals of Family Medicine, 12,* 573–576.

Carroll, R. (2009). *Risk management handbook for healthcare organizations* (Student ed.). Jossey-Bass.

Chang, C., Bynum, J. P. W., & Luri, J. D. (2018). Geographic expansion of federally funded health centers 2007–2014. *The Journal of Rural Health, 35*(3), 385–394.

Crema, V., & Vergana. C. (2013). Future developments in health care performance management. *Journal of Multidisciplinary Healthcare, 6,* 415–421.

Dam, R., & Siang, T. (2019). *5 stages of design thinking process/Interaction design*. https://www.interaction -design.org>literature>articles>5-stages-in-the-design-thinking-process-interaction-design

Department of Health and Human Services. (2011). *Performance management & measurement*. http://www.hrsa.gov/quality/toolbox/methodology/performancemanagement

DiCenso, A., Guyatt, G., & Ciliska, D. (2005). *Evidence-based nursing. A guide to clinical practice*. ElsevierMosby.

Groves, P., Finfgeld-Connett, D., & Wakefield, B. (2014). It's always something: Hospital nurses managing risk. *Clinical Nursing Research, 23*(3), 296–313.

Hall, H., & Roussel, L. (2014). *Evidenced-based practice: An integrative approach to research, administration, and practice*. Jones & Bartlett Learning.

Hasso, P., Meinel, C., & Weinberg, U. (2009). *Design thinking*. Springer.

Healthcare Information and Management Systems Society. (2015). *2015 HIMMS impact of the informatics nurse survey*. https://www.himiss.org/ni-impact-survey

Institute of Medicine. (1999). *To err is human: Building a safer health system*. National Academies Press.

Institute of Medicine. (2001). *Crossing the quality chasm: A new health system for the 21st century*. National Academies Press.

Institute of Medicine. (2003). *Health professions education: A bridge to quality*. http://www.iom.edu /Reports/2003/Health-Professions-Education-A-Bridge-to-Quality.aspx

Institute of Medicine. (2015). *Measuring the impact of interprofessional education on collaborative practice and patient outcomes*. https://www.ncbi.nlm.nih.gov/books/NBK338360/

The Joint Commission. (2008). *Health care at the crossroads: Guiding principles for the development of the hospital of the future*. https://www.jointcommission.org/-/media/deprecated-unorganized /imported-assets/tjc/system-folders/topics-library/hosptal_futurepdf.pdf?db=web&hash= BEDD225214DB9A1BB436C69A2E0C8123

Kelly, P., Vottero, B., & Christie-McAuliffe, C. (2014). *Introduction to quality and safety education for nurses: Core competencies*. Springer.

Lohr, K. (1990). *Medicare: A strategy for quality assurance*. National Academies Press.

Marzorati, C., & Pravettoni, G. (2017). Value as the key concept in the health care system: How it has influenced medical practice and clinical decision-making processes. *Journal of Multidisciplinary Healthcare, 10,* 101–106.

McLaughlin, C., & Kaluzny, A. (2005). *Continuous quality improvement in health care: Theory, implementations, and applications* (3rd ed.). Jones & Bartlett Publishers.

National Quality Forum. (2017). *What we do.* https://www.qualityforum.org/what-do-we-do.aspx

Nelson, E., Batalden, P., & Godfrey, M. (2007). *Quality by design: A clinical microsystems approach.* Jossey-Bass.

New England Journal of Medicine Catalyst. (2018). *What is risk management in healthcare?* https://www.catalyst.nejme.org

Newhouse, R. (2006). Selecting measures for safety and quality improvement initiatives. *Journal of Nursing Administration, 36*(3), 109–113.

Ott, K., Haddock, S., Fox, S., Shinn, J., Walters, S., Hardin, J., Durand, K., & Harris, J. (2009). The Clinical Nurse Leader: Impact on practice outcomes in the Veterans Health Administration. *Nursing Economics, 27*(6), 363–370.

Porter, M. E. (1985). *Competitive advantage—Creating a sustaining superior performance.* The Free Press.

Rusch, L., & Bakewell-Sachs, S. (2007). The CNL: A gateway to better care. *Nursing Management.* https://doi.org/10.1097/01.NUMA.0000266719.94334.96

Stavrianopoulos, T. (2012). The Clinical Nurse Leader. *Health Science Journal, 6*(3), 392–401.

Strome, T. (2013). *Healthcare analytics for quality and performance improvement.* John Wiley & Sons.

Tornabeni, J., Stanhope, M., & Wiggins, M. (2008). The CNL vision. *Journal of Nursing Administration, 36*(3), 103–108.

Weaver, S. J., Lukomksi, L. H., Wilson. R. F, Pfoh, E. R., Martinez, K. A., & Dy, S. M. (2013). Promoting a culture of safety strategy: A systematic review. *Annals of Internal Medicine, 158,* (502), 369–774.

White, K., Dudley-Brown, S., & Terhaar, M. (2016). *Translation of evidence into nursing and health care* (2nd ed.). Springer.

Williams, M., & Bender, M. (2015). Growing and sustaining the Clinical Nurse Leader initiative. *Journal of Nursing Administration, 45*(11), 540–543.

Wilson, D. (2013). Registered nurses' collective safety organising behaviours: The association with perceptions of patient safety culture. *Journal of Research in Nursing, 4*(18), 320–333.

Wilson, L., Orff, S., Gerry, T., Shirley, B., Tabor, D., Caizaao, K., & Rouleau, D. (2013). Evolution of an innovative role: The Clinical Nurse Leader. *Journal of Nursing Management, 21*(1), 175–181.

Suggested Readings

AHRQ. https://innovations.ahrq.gov/

AHRQ—Quality and Safety. http://www.ahrq.gov/professionals/quality-patient-safety/index.html

AHRQ. *Tools and strategies for quality improvement and patient safety.* http://www.ahrq.gov/legacy/qual/nurseshdbk/docs/HughesR_QMBMP.pdf

ASHRM. http://www.ashrm.org

Badawi, O., & Breslow, M. (2012). Readmissions and death after ICU discharge: Development and validation of two predictive models. *PLoS One, 7*(11). https://journals.plos.org/plosone/article?id=10.1371/journal.pone.0048758

Centers for Medicare and Medicaid Services. http://www.cms.gov

Daniels, C., Farmer, C., Gajic, O., Kashyap, R., Ofoma, U., & Pickering, B. (2012). Does implementation of a previously validated prediction tool reduce readmission rates into a medical intensive care unit? *Chest, 142*(4). http://journal.publications.chestnet.org/article.aspx?articleid=1376124

Greene, B. (2007). Tracking the six aims of the IOM report: Crossing the quality chasm—Healthcare in the 21st century. *Journal of Ambulatory Care Management, 30*(4), 281–282. https://doi.org/10.1097/01.JAC.0000290395.20672.34

Hughes, R. G. (2008). *Patient safety and quality: An evidence-based handbook for nurses.* NCBI. https://www.ncbi.nlm.nih.gov/books/NBK2681/

The Joint Commission. http://www.jointcommission.org/

National Quality Forum. http://www.qualityforum.org

Preventing VTE Core Measure Fallouts Toward Quality Outcomes

Jessica Kyles

Texas Health Resources instituted standardized anticoagulation discharge instructions to satisfy accountability requirements (The Joint Commission, 2015). Drug education, dietary restrictions, compliance issues, and potential adverse reactions are automatically inserted in discharge instructions for all patients discharging on warfarin therapy. However, the discharging nurse must make sure there is documentation of follow-up monitoring (appointment for international normalized ratio [INR] check).

During a microsystem assessment, the CNL identified that patients discharging to inpatient rehabilitation units or skilled nursing facilities were not routinely provided with hospital discharge instructions. The latter was identified as a system issue following an RCA that was performed after a near miss opportunity occurred within the microsystem. CNL interventions included collaborating with the risk management department to develop solutions to this issue and meeting with RNs and providing education on the importance of providing written discharge instructions to all patients regardless of discharge destination. The CNL provided hands-on training to staff members who did not know how to prepare discharge instructions for patients discharging to a facility. Presently, the CNL communicates the need for follow-up monitoring and dietary restrictions with clinical liaisons of outside facilities. Lateral integration is demonstrated by reaching out to facility liaisons to facilitate communication, improving patient outcomes, and ensuring care is continued across the continuum.

System analyst, risk anticipator, educator, client advocate, outcomes manager, and team manager skills demonstrated by the CNL enhance the safety of patients discharging from hospital to facility and prevent hospital readmissions related to anticoagulant therapy. Post intervention by the CNL has resulted in no venous thromboembolism (VTE) core measure fallouts in the CNL's microsystem.

Reference

The Joint Commission. (2015). *Facts about accountability measures*. http://www.jointcommission.org/accountability_measures.aspx

Integrating Evidence-Based Practice into Daily Clinical Practice

Beth VanDam

Catheter-associated urinary tract infections (CAUTI) are considered preventable; therefore, the CMS will no longer reimburse the healthcare organization for the care required to treat the acquired infection. CAUTI can lead to patient discomfort as well as lead to an increase in length of stay, mortality, and healthcare costs. Data collected on the 42-bed oncology/surgical unit indicated 5 CAUTI occurred on the unit in 2014. Since CAUTI are preventable, the goal for 4 Lacks was to decrease CAUTI to zero in year 2015.

The CNL and two unit RNs who served on the organizational CAUTI team worked together to identify the root cause. The team utilized a fishbone diagram to lead staff members to identify what may result in foley CAUTI. The next step was for the team to brainstorm with RN-PCA (patient care assistant) dyads for possible solutions. Many creative and unique solutions were discussed in an attempt to eliminate CAUTI on the unit. It was also identified that evidence-based practice involving a basic soap and water cleaning of the catheter once a day was not being done.

The CNL along with the two unit RNs worked to implement a process to ensure evidence-based care around CAUTI prevention was consistently part of patient care. The interventions included:

1. Daily soap and water cleaning of the catheter at the insertion site with morning care
2. Stabilization of catheter with stat loc
3. Catheter tubing without kinks
4. Documentation completed including catheter without kinks and off the floor

Implementing these measures of evidence-based practice care resulted in significant improvements. Baseline data included 1,766 foley catheter days and 5 CAUTI on 4 Lacks in 2014. Data for 2015 consisted of 2,474 foley catheter days and 0 CAUTI. The CNL developed a CAUTI-prevention audit tool the RN CAUTI unit representatives use to audit compliance with the previously mentioned interventions to monitor CAUTI rates going forward. It is the role of the CNL to ensure evidence-based practices are incorporated into the care of patients to improve safety and quality outcomes.

EXEMPLAR

Quality Improvement and Safety

Mary Harnish

Hypoglycemic episodes in hospitalized patients can lead to patient dissatisfaction and safety issues. Immediate treatment and timely rechecking of the blood glucose level are of vital importance to patient safety via hypoglycemic rechecks.

The CNL for diabetes receives daily reports from information systems on frequency of hypoglycemia, timeliness of treatment, and effectiveness of that treatment. These data are evaluated to assure the patient is receiving optimal care. Real-time analysis and evaluation allows "at-the-elbow" coaching of bedside nurses by the CNL for diabetes when the process is not followed. The closer to the event that the coaching is done, the greater the impact on the nurse's practice.

The CNL for diabetes integrates the data into ongoing reports of success and failures in following the protocol. This information is demonstrated in run charts, which are communicated to nursing unit managers and unit-based CNLs. This collaboration and partnering with managers and unit CNLs holds staff accountable for patient safety. An engaged team approach to best practices thereby reduces the risk of prolonged hypoglycemia. Sharing the unit-based data helps drive competition between units to improve their scores.

Implementation of the role of CNL for diabetes six years ago moved the protocol compliance scores from 50–60% to 78–92%. Continued efforts intend to increase that percentage to 92–95% or greater, improving patient safety and satisfaction.

EXEMPLAR

Looking for Risk

Rebecca Valko

Many CNLs work within microsystems that include 30 to 40 patients. As this becomes increasingly more common, knowing the *story* on every patient is impossible. Prioritizing your focus is a learned skill from our coursework and practice. A CNL has to listen carefully during report or interdisciplinary rounds and analyze the patient's risk. Keywords such as: *impulsive, pain out of control, refusing care, unsteady, multiple wounds, central line, foley catheter,* and *complex* guide me in my prioritization. I constantly scan the environment and continue to search out potential risks and address them before they become a major problem.

As a CNL, you not only anticipate risk, you mentor others to do the same, and, in turn, change to a proactive culture. One of the most memorable moments is when a few nurses came to me regarding a patient with a central line that had been placed prior to admission that appeared infected. As a unit, we had done extensive central line education after our unit had a central line associated bloodstream infection (CLABSI) a month earlier. Staff were very concerned about the tests or documentation needed to be done on admission to avoid having the unit "charged" with a CLABSI. This was a sign that a shift in thinking was occurring.

EXEMPLAR

Innovation/Collaboration

Rebecca Valko and Lauran Hardin

Patients with gastroparesis comprise a highly complex patient population that is at high risk for readmissions and emergency room visits. RCA showed that most patients were not following a gastroparesis diet. A literature review showed that diet modification is essential to controlling this disease. Through evidenced-based practice and collaboration with the dieticians from the hospital and the diabetes center, we created an innovative gastroparesis diet guideline.

This easy-to-read and informative patient education tool has been well received by patients and providers. A patient even told me that he kept it on his refrigerator! This was just the first step of an interdisciplinary complex-care-plan approach that decreased readmissions and the lengths of stays for this challenging patient population.

Hardwiring Hourly Rounding as a Team: A CNL Initiative to Improve Patient Satisfaction Scores by Developing a New Process to Complete Hourly Rounds

Catherine Delanoix

In November 2012, a CNL in the Adult Stem Cell Transplant unit of a comprehensive cancer center assessed the need to improve patient satisfaction scores. A comprehensive literature review illustrated the close correlation between patient satisfaction and hourly rounding.

The CNL assessed current rounding practice through direct observation, review of hourly rounding logs, and patient interview. Although hourly rounding was an institutional expectation, the assessment revealed that hourly rounding was not consistently being performed. A plan was developed to make hourly rounding the objective of all team members, rather than the responsibility of the RN assigned to the patient.

Initial implementation began on a 12-bed pod. A clock was placed outside each patient room and staff were educated to advance the clock each time a purposeful round was performed. In doing this, the clock would indicate the next time rounds were to be conducted on each patient. The clock served as a visual cue for all team members and allowed each person to be accountable for ensuring that rounds were completed on all patients every hour.

Compliance was measured through audits of rounding clocks and patient interviews. Unit-based HCAHPS scores specific to patient satisfaction were also measured. The CNL performed weekly patient satisfaction rounds to evaluate the effectiveness of the improved rounding.

Preliminary results collected during the initial phase of the intervention identified a significant improvement in patient satisfaction scores. Statistical analysis of the data was performed to identify a relationship between the improving patient satisfaction scores and improved hourly rounding. A Fisher's exact test was used to compare satisfaction scores yielding a score of 0.017. This finding significantly identifies a relationship between hourly rounding and patient satisfaction scores. Furthermore, a Spearman's correlation was performed with a result of 0.9487, which identifies a strong positive correlation between hourly rounding and patient satisfaction scores. This preliminary data justified disseminating team-based hourly rounding to the rest of the 48-bed unit. Evaluation of HCAHPS scores have shown sustained improvement in all questions related to patient satisfaction since dissemination.

Using the clocks as a visual tool to implement team-based hourly rounding not only improved rounding compliance and patient satisfaction scores but it also improved teamwork, accountability, and situational monitoring. Staff comments reflect improved collaboration and awareness of contributions of team members. The success of this innovative approach has been shared throughout the institution.

EXEMPLAR

Developing an Assessment Guide in the Management of Patients Receiving High-Dose Interleukin (IL-2)

Noel Mendez and Myrna Martinez

Since the transition of the CNL to a Melanoma/Sarcoma unit in 2012, there was a steady influx of new graduate nurses. It is important to note that the Melanoma/Sarcoma unit is the only non-ICU that administers high-dose IL-2 treatment in a 600-bed NCI-designated hospital. Assessment, monitoring, and management of infusion-related toxicities are critical in this population to ensure safe, optimal patient outcomes. Cognizant of how critical it is for new nurses to develop good assessment and critical-thinking skills, the CNLs collaborated with key stakeholders to develop an assessment guide in the management of patients receiving high-dose IL-2.

After the CNLs presented their process improvement plan for approval by the unit leadership, the CNLs reviewed the institutional high-dose IL-2 administration guidelines and protocol, as well as the evidence from the literature to provide a rationale for the different aspects of the protocol in relation to the required assessment. They collaborated with the unit nurse educator in developing the educational material to prepare the new nurses in managing patients receiving this specialty treatment, including an introductory course and an assessment guide.

After a didactic class with the CNL and/or nurse educator, the new nurses receive a copy of the assessment guide. The assessment guide consists of a body diagram that provides the new staff a visual guide illustrating each system and the corresponding required assessment. The diagram also helps nurses in communicating the required assessment to the primary physician prior to each dose of high-dose IL-2. This not only promotes the consistency of information communicated prior to each dose but also ensures safe administration and management of side effects associated with high-dose IL-2.

This collaborative initiative reflects the fundamental roles of the CNL as a clinician, client advocate, risk anticipator, and educator in promoting the delivery of quality patient care for this specialty population.

Decreasing the Occurrence of Heel Pressure Ulcers in the Critically Ill Oncology Patient: A CNL Initiative to Promote Quality Patient Care, Patient Advocacy, and Evidence-Based Practice

Amber Tarvin

Background

After trending unit-acquired pressure ulcers by anatomical location in a critical care oncology unit, the CNL noted unit-acquired deep-tissue injury (DTI) heel pressure ulcers were reported consistently every month. At the time of discovery, the current practice was the use of pillows and inflatable heel protector boots. These prevention methods were proven to be ineffective because in many cases the patient's heels would still touch the bed after applying inflatable heel protector boots and as well as with the use of pillows. According to the literature, the use of effective pressure-relieving devices for prevention has an inverse relationship with the amount of pressure ulcers reported. This, in turn, led the unit leadership to make the decision to use an evidence-based heel protector boot. Deep-tissue injury pressure ulcers are categorized with full thickness pressure ulcers stage 3, stage 4, and unstageable pressure ulcers. They are among the most costly pressure ulcers because they can lead to increased length of stay, sepsis, and mortality.

Aim

To reduce heel pressure ulcers in the oncology medical/surgical intensive care patient population by using an evidence-based heel protector boot.

Methods/Process

The CNL collaborated with the organization's Value Analysis Team (VAT) to pilot pressure-relieving heel protectors on a 10-bed pod in a 54-bed ICU. During the trial, the vendor provided education on use of the boots and obtained employee feedback. A vendor decision tree was introduced to staff for assistance in delineating the benefit between the new boots or pillows for heel pressure relief.

After compiling the staff survey, the CNL worked with VAT to facilitate the acquisition of the pressure boots for use in the organization. The CNL then coordinated the staff education for both shifts to prepare the nursing staff in this change of practice. In addition, the heel protector process map was changed to address the unique patient population, after which the information on the boot and process map was sent to the faculty multidisciplinary education committee.

Outcome

Prior to implementation, the heel pressure ulcer trend continued to rise from one to at least two a month. Post implementation of the heel pressure ulcer rate decreased 50%. Moving forward the goal is to sustain the downward trend in unit-acquired heel pressure ulcers until there are zero unit-acquired heel pressure ulcers.

Conclusion

The CNL championed the introduction of an evidence-based heel protector boot to prevent heel pressure ulcers, assisted with the development of criteria through a decision tree, disseminated education, and making the boot accessible to all unit staff. The effects of this change in practice resulted in more effective, equitable patient care.

Reference

Institute for Healthcare Improvement. (2011). *How-to guide: Prevent pressure ulcers.* Author.

EXEMPLAR

Reducing Electrolyte Boluses Utilizing an Interdisciplinary Approach

Kristi Alexander

Electrolyte imbalance can be profound in the leukemia population and is closely associated with the disease process and pharmacologic interventions, including chemotherapy. Leukemia patients consistently require electrolyte replacement, most commonly with potassium and magnesium. On an inpatient adult leukemia unit, it was observed that patients were receiving an average of 78 milliequivalents (mEq) potassium bolus and 18.6 mEq magnesium bolus daily. In addition, providers were prescribing multiple intravenous fluids (IVF) mixtures with varying doses of additional electrolytes resulting in higher costs for the pharmacy, because IVF orders were changed frequently, requiring additional time and effort for the pharmacy and wasting of partially completed fluids.

The CNL, acting as a coordinator, in collaboration with the pharmacy, formed a task force comprised of clinical nurses, clinical and operational pharmacists, and advanced practice providers. The primary aim of the group was to develop and standardize the clinical guidelines for electrolyte replacement for the leukemia population.

After reviewing the literature and current clinical guidelines, the group came up with a standardized IVF that would benefit the majority of the leukemia population—0.45% normal saline with 40 mEqs potassium chloride and 8 mEqs of magnesium sulfate. A standardized clinical guideline that incorporated an electrolyte replacement algorithm was developed. All advanced practice providers, pharmacists, and nurses were educated on the guidelines. A copy of the algorithm was also posted in the team and medication rooms as a quick guide and reference.

Preliminary results showed a 21% decrease in the average amount of potassium replacement from 78 mEq to 62 mEq of potassium daily. Magnesium boluses were decreased by 2% from 18.6 mEq to 18.2 mEq. There were no episodes of hyperkalemia, hypomagnesaemia, or hyponatremia, demonstrating that in this population, electrolytes can be safely given in IVF.

The process change received enthusiastic support from nurses and pharmacists. There was also a perceived benefit from the nurses as workflow improved and fewer calls to the pharmacy were required. A challenge with antibiotic compatibility with the IVF composition was discovered and is being investigated further.

EXEMPLAR

Implementing Evidence-Based Practice in an ICU: A CNL Initiative to Implement an Evidence-Based Project in Assessing and Monitoring Pain in Critically Ill Patients Who Are Sedated, Intubated, or Have a Decreased Level of Consciousness

Neetha Jawe

In November 2013, a new CNL evaluated the pain assessment of critically ill patients and compared it with the AACN's gold standard for assessment, which is patient self-reporting. The CNL recognized that many patients requiring intensive care were unable to express their pain verbally due to sedation, intubation, and decreased levels of consciousness, making effective pain assessment and management challenging. Cognizant of the need for a valid and reliable instrument to assess the presence of pain in nonverbal patients, the CNL met with the unit leadership to embark on an evidence-based project. The aim of this evidence-based practice project was to identify and implement a valid and reliable pain assessment tool for use with intubated and sedated critically ill patients.

To establish a standardized pain assessment tool for intubated and sedated critically ill patients, a literature review was conducted using the following keywords; *pain assessment, pain management, intubated, critical care,* and *nonverbal*. CINAHL, Ovid, Scopus, and PubMed databases were searched using these keywords. Twenty-two relevant articles were reviewed and eleven were found to meet the inclusion criteria, including three systematic review articles published in 2008 and subsequent studies published after 2008. After reviewing the literature and evaluating the institutional practice setting, the Behavioral Pain Scale (BPS) was selected as the most appropriate tool for pain assessment in sedated and intubated patients. The CNL facilitated educational sessions for nurses throughout the unit to discuss this practice change in January 2014. She also collaborated with information technology colleagues to integrate the BPS into the existing electronic health record (EHR).

The use of the BPS was adopted by ICU nursing staff. By April 2014, nursing pain assessment documentation of "Unable to assess" or "Patient unable to verbalize" decreased from the baseline of 93% to 0%, reflecting a significant increase in pain assessment and documentation for nonverbal patients from a baseline of 7% to 100%. The CNL worked in partnership with the physicians and APPs in integrating BPS into the Adult Analgesia Order set in January 2015. The CNL and her collaborators have met with the chair of the Nursing Policy and Procedure Committee and provided the evidence to support the changes in the policy.

The processes involved in this initiative truly reflected the fundamental aspect of the CNL's role in the provision of evidence-based practice, patient advocacy, and delivery of quality patient care for this specialty population.

EXEMPLAR

Reducing Falls in the ED: Strategies and Outcomes

Laurie A. Schwartz

Patient falls are considered a nursing-sensitive indicator and have been a focus for research and performance improvement within inpatient units for many years. The impact of a fall can increase the cost of a patient's stay by up to $15,000 or lead to death. Benchmarking ED falls data in the literature has been difficult; however, starting February 2014, falls in the ED are being reported voluntarily through National Database of Nursing Quality Indicators (NDNQI). A patient's ED course can be impacted greatly by a fall causing an unnecessary admission, an injury, and delays in discharge from the ED, or death. Nationally, many organizations and payers consider falls to be a *never event*.

The ED began to review each fall and conduct root-cause analyses in July 2011. We reviewed the data by looking for themes according to shift, gender, age, and commonalities in reasons for falls. Commonalities included males, ages 40 to 64, and often having a chief complaint concerning intoxication.

CNL interventions included meeting with nursing staff and the ED CNS to determine root causes, develop nursing care guidelines (reflecting standard and targeted interventions utilized by inpatient nursing units), and review additional equipment needs (bed pad alarms). The CNL provided at-the-elbow mentoring of the nursing staff and collaborated with the ED manager to include patient fall reduction as a staff goal on performance evaluations. To share information and updates on ED falls, a monthly summary of falls was posted in the department.

Falls have been reduced as below over the past five fiscal years:					
	FY11	**FY12**	**FY13**	**FY14**	**FY15**
Fall rate	0.051%	0.069%	0.056%	0.034%	0.034%

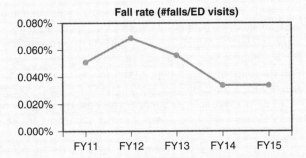

Our highest number was 43 falls in one fiscal year has been decreased to our current number of 22 falls each in the past two fiscal years representing a savings of $315,000/year.

EXEMPLAR

Impact of Chlorhexidine Bathing on Hospital-Acquired Infections and Skin Tolerance Among Stem Cell Transplant Patients

Glemen Banaglorioso

Hospital-acquired infections (HAIs) pose a significant threat to patient safety and outcome, and a significant cause of mortality and morbidity in the stem cell transplant (SCT) population. CLABSI and VRE colonization is not uncommon among SCT patients by nature of their underlying disease process, therapy-induced immunodeficiency, and prolonged neutropenia. VRE colonization is a significant risk factor for infection with VRE. Chlorhexidine gluconate (CHG) bathing has been extensively researched in the intensive care and medical/surgical units, but there is minimal literature regarding the oncology population, specifically SCT patients. Results of a literature review suggest that daily bathing with CHG may prevent hospital-acquired bloodstream infections and VRE colonization among SCT patients.

The purpose of this quality improvement initiative was to evaluate the operational efficacy of a pilot implementation of daily CHG bathing in SCT patients. The secondary goal was to evaluate patient compliance and to monitor the frequency and severity of CHG skin reactions.

Sixteen patients on a 12-bed pod SCT unit were instructed to bathe daily with CHG wash during their admission from October through November 2013. The nurses and nursing assistants on the unit were educated on the use of the CHG solution. All patients without known sensitivity to CHG 4% solution were educated by an RN during admission class, and given instructions regarding CHG bathing and possible skin reactions. Active surveillance testing for VRE was obtained within 48 hours of admission and repeated weekly through rectal swabs. Blood cultures were obtained weekly and during episodes of neutropenic fever. The infection-control preventionist investigated all suspected HAIs.

Although CLABSI and VRE colonization rates post implementation of daily CHG bathing was statistically not significant, the VRE infection rate remained low at 0.12 per 1,000 patient days. Compliance rate with CHG bathing was 90% whereas incidence of skin reactions among 16 patients was 0.06%.

Results from this pilot demonstration suggest that CHG may be an effective strategy in reducing VRE colonization and preventing CLABSI and other infections in SCT patients. CHG is a well-tolerated solution and patient compliance is high. As a result, daily CHG bathing has been implemented throughout the 48-bed SCT unit.

During initial data collection and analysis, the amount of CHG solution to be used was modified according to the manufacturer's recommendation because of skin dryness. Some patients preferred soap and water baths and refused to shower or bathe on sick days. Inconsistent patient education was also observed from the bedside nurses. Repeated in-services and education programs helped overcome some of the obstacles.

EXEMPLAR

Hourly Rounding Initiative: The Impact on Measurable Outcomes

Jennifer H. Towery

Literature shows that with an increased presence of nursing staff to anticipate patient needs, there is often an opportunity to put measures in place to improve patient satisfaction, prevent the risk of falls, and prevent the occurrence of pressure ulcers through early interventions (Brosey & March, 2015). One way to do this would be to implement purposeful hourly rounds; whereas, the rounds would also aid the nursing staff in anticipating patient needs before they arise. Employee satisfaction may also improve through the reduction of call light interruptions, which may lend improvement to inpatient satisfaction scores as well.

During the assessment of a medical/surgical unit, there was noted to be a significant amount of delay in responding to patient call lights, thereby impacting the unit's patient satisfaction scores. A project was implemented involving purposeful hourly rounding from September 2015 to April 2016. Anticipation of patient need is influential in reducing the potential for adverse events occurring in the healthcare setting; it was agreed on that these rounds might also help in improving outcome measures associated with hospital-acquired pressure ulcers (HAPUs), as well as patient fall rates.

The aim of this project was to compare the impact that purposeful hourly rounding, as opposed to the previous practice of rounding when called on, had on patient satisfaction, patient fall rates, and HAPU rates. A change was noted by comparing baseline data to post-intervention data for the following: patient satisfaction survey results, fall rates, and the incidence of HAPUs. The post-implementation goal was to be a 10% improvement in patient satisfaction survey results, a 50%

reduction in the number of patient falls, and a goal of zero for the incidence of HAPUs.

A multidisciplinary lead team agreed on a definition of purposeful hourly rounding. A means to capture that rounding was also agreed on with the use of electronic sensors that the nursing staff wears that are able to communicate with a technological mainframe to identify when a staff member enters and leaves a patient's room. Education was then provided to all the nursing staff prior to implementation of the project, weekly for the first month of implementation, and then biweekly thereafter to promote continued engagement and identify potential barriers to the process.

The findings of the project revealed that overall patient satisfaction scores declined during this time; however, the "responsiveness of staff" section of the survey revealed a score of 57.1% quarter to date (QTD). This percentage is approximately a 26% increase from the last quarter of 2015, which was 45.2%. The number of HAPUs, quarter to date for 2016, totals 3, compared to the prior quarter results of 1. The number of falls, quarter to date for 2016, totals 12, compared to the prior quarter results of 14. Although the number of falls do not reveal a significant decline, per month fall rates had dropped considerably since implementation; this is noted when comparing the first month of the fourth quarter for 2015, where there was a documented 8 falls versus the first quarter of 2016, which had a 50% reduction in fall rates to a rate of 4.

This project hoped to reveal to the staff, and leadership team, the benefit of proactively anticipating patient needs, improving nursing staff response times, decreasing existing fall rates, and reducing the risk of HAPUs within the unit. Based on the data provided prior to implementation and post implementation, there appears to be a positive link between staff compliance with purposeful hourly rounding and outcome improvements; however, a true measure of this data may be better interpreted over a longer time frame to determine the overall impact.

Reference

Brosey, L. A., & March, K. S. (2015). Effectiveness of structured hourly nurse rounding on patient satisfaction and clinical outcomes. *Journal of Nursing Care Quality, 30*(2), 153–159. https://doi .org/10.1097/NCQ.0000000000000086

EXEMPLAR

Secretarial Daily Rounding: It Works!

Courtney D. Edwards and Kristen Noles

Introduction

HCAHPS is a metric that represents the patient's perception of quality care received. Data supports that the patient's experience is linked to great clinical care, reduced medical error, and improved patient outcomes. Each individual patient's survey results matters. These questions measure frequency on a scale of never, sometimes, usually, and always. Of the six categories, two measure the responsiveness of hospital staff and patient overall satisfaction with care. The purpose of this presentation is to describe the innovation of incorporating daily secretarial rounds on a trauma and burn unit and its impact on overall patient satisfaction and their view of staff responsiveness.

Methods

With the idea of increasing HCAHPS in patient satisfaction and improving response time in mind, an innovative approach was taken to utilize the frontline staff responsible for communicating the patient's needs—the unit secretaries. A multidisciplinary team was formed. A review of current literature was completed and best practices identified. The team decided to incorporate daily secretarial rounding as a part of the patient and family-centered care model. Education was provided; a script highlighting key points was developed and distributed to staff. The objectives of the secretarial rounding are to inform the patients on who will be answering their calls, what needs they can and cannot assist with, and ensuring the patients that they will communicate any other needs to the nurse and/or PCTs.

Results

HCAHPS scores in responsiveness of staff and patient satisfaction improved. Patients provided positive feedback on how good it was to place a face with the voice on the other end. Unit secretaries also provided positive qualitative information on the increased satisfaction they have for their position due to the amount of gratitude the patients have shown them as a result of the rounding. The process has been largely accepted on the unit and stands to spread hospital-wide soon.

Conclusions

Secretarial rounding can have a positive influence on patient satisfaction and personal views of staff response because it gives the patients confidence in knowing that the staff is doing all they can to provide quality patient-centered care.

EXEMPLAR

The Use of a CNL as a Nurse Navigator to Decrease Length of Stay and Hospital Cost of Complex Trauma Tracheostomy Patients

Meridith Gombar

Trauma patients requiring tracheostomy have significant injuries that require substantial clinical knowledge and assessment skills, hospital resources and high-level coordination. In 2013, the observed length of stay in this patient population in our

Level 1 trauma center was higher than expected based on risk-adjusted modeling. As a result, Lean methodology was implemented to improve processes and minimize waste with the creation of a Lean team (LT), which was led by a CNL acting as a nurse navigator. The purpose of this study was to evaluate the effectiveness of the LT on length of stay and hospital costs in this complex patient population.

In 2014, the team developed a value stream map of the trauma tracheostomy patient, looking at people, processes, and the purpose. The multidisciplinary team, including physicians, nurses, respiratory care therapists, physical therapists, care managers, and a CNL identified barriers to optimal patient care. Three focus areas were identified to impact patient care: standardized rounding process, tracheostomy clinical pathway, and a navigator to guide the patient through the care delivery system. The initial implementation of a CNL as the nurse navigator showed improvements in length of stay and cost, but something more needed to be done. In 2015, the team completed a rapid improvement event consisting of an 11-week trial with a consistent multidisciplinary LT working collaboratively with this specific population across the continuum of care from admission to discharge. Demographics, care variables, and true cost (not charge) data was collected prospectively and compared with a historical control group of all the 2014 tracheostomy patients (CON).

During the trial period, 14 patients were followed by the LT from admission to discharge. The CON group consisted of 117 patients. Both groups were severely injured with median injury severity scores greater than 25 (LT: 30, CON: 26, $p = 0.97$). Continued work is currently being focused in the area of readmissions concerning this initiative, but recent data reveals lower readmission results of the LT group as compared to the CON group. Additionally, the LT group resulted in a significant reduction in ventilator days (LT: 12, CON: 17, $p = 0.01$), overall length of stay (LT: 16, CON: 25, $p = 0.05$), and total costs (median LT: \$57,894, median CON: \$77,692, $p = 0.04$).

Utilizing Lean methodology resulted in a 36% reduction in length of stay and a 25% reduction in hospital costs for care of the trauma tracheostomy patient. Although there was an increase in the readmission rates of the LT group, through process evaluation and real-time action planning, recent data already reveals an improvement in this metric.

Successful implementation of an LT led by a CNL as a nurse navigator resulted in an annual savings of more than \$2.3 million. This example highlights the added success any healthcare-related initiative or project is destined to have as a result of including a CNL.

EXEMPLAR

Reducing Readmissions: Application of the CNL Role in an Inpatient Hospital Setting

Heather Galang

CMS defines readmissions as admissions to a hospital within 30 days of discharge from the same or similar hospital (CMS, 2016). The Hospital Readmissions Reduction Program (HRRP), a component of the Affordable Care Act (ACA), established financial incentives to avoid reimbursement penalties for hospitals with higher than expected readmission rates (Kripalani et al., 2014). Thus, interventions aimed at reducing readmissions have increased in importance and frequency. Interventions aimed at reducing care fragmentation, specifically enhancing awareness, risk identification, and meaningful communication among community partnerships is of particular interest.

The leadership team in an acute care hospital completed an RCA, isolating possible causes for higher than expected readmission rates. Fragmented communication among patient resources was a contributing factor for high readmission rates. Therefore, an interdisciplinary team, led by a CNL, was formed to address fragmented communication for highly vulnerable populations, identified as most at risk for readmission. Using the PDSA cycle of change model, the team developed a weekly complex case review. The purpose was for the team to communicate care plans for identified readmission patients, adequate follow-up and community resources, and what barriers exist, preventing patients from successful transition (Health Research & Educational Trust [HRET], 2015; Kleinpell, 2013). Different from multidisciplinary rounding, this complex case weekly review would provide a separate opportunity to communicate and resolve barriers appearing in complex cases, such as frequency of readmission, high length of stay, or high hospitalization costs. The group planned the meeting structure, including whom to include, location, and time. The initial team consisted of case managers, inpatient physicians, social workers, and clinical performance improvement.

Each week, prior to this review, the CNL generated a complex case list and distributed this to all team members. At the start of a weekly complex case review, current readmission data was provided by the CNL. In roundtable fashion and by unit, each patient is reviewed, highlighting patient barriers, identifying risk factors for future readmissions, and learning the reason for current readmission. After the first review, the team realized it would be helpful to have outpatient case managers included and provide an audio conference line for when offsite team members, like primary care and community representatives, are unable to attend in person. The team believed it would be important to have all team members stay for the entire review, learning from other case study reviews and contributing ideas to complex cases. Feedback received was evaluated, adopted, and then implemented for subsequent weekly reviews.

Since the implementation of this PDSA cycle for change, regular discussion of readmitted patients occurs. Increased awareness of readmitted patients yields increased opportunities to discuss specific strategies to mitigate risk and reduce readmissions. Staff and leadership feedback regarding the process of identifying highly vulnerable patient populations occurs routinely. On a regular basis, the CNL monitors all-cause 30-day readmission rates, in search of trends in patient population and readmission cause. Furthermore, the CNL facilitates ongoing performance improvement initiatives with interdisciplinary teams, assessing effectiveness, and sustainability of reducing readmission efforts.

References

Centers for Medicare & Medicaid Services. (2016). *Hospital readmissions reduction program (HRRP)*. https://www.cms.gov/medicare/medicare-fee-for-service-payment/acuteinpatientpps/readmissions-reduction-program.html

Health Research & Educational Trust. (2015). *Preventable readmissions change package.* http://www
.hret-hen.org

Kleinpell, R. M. (2013). *Outcome assessment in advanced practice nursing* (3rd ed.).Springer.

Kripalani, S., Theobald, C. N., Anctil, B., & Vasilevskis, E. (2014). Reducing hospital readmissions:
Current strategies and future directions. *Annual Review of Medicine, 65,* 471–485.

Antibiotic Stewardship in Patients with Sepsis

Valerie Heinl

Background

Overuse and misuse of antimicrobials leads to increased antibiotic-resistant organisms (Harbarth et al., 2007). Patients experiencing sepsis require rapid, appropriate antibiotic selection in order to prevent the progression of sepsis. The organization's sepsis mortality was approximately 20% in 2013. The goal of an antibiotic stewardship program (ASP) is to use antimicrobials that are best suited to the clinical presentation of the patient and clinical situation. The Surviving Sepsis Campaign outlines multiple goals and provides a toolkit for organizations to pursue best practice recommendations in the management of sepsis (Dellinger et al., 2013). One of the elements to reduce sepsis mortality is early and appropriate antimicrobial therapy. This project's focus rested on the identification of sepsis and timely, appropriate antibiotic selection in patients meeting sepsis criteria.

Reproduced from Department of Emergency Medicine, University of South Alabama.(2013). *Sepsis protocol.* Mobile, AL: Author.

First Line Antimicrobial Therapy for Sepsis

Purpose

The purpose of this project was to first examine and later improve the timeliness and accuracy of initial antibiotic administration. By using the sepsis protocol currently in place in the ED, the project leader evaluated how and when patients are identified as meeting the criteria for sepsis. This project included implementation of an algorithm that guides providers to choose an appropriate first dose of antimicrobial. If practitioners intervene early and appropriately, sepsis, and therefore sepsis mortality, can be reduced.

Methods

Based on a 30-day retrospective data collection, 24 admitted or transferred patients to medicine units were identified as potentially having a diagnosis of sepsis. Of those patients, 12.5% received antimicrobial therapy within one hour of screening positive for sepsis criteria. Only 37.5% of additional patients meeting the criteria for sepsis received antibiotic therapy within three hours. It took greater than three hours for 50% of patients meeting the sepsis protocol criteria to receive the first dose of antibiotic. An expanded review was conducted on a 60-day retrospective period; 64 admitted

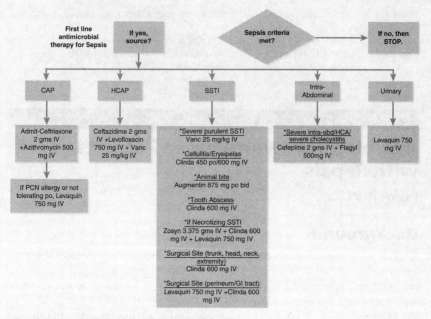

First Line Antimicrobial Therapy for Sepsis

Reproduced from Department of Emergency Medicine, University of South Alabama. (2013). Sepsis protocol. Author

or transferred patients to medicine units were identified as meeting the sepsis criteria per protocol. Of those patients, 18% received antimicrobial therapy within one hour, and 38% received antibiotic therapy within three hours. It took greater than three hours for the remaining 44% of patients to receive the first dose of antibiotic.

Initial interventions aimed to improve antibiotic selection, sepsis recognition, and antibiotic first dose administration. Reeducation of staff at triage was completed to reinforce the importance of accuracy in vital sign collection. The ED pharmacist coordinated the stocking of additional antibiotics in the ED automated dispensing cabinet not previously available to nurses.

An algorithm was developed using the organization's antibiogram and current literature to choose first dose antibiotics. The project leader and key stakeholders collaborated to develop an algorithm based on source of infection to guide first dose antimicrobials.

Results

The baseline sepsis mortality rate from January to May 2013 was 20%. The algorithm for antibiotic selection was implemented in late 2015. The sepsis mortality rate for October 2015 to February 2016 fell to 11.8% resulting from this effort along with the implementation of core measure standards and improved documentation.

Conclusions

The antibiotic algorithm has been implemented as part of the sepsis bundle to encourage best practice selection of antibiotics. Reducing mortality and improving patient outcomes continues to be the goal of the organization's antibiotic stewardship program.

References

Dellinger, R. P., Levy, M. M., Rhodes, A., Djillali, A., Gerlach, H., Opal, S. M., & Angus, D. C. (2013). Surviving sepsis campaign: International guidelines for management of severe sepsis and septic shock: 2012. *Critical Care Medicine, 41*(2), 580–637. https://doi.org/10.1097/CCM.0b013e31827e83af

Department of Emergency Medicine University of South Alabama. (2013). *Sepsis protocol.* Author.

Harbarth, S., Nobre, V., & Pittet, D. (2007). Does antibiotic selection impact patient outcome? *Healthcare Epidemiology, 44,* 87–93. http://cid.oxfordjournals.org

Counting on Moms: Addressing Postpartum Hemorrhages

Lisabeth Emley and Claudia Reed

Introduction

Postpartum hemorrhage (PPH) is an obstetrical emergency and accounts for one of the top five causes of maternal mortality. As an obstetric emergency, PPH increases maternal morbidity and mortality (D'Alton et al., 2017). Recognition, diagnosis, and treatment are necessary to prevent injury and death (Belfort, 2018). As such, The Joint Commission in 2010 issued a sentinel event alert to identify, report, and develop strategies to prevent pregnancy-related mortality and morbidity (The Joint Commission, 2010).

As part of the requirements for completion of a CNL program, a gap analysis was completed at an obstetrical clinical site that revealed the facility had adopted the California Maternal Quality Care Collaborative Toolkit (CMQCC, 2011) and availability of the recommended hemorrhage cart. However, two additional parts of the toolkit were absent, a massive transfusion protocol and adoption of a policy specifying how to measure blood loss and the accompanying computerized calculation option for documentation in the medical record.

The Improvement Plan

Based on findings from the gap analysis, The Johns Hopkins Nursing Evidence-Based Model (JHNEBPM; practice, evidence, translation) guided the project. Specifically, the practice (P) question regarding how to use evidence in recognition of a (PPH); evidence (E): re-educate staff about PPH and evidence presented in the CMQCC toolbox; and translation (T): the staff will assess for PPH risk factors, improved recognition of hemorrhage, increased response to PPH, and standardized reporting (Newhouse & Johnson, 2009).

Findings from RCAs also assisted in identifying causes or factors of near misses or adverse events. Causes or contributing factors were identified and analyzed to develop action plans regarding the potential systems failure. Utilizing a fishbone diagram, the healthcare team was able to discuss the identified problem related to PPH. Brainstorming followed to identify other related issues or practice problems. Debriefing followed using the AWHONN Postpartum Hemorrhage Project's algorithm (AWHONN, 2014).

Project Outcome

Throughout the project, a series of activities occurred beyond identifying the problem(s) and debriefings. A slogan was proposed at the institution: Counting on Moms. The blood loss calculator and a policy to measure blood loss was completed awaiting approval that included documentation in the medical record. A pilot program of a modified early warning system (MEWS) instituted for ICU units and pending approval for labor and delivery was also initiated. All patients were assessed on admission, during labor, and after delivery for risk of hemorrhage and a debriefing form was in the development process in order to evaluate situations, discover gaps in care, and provide future improvement processes. The massive transfusion protocol (MTP) awaits approval.

While the student was unable to measure specific outcomes and assist in the implementation of new processes due to the duration of the experience, improvement processes were introduced at the facility. Opportunities to use evidence and methods to guide the project offered the student an opportunity to gain new skills in improvement. Staff also were able to recognize the value of improvement processes and how evidence guides practice change.

References

The Association of Women's Health, Obstetric, and Neonatal Nurses. (2014). *Postpartum Hemorrhage Project: Recognition, readiness & response.* http://www.pphproject.orgpdg?dmc=1&ts-20180210T1723584413

Belfort, M. (2018). Overview of postpartum hemorrhage. *Up-to-date.* https://www.-up-to-date-lib-proxy.usothal.edu/contents/overview-of-post-partum-hemorrhage#H9

California Maternal Quality Care and Collaborative. (2011). *Obstetric hemorrhage: New strategies.* https://cmqcc.org/resources-tool-kits/toolkit/Ob-hemorrhage-toolkit

D'Alton, M. E., Cohen, J. S., Weinstein, D. C., Dweck, M. F., & Kober, S. (2017). Best practice in the management and treatment of postpartum hemorrhage. *Contemporary OB/GYN, 8.* http://contemporaryobgyn.modernmedicine.com/contemporary-ob/gyn/new/best-practices-management-andtreatment-postpartum-hemorrhage

The Joint Commission. (2010). Preventing maternal death. *Sentinel Event Alert, 44,* 1–4. http://www.jointcommision.org/assest/1/18/SEA_44PDF

Newhouse, R. P., & Johnson, K. (2009). A case study in evaluating infrastructure for EBP and selecting a model. *Journal of Nursing Administration, 3*(10), 409–411.

EXEMPLAR

Improving Fall Outcomes: A CNL's Patient Safety Collaborative Initiative

Patricia Baker

The literature confirms that the population of elderly persons (age 65 and older) is growing rapidly, and this growth corresponds with an increased risk of injury from falling. The number of elderly persons is expected to increase from 31 million in 1990 to 68.1 million by 2040. This 45-bed medical telemetry unit averages 72%

"high fall risk" patients, as shown by an EBP fall assessment tool. The facility and unit-based leadership's top priority is to improve fall outcomes, as illustrated by the NDNQI's first and second quarter FY 2010 data, with 7.18 and 6.74 falls per 1,000 patient days, respectively, and 0.94 and 1.18 falls with injury per 1,000 patient days. This negatively impacts patient safety outcomes and detracts from the clinical excellence of the institution. Falls are considered a potential hazard of hospitalization for the frail, elderly individual. Annually, elderly persons fall at a rate that is three times higher in nursing homes and hospitals.

The microsystem's interdisciplinary team's specific aim was to decrease the number of total falls by 50% by the end of the third quarter of FY 2010, which would meet NDNQI's 50th percentile. A strengths, weaknesses, opportunities, and threats (SWOT) analysis showed an insufficient supply of bed alarms. The team submitted a business proposal that suggested 100% of "high fall risk" patients be guaranteed a bed alarm in addition to the facility's other EBP fall precaution interventions, including patient/family-centered education. Utilizing the continuous quality improvement of PDSA monitoring, third-quarter data revealed a marked improvement; there was a 2.98 fall rate and 0.32 falls with injury rate, exceeding NDNQI's 50th percentile. The return on investment was a benefit of $251,152.

EXEMPLAR

Closing the Loop: The Need for Resolution Feedback in Patient Safety Event Reporting

Megan T. Dickinson and Rebecca Pomrenke

Event reporting in healthcare that highlights safety events and near miss situations has the potential to substantially impact patient care and safety when utilized to its full extent. The 2001 IOM report, *To Err Is Human*, and the UK Department of Health report, *An Organization with Memory*, recognized the vital need for healthcare organizations to monitor patient safety events and learn from those events. Subsequently, healthcare systems globally have established strategies to accomplish the need through implementation of electronic safety event reporting systems (Hutchinson et al., 2007). Electronic safety reporting provides a structured format for collecting data that tracks trends, patterns, and underlying factors. This allows patient safety researchers to accurately analyze data directed at continuous quality improvement (Gong et al., 2015). However, electronic event reporting systems only produce data when incidents are reported. Several reasons for underreporting include time constraints, lack of knowledge about what should be reported, fear of retaliation, and a lack of feedback that leaves reporters feeling as if there is little value in the process (Hutchinson et al., 2007). Healthcare systems have opportunities to enhance patient safety by ensuring that all staff are aware when reported events contribute to improved safety measures. According to the AHRQ (2019), event-reporting systems are a great way to identify issues that require further investigation, and consistent use can indicate a positive safety culture. Organizations should resist encouraging event reporting without a defined plan for action.

Innovative approaches are needed to accelerate the progress in healthcare systems for successful implementation of an electronic patient safety reporting system. Meaningful feedback in patient safety event reporting is vital to the effectiveness of reporting systems. Reporting event systems have the potential to become much more effective at improving patient safety if staff can more easily recognize the outcomes of reporting via resolution feedback. The goal to provide safe, high-quality care to patients can be accomplished by increasing the number of reported patient safety events through the implementation of a resolution feedback program.

Conducting an annual engagement survey to elicit employee feedback is a common approach. Survey questions related to the topic of safety, including patient safety, worker safety, perceptions about safety culture, and the perceived effectiveness of safety event reporting provide meaningful data. Focus groups with staff using a third-party consulting company allow staff to speak freely about concerns and observations of safety culture in systems. The results of the survey and focus groups can provide data specific to misconceptions about event reporting and a desire for feedback throughout the system. A patient safety team comprised of nursing leaders and led by a CNL who meets with nurse managers is also useful when implementing a feedback mechanism such as an electronic report that staff members would have access to view. The patient safety team can use the information when assisting creators of an electronic event reporting system that includes a "turn-on" feature within any current system for a generic feedback option to be chosen from a drop-down list available to view by the reporter. The feature may be implemented in two departments initially to identify any issues and make corrections. Using the PDSA method of evaluation will assist in determining the effectiveness of the feedback mechanism. The patient safety team can also analyze the data that is generated from implementing the feedback feature in one or more microsystems and use the information to make changes or additions to the feedback mechanism before implementing it system-wide. This initial step to implement a feedback mechanism can increase safety event reports.

The ultimate goal of any patient safety team is to capture event feedback on a larger scale initiative and use a variety of tools such as a routine newsletter, emailed tips, or other strategies that will reach staff and keep them engaged in upholding a culture of safety. Success in improvement projects impacts workflow, but requires new education for all staff and department managers/directors. It also requires a commitment by both staff and leaders to a culture of safety. A patient safety team dedicated to closing the loop on safety events and ensuring that feedback occurs in timely and meaningful ways promotes quality, value, and ultimately a culture of continuous improvement directed at patient and worker safety.

References

Agency for Healthcare Research and Quality. (2019). *Reporting patient safety events.* https://psnet
.ahrq.gov/primer/reporting-patient-safety-events

Gong, Y., Song, H., Wu, X., & Hua, L. (2015). Identifying barriers and benefits of patient safety event reporting toward user-centered design. *Safety in Health, 1*(7). https://doi.org
/10.1186/2056-5917-1-7

Harris, J. L., Roussel, L., Dearman, C., & Thomas, P. L. (2020). *Project planning and management* (3rd ed.). Jones & Bartlett Learning.

Hutchinson, A., Cooper, K. L., McIntosh, A., Karnon, J. D., Scobie, S., & Thomson, R. G. (2007). Trends in healthcare incident reporting and relationship to safety and quality data in acute hospitals: Results from the national reporting and learning system. *BMJ Quality & Safety, 18*(1), 5–10. http:// doi.org/10.1136/qshc.2007.022400

Improvement and Implementation Sciences: Links to Innovation, Effectiveness, and Safety

Kathleen R. Stevens

*Acknowledgments: Portions of this work are supported by a federal grant from the National Institute for Nursing Research (NIH 1RC2 NR011946-01).

LEARNING OBJECTIVES

1. Define improvement science and implementation science and roles in ensuring effective and efficient care delivery.
2. Describe the goals of improvement and implementation sciences in promoting EBP for CNLs.

KEY TERMS

Effectiveness

Evidence-based practice

Innovation

Implementation science

Quality

Safety

CNL ROLES

Advocate

Clinician

Educator

Information manager

Lifelong learner

Member of a profession

Outcomes manager

CNL PROFESSIONAL VALUES

Accountability
Evidence-based practice
Integrity
Interprofessional teams
Microsystems management

Outcome measurement
Quality improvement
Quality patient care and safety
Social justice

CNL CORE COMPETENCIES

Assessment
Assessment environment of care
   manager
Communication
Critical thinking
Design/Management/Coordination
   of care

Ethical decision-making
Healthcare systems and policy
Member of a profession
Team leader

Introduction

Heightened interest in evidence-based quality and safety of healthcare has created a sense of urgency around developing a focused program of improvement science that can guide the transformation of healthcare. CNLs, in roles as clinician, advocate, and outcomes manager, use the highest level of evidence to support patient-centered care. Improvement and implementation sciences have raised the bar in translating research evidence at the bedside and at the point of care. Consensus priorities for these fields ensure that research resources are first applied to the nation's most urgent knowledge gaps in improvement science (Powell, Fernandez et al., 2019; Stevens & Ovretveit, 2013). This chapter explores these evolving fields and presents the priority topics in new sciences that direct the CNL role in improving care. The role of healthcare improvement for the CNL is in relationship to evidence-based quality improvement and collaboration for change.

Background

Healthcare quality problems are widespread and often glaring, but the underlying causes of these problems remain unclear (McGlynn et al., 2003). Since the alarm in 1999 regarding deaths due to poor quality care (IOM, 1999), quality problems continue to be the third leading cause of death in the United States (Makary & Daniel, 2016). Attempts to achieve optimal care have been expressed in a wide array of approaches, including translational research targets, evidence-based care, accreditation and external accountability for quality and safety, risk management, error prevention, organizational development, leadership and frontline enhancement, and complex adaptive systems frameworks (Grol et al., 2004). Nevertheless, effective methods of achieving improvement have not been confirmed by the simple tests pursued in the context of approaches; more complex, well-designed interventions and testing strategies are required. The CNL's understanding of improvement underscores their role in evidence-based care and innovation. Skills such as use of measurement tools as the foundation for assessment and clinical decisions and applying clinical judgment and decision-making skills to design, coordinate, implement, and evaluate client-focused care are the cornerstones to improvement science for the CNL (King, 2013). Guided by the revised Essentials of Master's Education in Nursing (Essential IV), the master's-prepared CNL recognizes the critical nature of applying research outcomes within the practice setting, mitigates practice problems, functions as a change agent, and evaluates and disseminates results (AACN, 2011, p. 2). The CNL translates evidence to design and direct system improvements addressing complex issues in safety and quality. The CNL is prepared to implement quality improvement strategies based on sound science and the highest levels of evidence, analytics, and risk anticipation. By promoting a culture of continuous quality improvement within a system, the CNL leads microsystem's change (AACN, 2013).

The Importance of Improvement Science

Quality improvement and patient safety are imperative clinical targets supported by policy, patient advocacy, and healthcare professional groups; yet, research to determine which improvement strategies has not filled the need. Despite the critical need for improvement research evidence, corresponding infrastructure, and capacity among health scientists to conduct rigorous, well-designed, and action-oriented studies are often absent.

The gap is caused, in part, by the lack of rigorous research approaches in the field of improvement science. Shojania and Grimshaw (2005, p. 74) questioned, "Why would we exempt research in quality improvement from scientific standards that we routinely apply to the leading causes of morbidity and mortality?" Research approaches remain to be invented. In addition, the science is developing theories, methods, and designs for achieving rigorous research in these new fields. While the sciences are progressing, both healthcare scientists' capacity and dedicated research resources are yet in short supply. Training programs are only beginning to include these topics in the education of future healthcare scientists (Dolor et al., 2019; Rubio et al., 2010).

CNLs understand that there are critical barriers to progress in improvement research and seek to develop their knowledge base of implementation and translational science. Barriers recently underscored by an expert panel of the IOM include the following (IOM, 2007):

1. Improvement initiatives are conducted for different purposes than scientific research, instead emphasizing experiential learning and compromising the understanding of generalizable truths.
2. Specific contexts of improvement initiatives limit generalizability.
3. Improvement science does not have a scientific home and requires interdisciplinary research.
4. There is a mismatch between training and practice—those conducting improvement projects have little research training.
5. Ethical oversight principles are not clear-cut.
6. Improvement studies are not subject to rigor, and causality is difficult to establish.

7. In the rare instance when improvement studies are published, they are often poorly conducted and not generalizable.
8. Lack of a common vocabulary and taxonomy for improvement research terms hinders progress.

The discipline of nursing is well positioned to lead improvement initiatives across multiple professions and urged to do so (Altman et al., 2016; IOM, 2011c). CNLs can effectively lead initiatives if prepared with knowledge of which change strategies are effective in implementing best practices and assuring patient safety. However, widespread improvement is hampered by insufficient skills within the profession (Saunders et al., 2016).

Improvement research has the potential to transform healthcare, and barriers can be overcome. Exploration of terminology and establishing research priorities will help clarify collective thinking about the most fruitful first steps. These are important steps as CNLs implement, measure, and sustain evidence-based quality improvement.

Several terms have emerged related to discovering what is effective in making changes that are intended to improve care and outcomes. In this discussion, the umbrella term *improvement science* is used to refer to the collection of terms. Terms in the field are often interrelated and overlapping (e.g., complexity science, science of change, implementation science, systems research, and improvement science). None is adequately defined by experts in the field; hence the IOM's reference to barrier 8.

The paradigm shift to emphasizing the science underlying healthcare quality improvement is a recent one (Stevens, 2013). Research directions began to change around 2005 (Zerhouni, 2005) and were heavily influenced by the IOM's quality initiative reports (IOM, 1999, 2001, 2008a, 2008b, 2011a, 2011b). The escalating movement has spawned several terms and approaches, adding to the initial scatter of the effort. Among the terms used are *improvement science* (preferred in this discussion and provided as a term to include others), *translational science, science of change,* and *implementation science.* Evolution and final determination of terminology in the field is beyond the scope of this discussion, but the term *improvement science* will be discussed in juxtaposition to the other terms, such as *implementation* and *translational science.*

Health sciences have traditionally focused on determining whether a clinical intervention is efficacious in resolving a specific health problem. For example, how efficacious is diabetes self-care training in controlling hemoglobin A1C? Once efficacy is shown, the evidence-based intervention must be put in place across all patient care to broadly impact population health. The chasm is wide between knowing which clinical intervention works and putting it into routine practice. This challenge stimulated interest in "what works in improvement strategies" and "how it works" has rapidly grown. This major shift was catapulted forward with the issuance of the NIH Roadmap, which set new directions and created new scientific foci. The term *translational science* was used in this 2005 report (Zerhouni, 2005). Following this, the establishment of the NIH's Clinical Translational Research Awards (CTSA) program firmly linked bench research to bedside care by setting requirements (e.g., translational science and community outreach) that are intended to focus on the full spectrum of the clinical research-to-care enterprise (Leppin et al., 2019).

With effective clinical interventions, the CNL role assists clinicians and microsystems to adopt best practices in routine care. This chapter's definition of improvement science frames it within translational science, a science that seeks to discover the "how to" of embedding best practice into care delivery so that "evidence-based treatment, prevention, and other interventions are delivered reliably to all patients in all settings of care and improve the health of individuals and populations" (Dougherty & Conway, 2008, p. 2320). As one of the phases of translational science, implementation science focuses on evaluation of strategies that stimulate the uptake, adoption, and integration of evidence-based clinical interventions into routine care; it also includes understanding the barriers and facilitators that influence implementation of effective interventions.

The CNL focuses on the "why" and "how," thus supporting evidence-based care in collaborative teams. The CNL provides clinical leadership for changing practice based on evidence-based research and improvement science methods. Through assessment, critiquing, and analysis of information sources, the CNL becomes an informed consumer, thus enhancing synthesis of knowledge to evaluate and achieve optimal client outcomes.

In this schema, translational science engages multidisciplinary collaboration to accelerate application of the discoveries across all stages and moves toward improved healthcare quality and value and population health (Dougherty & Conway, 2008; IOM, 2011c). The CNL is truly primed for this function. Improvement through implementation represents the practice-oriented stage and answers questions about whether the effective practices are commonly used in practice. Implementation research questions include: What is the best method to reach clinicians and patients with a policy concerning a given treatment so that they will (1) understand the new treatment and (2) start to use it? Also, in EBP implementation, new practices are standardized as scientific and new policies are formulized. Additional questions focus on effective ways to achieve systems changes and create organizational cultures of quality. Implementation for improvement moves what is discovered in a lab into the common care of the general population.

In their microsystem, the CNL assesses the gap between current care and best care, engages stakeholders, then develops change strategies to improve care. Implementation science develops the base for knowing which change strategies work.

Research methods in this stage of translational science are embryonic. The methods more closely follow the broad field of health services research and incorporate theory and design from human factors, organizational development, and change management. Two paradigmatic shifts will be necessary to hasten the evolution of improvement science methods. The first shift is from quality improvement strategies to the science of improvement and implementation that tests the improvement strategies. The second shift is from classic experimental research with highly controlled variables to research about complex and dynamic phenomena. Relatively highly controlled designs, such as randomized controlled trials (RCTs), are ill fitted to provide explanations for phenomena within complex adaptive systems (such as change within clinical care units); designs that include triangulation of qualitative and quantitative data within such frameworks will provide greater explanation of the dynamics of improvement.

The CNL is prepared to critically appraise research evidence, while focusing on a microsystem's change during the CNL immersion experience. Knowing the "metrics that matter" will further help the CNL determine the best qualitative and quantitative data to collect. Evaluation of the process goes hand in glove with quality improvement initiatives. The collaborative nature of the work further provides the strategies to achieve local improvement.

Following the IOM report, *Knowing What Works in Health Care*, scientists have furthered the science of systematic reviews and systematic development of evidence-based clinical practice guidelines (IOM, 2008b, 2011a, 2011b). The scientific methods raised rigor in systematic reviews and increased the trustworthiness of clinical guidelines. These two forms of knowledge are noted to be "bridges to quality improvement" in healthcare (IOM, 2008b).

Experts have asserted that unique research designs are required to capture cause and effect from improvement interventions (Pawson & Tilley, 1997). A series of articles highlighted the specific aspects necessary to adequately study improvement. Indeed, some suggest that new academic posts, "translationally oriented," are urgently needed to raise awareness and accomplish reorganization of academic teams to address translational research (Kermaris et al., 2008). The CNL as a lateral integrator is important to this end. The CNL identifies relevant outcomes and measurement strategies that will improve patient outcomes and promote cost-effective care.

As improvement and implementation sciences grow, greater knowledge will be available to CNLs as they transform and improve microsystems. Scientific principles will become available to apply in improvement initiatives. To that end, CNLs have an interest in priorities that have been set for these sciences and have the opportunity to guide such priorities.

An example of broad collaboration to advance improvement science is the national Improvement Science Research Network (Stevens, 2013). This AHRQ-registered practice-based network generated collaboration to increase the quantity and quality of improvement research in acute care settings. As part of the network, national healthcare leaders guided activities to advance improvement science through multiple interprofessional venues, including this proposed scholarly work.

The Need for Priorities in Improvement and Implementation Research

The overriding goal of improvement and implementation sciences is to ensure that improvement efforts are based as much on evidence as the best practices they seek to implement (Shojania & Grimshaw, 2005). Strategies for implementing evidence-based quality improvement need an evidence base of their own. Experts point to the increasing challenge of translating and disseminating improvements in a way that makes them useful in decision-making processes that strive to improve health and healthcare. Indeed, research is considered a driving force for change in healthcare improvement and is at the core of the business case for quality improvement. The revolutionary direction outlined in the NIH's Roadmap brought with it the impetus to redesign the very foundation of the health research enterprise—the CTSAs (Zerhouni, 2005). The goal of these awards was to create research infrastructure that would translate basic research through clinical trials into widespread use in patient care, thus impacting patient outcomes. Included in the redesign was the requirement to effectively involve the public and clinicians in clinical and translational research priority setting and participation through community engagement groups (NIH, 2007). Taken together, these recommendations and funding directions have launched improvement and implementation sciences and pointed to the need for research agenda for the fields.

There is a limited cadre of improvement and implementation scientists, a situation that may not be remedied soon because current training is inadequate and often unrelated to improvement research (IOM, 2008c). In addition, research dollars in the field are constrained. Federal and foundation spending for implementation and quality improvement research is estimated to be only 1.5% of total biomedical research funding (Dolor et al., 2019; Moses et al., 2005). CNLs sitting at the table are important to this ongoing discussion, because they are translational in their role.

Priorities in Improvement Science

The call for quality improvement research to be relevant, useful, and practical to decision makers anchors the development of improvement science priorities. This situation accentuates the need for a well-targeted agenda for improvement science. Clear priorities can pave the way for today's limited brain trust and fiscal capacity to be focused on the most urgent improvement topics, enabling research to become a driving force in quality improvement. Among the recommendations to advance improvement research is an improved infrastructure involving multiple institutions from a variety of regions and practices. The ideal infrastructure would enable cross-institutional studies, multidisciplinary studies, researcher training, and funding, all of which are necessary to enrich the improvement research infrastructure. Along with these new directions, experts emphasize that a priority agenda for quality improvement research would stimulate and validate such research efforts (IOM, 2008a). The great need for improvement science carries with it the opportunity for myriad priorities to be defined. Consensus priorities can highlight the most important and urgent gaps in improvement knowledge as identified by clinical and academic scholars, leaders, and change agents in healthcare settings. The need for improvement research is great, yet today's resources are limited. Advancements could be made by focusing on the clinician's highest needs for knowledge. Consensus will help to systematically build the knowledge for how to transform improvement in healthcare delivery and care. CNLs recognize the importance of this work and are front and center to these efforts to improve patient-centered care in a collaborative way. With a heightened interest in the quality of healthcare comes a burgeoning concern about the science underlying practices and delivery of care. However, insufficient progress has been made in improvement science.

In characterizing the current status of improvement research, the following shortcomings were noted: studies are performed in single organizations and do not yield generalizability information; imprecise measurement and insufficient description of the improvement intervention are apparent; studies do not produce information about sustainability of changes; contexts affecting implementation are not considered; cost or value are not estimated; and such research tends to be opportunistic rather than systematically planned (IOM, 2008a). The nascent field has many challenges in moving forward. One of the most urgent is to set a course toward highly relevant improvement research studies. This discussion presents the first major action of the International Scholarly Research Network (ISRN)—to establish consensus for priorities in improvement research (Stevens, 2013; Stevens & Ovretveit, 2013). The ISRN research priorities defined the most urgent clinical issues and pointed to research studies needed to determine effective strategies in quality improvement and patient safety. The clinical issues presented in **Table 5-1**

Table 5-1 Research Priorities of the ISRN

A. CARE COORDINATION AND TRANSITIONS OF CARE—Investigate strategies for improvement in care processes for specific clinical conditions.

Evaluate strategies and methods to assure coordination and continuity of care across transitions in given clinical populations.

Test and refine methods of handoffs and other strategies to assure safe, effective, and efficient transitions in given clinical populations.

Examples of Improvement Strategies and Research Issues:

Team performance, medication reconciliation, discharge for prevention of early readmission, patient-centered care, measurement of targeted outcomes.

B. HIGH-PERFORMING CLINICAL SYSTEMS AND MICROSYSTEMS APPROACHES TO IMPROVEMENT—Investigate structure and process in clinical conditions.

Determine effectiveness and efficiency of various methods and models for integrating and sustaining best practices in improving care processes and patient outcomes.

Investigate strategies to engage frontline providers in improving quality and patient safety.

Evaluate strategies for preventing targeted patient safety incidents.

Establish reliable quality indicators to measure the impact of improvement and isolate nursing care impact on outcomes.

Examples of Improvement Strategies and Research Issues:

Frontline provider engagement, factors related to uptake, adoption, and implementation, sustaining improvements and improvement processes.

C. EVIDENCE-BASED QUALITY IMPROVEMENT AND BEST PRACTICE—This category emphasizes developing methods to identify and close the gap between knowledge and practice through translating knowledge and designating and implementing best practices.

Evaluate strategies and impact of employing EBP in clinical care for process and outcomes improvement.

Determine gaps and bridge gaps between knowledge and practice.

Transform evidence for practice through conducting systematic reviews, developing practice guidelines, and integrating into clinical decision-making.

Develop new research methods in evidence-based quality improvement, including comparative effectiveness research and practice-based evidence.

Examples of Improvement Strategies and Research Issues:

Develop and critically appraise clinical practice guidelines, adoption and spread of best practices, customization of best practices, institutional elements in adoption, defining best practice in absence of evidence, consumers in EBP, technology-based integration.

(continues)

D. LEARNING ORGANIZATIONS AND CULTURE OF QUALITY AND SAFETY

Examine human factors and systems aspects related to organizational culture and commitment to quality and safety.

Investigate strategies for creating organizational environments, processes that support cultures fully linked to maintaining quality, and patient safety to maximize patient outcomes.

Determine effective approaches to developing organizational climates for change, innovation, and organizational learning.

Examples of Improvement Strategies and Research Issues:

Professional practice environments, protecting strategy from culture, shared decision-making and governance, patient-centered models, leadership to instill values and beliefs for culture of patient safety, and organizational design (e.g., mitigating of first-order failures).

Reproduced from Improvement Science Research Network. (2010). Research priorities. http://www.improvementscienceresearch .net/research

---

point to the nation's highest knowledge needs to improve care and have been used to drive research priorities (Stevens & Ovretveit, 2013).

This agenda for improvement science represents the first in the nation. Collaborative research teams of academic and clinical partners come together to conduct improvement studies reflecting these priorities (Stevens & Ovretveit, 2013). This will provide a science base for CNL initiatives.

Research Priorities in Implementation Science

Implementation science seeks to evaluate the impact of implementation strategies, which are methods or techniques used to promote adoption, implementation, sustainment, and scale-up of proven clinical interventions. Such strategies vary in complexity, from single component strategies (e.g., computerized reminders; audit-feedback loops), to multicomponent strategies that combine two or more discrete strategies. Strategies are designed to address multiple stakeholders and multiple contexts across various phases of implementation. These include providers, patients, organizational systems, community, policy, and economics. Upon review of progress in implementation science, a panel of experts recommended five priorities in investigating the public health impact of implementation strategies (Powell et al., 2019). **Table 5-2** lists the five priorities in implementation science.

These experts suggested that "pursuing these priorities will advance implementation science by helping us to understand when, where, why, and how implementation strategies improve implementation effectiveness and subsequent health outcomes" (Powell et al., 2019, p. 6).

The directions established through these research agenda will advance knowledge translation, clinical decisions, and ultimately inform policy related to quality improvement, thereby driving healthcare transformation. By making substantial progress in these areas over the next three to five years, implementation and improvement sciences will contribute significantly to address patient outcomes in our nation.

Table 5-2 **Research Agenda to Enhance the Impact of Implementation Strategies**

(1) Enhance methods for designing and tailoring implementation strategies.
(2) Specify and test mechanisms of change.
(3) Conduct more effectiveness research on discrete, multifaceted, and tailored
   implementation strategies.
(4) Increase economic evaluations of implementation strategies.
(5) Improve the tracking and reporting of implementation strategies.

Powell, B. J., Fernandez, M. E., Williams, N. J., Aarons, G. A., Beidas, R. S., Lewis, C. C., McHugh, S. M., & Weiner, B. J. (2019). Enhancing the impact of implementation strategies in healthcare: A research agenda. *Frontiers in Public Health, 7,* 3. https://doi. org/10.3389/fpubh.2019.00003

CNLs play a crucial role in responding to public demand for moving new knowledge into practice as part of quality improvement. Emerging sciences emphasize *how* to move research findings into everyday practice. Researchers across all health disciplines are investigating strategies to move evidence into practice through the new field of implementation science, evaluating strategies that overcome organizational, individual, and policy barriers to the adoption of EBP. Evidence-based quality improvement initiatives call on collaboration between nurse scientists and CNLs to extend and apply what is known about system change strategies to support quality healthcare. To evolve this science, systematic reviews (SRs) and knowledge of new models such as complex adaptive systems (CASs) place nurses at the forefront of advancing healthcare improvement.

Implementation science is important to improvement initiatives because it evaluates ways to link evidence into practice; it adds to our understanding of strategies to "adopt and integrate evidence-based health interventions and change practice patterns within specific settings" (National Institutes of Health [NIH], 2019). Together, improvement and implementation sciences add to an increased understanding of the *system* aspects of the care.

One definition of *quality of healthcare* emphasizes that patient care is guided by "conscientious, explicit, and judicious use of current best evidence" (Sackett et al., 1996, p. 3). Unless patient care is based on the most current and best evidence, it lacks quality. EBP is defined as "integration of best research evidence with clinical expertise and patient values" (Sackett et al., 2000, p. ii). Current thinking is that evidence-based quality improvement melds research evidence with clinical expertise and patient preferences *within the circumstances of the setting.*

However, the EBP movement has met several challenges; implementation science is developing strategies to overcome these challenges. A key requirement in science is the explanatory power offered by theories, models, and frameworks. The EBP movement produced several models and techniques to meet the challenges of adopting research into care to improve quality and patient safety (Nilsen, 2020). The widely adopted Stevens Star Model of Knowledge Transformation is among 47 EBP models (Mitchell et al., 2010). The following discussion expands on the Star Model as a helpful organizer to explain important aspects of the CNL's role in evidence-based quality improvement.

The Star Model explains how to overcome two key challenges in moving evidence into action. First, research results from multiple studies must be combined and repackaged to maximize utility at the point of clinical care. Second, systematic facilitation is requisite for successful implementation of the EBP. As depicted in

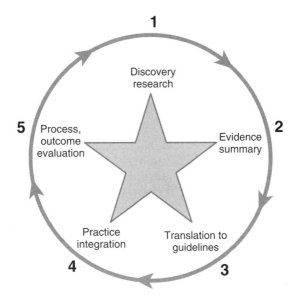

Figure 5-1 Stevens Star Model of Knowledge Transformation

Reproduced from Stevens, K. R. (2015). *Stevens star model of knowledge transformation*. Academic Center for Evidence-based Practice, The University of Texas Health Science Center at San Antonio. https://www.uthscsa.edu /academics/nursing/star-model

Figure 5-1, the stages represented in the Star Model are arranged around a five-point star representing (1) discovery research, (2) evidence summary, (3) translation into clinical guidelines, (4) integration into practice, and (5) evaluation of impact on outcomes (Stevens, 2013, 2015).

To offer a full perspective of "improving with evidence," each of the five Star points are briefly described next. Of particular interest to CNLs are the forms of knowledge described on points 3, 4, and 5 of the Star Model. Point 3 makes clear the evidence-based recommendations; point 4 explains the field of implementation science as it evaluates strategies and explains the "how to" of changing practice and promoting uptake of CPGs; and point 5 outlines the purpose of evaluating improvement in process and patient outcomes as well as return on investment and sustainment decisions.

Point 1: Discovery Research

The number of nursing research studies continues to expand rapidly. This large number of single research studies is not manageable to inform clinical choices at the point of care. In addition, the results from various studies may point to different conclusions about the efficacy of a clinical intervention (e.g., skin-to-skin neonatal care); one study may demonstrate efficacy, and another may show no difference. While it is vital that scientists continue to conduct discovery research, a single research report is not useful in clinical decision-making nor should it be directly applied in improving care.

Point 2: Evidence Summary

To manage the large volume of single research studies, a new approach to synthesizing knowledge was developed in the mid-1990s. The new approach systematically summarizes research results from multiple studies. The most rigorous scientific method for synthesizing all research into a single summary is an SR, which is defined as a scientific investigation that focuses on a specific question and uses explicitly preplanned scientific methods to identify, select, assess, and summarize similar but separate studies (IOM, 2008b, 2011b).

From an SR, a concise, comprehensive, comprehensible statement about the state of the science regarding clinical effectiveness is produced. SRs are identified as the cornerstone to understanding whether a clinical intervention works (IOM, 2008, 2011b) and are requisite to "getting the evidence [about intervention efficacy] straight" (Glasziou & Haynes, 2005). The somber other side of this logic is that *not* conducting a rigorous evidence summary or conducting a non-SR will likely result in *not* getting the evidence straight, leading to a misinformed clinical decision and poor patient outcomes. If not driven by synthesized research evidence, nursing care may be ineffective, unnecessary, or even harmful. With this realization, the focus of evidence-based quality improvement has turned away from using single research studies to using a much more rigorous form of knowledge—the evidence summary. A prime advantage of an evidence summary, such as an SR, is that all research results on a given topic are transformed into a single, harmonious efficacy statement about the clinical intervention (Mulrow, 1994).

With an SR, the state of the science on a given topic is placed at the fingertips of the CNL in terms of what is known and what remains to be discovered. Systematic reviews are deemed one of the two ways of *knowing what works* in healthcare (IOM, 2008b, 2011b). Regarding providing evidence-based direction for clinical care, an SR offers other advantages (Mulrow, 1994) as outlined in **Box 5-1**, which illustrates a systematic review of a topic of high interest to individual clinicians, healthcare organizations, and patients: falls prevention.

Point 3: Translation to Guidelines

As useful as SRs seem, knowledge transformation can be taken to the next step to increase usefulness to the CNL: producing evidence-based CPGs. In the Star Model,

---

Box 5-1 Example of a Systematic Review

A recent systematic review identified 62 randomized clinical trials ($N = 35,058$), which investigated seven types of fall prevention interventions. The conclusions were:

- Multifactorial and exercise interventions were associated with fall-related benefit.
- Evidence was most consistent across multiple fall-related outcomes for exercise.
- Vitamin D supplementation interventions had mixed results, with a high dose being associated with higher rates of fall-related outcomes.

Guirguis-Blake, J. M., Michael, Y. L., Perdue, L. A., Coppola, E. L., & Beil, T. L. (2018). Interventions to prevent falls in older adults updated evidence report and systematic review for the US Preventive Services Task Force. *JAMA, 319*(16), 1705–1716. https://doi.org/10.1001/jama.2017.21962

Box 5-2 Characteristics of a Trustworthy Clinical Practice Guideline

- Based on a systematic review of the existing evidence
- Developed by a knowledgeable, multidisciplinary panel of experts and representatives from key affected groups
- Considers important patient subgroups and patient preferences
- Based on an explicit and transparent process that minimizes distortions, biases, and conflicts of interest
- Provides a clear explanation of the logical relationships between various care options and health outcomes
- Provides ratings of the quality of evidence and the strength of the recommendations
- Reflects revisions when important new evidence warrants modifications of recommendations

Reproduced from Institute of Medicine. (2011a). *Clinical practice guidelines we can trust.* The National Academies Press. https://doi.org/10.17226/13058

CPGs offer *recommendations* for clinical practice. Evidence-based CPGs have the potential to reduce illogical variations in practice by defining clinically effective practices (IOM, 2008b, 2011a, 2011b). CPGs express the *likelihood* that a chosen intervention will produce the intended patient outcome, or more succinctly, CPGs are recommendations of "what works in healthcare" (IOM, 2008a, 2008b).

CPGs can promote the uptake of evidence-based improvements by presenting trustworthy recommendations that are directly applicable in clinical care. CPGs are "systematically defined statements that are designed to help clinicians and patients make decisions about appropriate healthcare for specific clinical circumstances" (IOM, 1990, p. 38). The definition is: "CPGs are statements that include recommendations intended to optimize patient care that are informed by a systematic review of evidence [Star point 2] and an assessment of the benefits and harms of alternative care options" (IOM, 2011a, p. 4). A guideline is a convenient "package" of evidence and clinical expertise in the form of intervention recommendations to healthcare decision makers. A trustworthy CPG is built using a standard, a transparent process for making recommendations and appraising reliability of evidence; the evidence is both specified and rated as the foundation for the recommendations. Characteristics of trustworthy guidelines are included in **Box 5-2**.

Nurses are engaged in guideline development in the US Preventive Services Task Force. The Task Force works to improve health by making evidence-based recommendations (CPGs) about clinical preventive services such as screenings, counseling services, and preventive medications. **Table 5-3** presents two examples of "Grade A or B" guidelines (U.S. Preventive Task Force, 2020).

When developed in a methodical and transparent way, CPGs are a critical form of knowledge (Star point 3) at the point of care, making evidence far more accessible for clinical decision-making.

Point 4: Integration

The CNI's role fits well with the process of "integrating best practices into routine care." Once evidence-based guidelines have been developed, routine practice

Table 5-3 Two Examples of "Grade A or B" Guidelines

Population	Recommendation
Pregnant women	Grade A "The USPSTF recommends screening for hepatitis B virus (HBV) infection in pregnant women at their first prenatal visit." https://www.uspreventiveservicestaskforce.org /uspstf/recommendation/hepatitis-b-virus-infection -in-pregnant-women-screening
School-aged children and adolescents who have not started to use tobacco	Grade B "The USPSTF recommends that primary care clinicians provide interventions, including education or brief counselling, to prevent initiation of tobacco use among school-aged children and adolescents." https://www.uspreventiveservicestaskforce.org/uspstf /recommendation/tobacco-and-nicotine-use-prevention -in-children-and-adolescents-primary-care-interventions

US Preventive Task Force. (2020). Home page. https://www.uspreventiveservicestaskforce.org/uspstf/

and clinical decisions can be realigned to this new standard to improve healthcare processes and outcomes. Introduction of EBP into routine care is accomplished through change management to promote uptake and sustainment at the individual clinician, organizational, and policy levels. The challenges of changing provider practices within an organizational context are many and complex.

Rapid advancement in the new field of implementation science contributes to our understanding of how to change practice and promote uptake of EBP. Implementation science has quickly expanded to invent new models, frameworks, methodologies, and metrics. As in most new sciences, the number of terms, models, and frameworks increase. Over 100 theories, models, and frameworks (TMFs) are identified in implementation science (Nilsen, 2020; Tabak et al., 2012). Many are grounded in Rogers's diffusion of innovations theory (Rogers, 2003), describing how innovations diffuse and the elements that speed innovation adoption (Nilsen, 2020; Rogers, 2003). Given the CNL's role in improvement, theories are especially useful as practice models for implementing evidence-based quality improvement and support successful uptake of evidence into clinical care.

In Star Model point 4, other models and frameworks are useful in planning integration with some defining domains connected with adoption, implementation, and maintenance of evidence-based interventions. Two that are helpful in planning for complex adaptive systems are (1) consolidated framework for implementation research (CFIR; Damschroder et al., 2009), and (2) the i-PARIHS model (Harvey & Kitson, 2015). Both consider the importance of "context" or organizational setting of the proposed practice change to explain or predict adoption of evidence into practice. The widely applied CFIR model provides a comprehensive framework to systematically identify factors in multilevel contexts that may influence implementation of EBP. The CFIR model identifies the following characteristics that can help or hinder adoption of the EBP improvement: intervention characteristics, outer setting, inner setting, characteristics of individuals, and process of implementation

(Damschroder et al., 2009). Similarly, core constructs of the i-PARIHS model are facilitation, innovation, recipients, and context; facilitation is a process that assesses, aligns, and integrates the other three constructs (Harvey & Kitson, 2015). As implementation research provides principles to direct integration into practice, reliable tools are also developed, such as those that assess organizational readiness for change (Weiner et al., 2020).

Implementation efforts can be maximized by applying these theories and tools in practice change projects to promote adoption and improve patient outcomes and to plan project evaluation. A focus on implementation has grown what is known about successful implementation strategies. These strategies often target multiple outcomes, including outcomes related to implementation (e.g., feasibility, fidelity, sustainment); service outcomes (the IOM standards of care—safe, timely, effective, efficient, equitable, and patient centered); and client outcomes (health status and satisfaction; Proctor et al., 2011). To be successful in a complex adaptive system, implementation strategies must target a range of stakeholders and include multi-level contextual factors across multiple phases of implementation. For example, strategies may include factors related to patients, providers, organizations, community, and policy and financing levels.

Implementation strategies are described as those methods and techniques used to enhance adoption, implementation, and sustainment of a clinical program or practice (Proctor et al., 2013). Such strategies overcome barriers to adoption of evidence-based quality improvement changes. Examples of implementation strategies include audit-feedback loops, reminders, decision support, communication technology, incentives, and disincentives. Other commonly used strategies include pay-for-performance, professional education, printed educational materials, educational meetings, educational outreach, facilitation and championing, opinion leaders, local opinion leaders, computerized reminders, and tailored implementation strategies. Strategies vary by their impact; it should be noted that some of the most commonly used strategies (e.g., professional education) have minimal impact on adoption. An initial discussion of effectiveness of implementation strategies was offered by Grimshaw and colleagues (2012). This work was extended through the project on Expert Recommendations for Implementation Change (ERIC; Powell et al., 2015). The ERIC project compiled 73 implementation strategies; examples of these are presented in a previous table.

Examples of Discrete Implementation Strategies (16 of 73 Strategies)	
Assess for readiness and identify barriers and facilitators	Involve executive boards
Build a coalition	Make training dynamic
Change physical structure and equipment	Organize clinician implementation team meetings
Conduct cyclical small tests of change	Provide clinical supervision
Conduct local needs assessment	Remind clinicians
Develop academic partnerships	Stage implementation scale-up
Develop and organize quality monitoring systems	Use an implementation advisor
Facilitation	Use train-the-trainer strategies

Data from Powell, B. J., Waltz, T. J., Chinman, M. J., Damschroder, L. J., Smith, J. L., Matthieu, M. M., Proctor, E. K., & Kirchner, J. E. (2015). A refined compilation of implementation strategies: Results from the Expert Recommendations for Implementing Change (ERIC) project. *Implementation Science, 10*(1), 21.

An example of an evidence-based program that is packaged along with implementation strategies is the program called Team Training for Enhancement of Performance and Patient Safety (TeamSTEPPS). TeamSTEPPS is a comprehensive EBP aimed at increasing patient safety through enhancing communication performance in healthcare professional teams, thereby reducing adverse events (AHRQ, 2016). While the program is evidence grounded and includes detailed curriculum, implementation guidance, and tools such as posters and flip cards, a few microsystems/systems have found that integrating the program into practice is challenging. A recent project used the CFIR model to design implementation of TeamSTEPPS into school mental health services. Implementation challenges were those that are common in implementation projects, including leader and staff turnover, agency policies, and logistical barriers (e.g., securing private space for interviews in schools). Strong implementation plans include consideration of stakeholder and organizational features within a complex organization (Wolk et al., 2019).

Research efforts in implementation science (e.g., Brownson et al., 2017) have overshadowed the *practice* of implementation. Greenhalgh (2018) is a definitive reference for CNLs who lead improvement initiatives through implementing evidence-based quality improvement (rather than study IS). This resource offers a comprehensive capture of the scientific principles discovered to date. In her book, she explains *how to successfully apply* evidence-based healthcare to practice to improve safety and practice effectiveness. CNLs will need to master a breadth of skill, including evidence, people, groups and teams, organizations, citizens, patients, technology, policy, networks, and systems (Greenhalgh, 2018). This definitive practice resource includes tools and techniques across each of these factors.

Point 5: Evaluation

Evaluation is a critical step in the change process as EBPs are implemented. Quality improvement projects must also estimate costs and savings over time, for the customer and other stakeholders. Once the practice change is integrated, it is evaluated for its impact on multiple outcomes, including care processes, healthcare services, and patient and population health outcomes. A major point in implementation science is how to evaluate successful implementation. Proctor and her associates (2011) list the types of outcomes in implementation research as shown in **Table 5-4**.

Success of implementation is measured in terms of feasibility, fidelity, cost, and sustainment of the EBP as it moves into care. Improvement in healthcare service is assessed in terms of safety, timeliness, effectiveness, efficiency, equitability, and patient-centeredness resulting from the change. Client, patient, family, and population outcomes are evaluated in terms of health status, symptomology, and satisfaction (Proctor et al., 2011). Building on this conceptual map, implementation scientists have developed implementation outcome measures to monitor and evaluate success of implementation efforts. This resulted in three noteworthy measures to evaluate implementation outcomes: acceptability of intervention, intervention appropriateness, and feasibility of intervention (Weiner et al., 2017). **Table 5-5** further defines each construct.

CNL projects will include evaluation designed around a systematic model. A frequently applied evaluation framework, the research-effectiveness-adoption-implementation-maintenance (RE-AIM) framework is useful not only in public health behavior change, but also in clinical settings (Glasgow et al., 2019). RE-AIM

Table 5-4 Types of Implementation Outcomes

Implementation Outcomes	Service Outcomes (IOM "STEPPS" Standards of Care*)	Client Outcomes
Acceptability	Safety	Satisfaction
Adoption	Timeliness	Function
Appropriateness	Effectiveness	Symptomatology
Costs	Efficiency	
Feasibility	Equity	
Fidelity	Patient-centeredness	
Penetration		
Sustainability		

*IOM, 2001

Table 5-5 Three Concepts of Fit and Match of an EBP Intervention

Concept Definition	4 Likert-Type Questions for Each Concept
Acceptability—Personal views of stakeholder (e.g., clinicians, administrators) perception that a given treatment, service, practice, or evidence-based innovation is agreeable, palatable, or satisfactory	Approval Appeal Preference Openness
Appropriateness—Technical or social views on perceived fit, relevance, or compatibility of the innovation for a given practice setting, provider, consumer for a given problem	Fitting Suitable Applicable Good match
Feasibility—Practical views on the extent to which a new treatment or evidence-based innovation can be successfully used or carried out in a given setting	Implementable Possible Doable Easy to use

identifies metrics to evaluate implementation success, that is, high reach and effectiveness, resulting in practice change.

The field of implementation science has greatly advanced, and several priorities have been identified for continuation. It is notable that one priority is economic evaluations of implementation strategies (Ovretveit, 2017; Powell et al., 2019). The goal of EBP is to improve healthcare, and the cost of the change is central in the value equation (Kilbourne et al., 2019). Every practice change requires an investment of time and resources, with the intent of improving patient and service outcomes. Process costs (e.g., clinician orientation to the new practice, supplies) are examined considering outcomes. Examples of outcomes are shortened length of hospital stay, reduced injurious falls, and avoidance of unplanned readmissions. Cost analysis is an approach to examine the return on investment of EBP, including implementation. Such analysis often includes determining the costs avoided and cost of implementing the change to estimate the return on investment. Organizational and individual endorsement of the change is enhanced when the benefits of the investment are demonstrated.

Growing CNL Capacity in Evidence-Based Quality Improvement

Implementing microsystem improvements is a critical activity to transform our healthcare system to deliver safe, effective, efficient, equitable, and patient-centered care (IOM, 2001). Several skill sets come together for CNL success as frontline managers in improvements. These include understanding EBP, translational and implementation sciences, change management, and evaluation. While education programs included these competencies for some time, there remains a limited capacity for improvement skills at the front line. One study indicated that frontline managers were not sufficiently equipped nor supported to complete the implementation process satisfactorily; they were torn between various commitments, lacked the autonomy to act as process drivers or facilitators, and did not take the necessary leadership role (Pedersen, 2019). By preparing the CNL workforce with this broad set of competencies, these shortfalls can be overcome.

Clarity on what comprises EBP competencies has been established. National consensus was developed around three levels of nursing competencies in evidence-based quality improvement (Stevens, 2009). These competencies are organized around the Star Model for Knowledge Transformation. CNL preparation enables the CNL to demonstrate the 32 competencies in the "intermediate" EBP role. Educational programs are available to enable nurses to achieve EBP competencies. To further advance these skills, leaders developed, tested, and made available in-depth online learning programs. The web-based evidence-based research (EBR) program (Long et al., 2016) incorporates sound instructional design, theoretical basis, including the Stevens Star Model of Knowledge Transformation (Stevens, 2015), and broad EBP skills. The EBR program is usable on multiple devices and is effective in helping interprofessional clinicians acquire skills and tap into important EBP resources. The e-learning strategy places evidence-based resources at the fingertips of users by addressing some of the most cited barriers to research utilization while exposing users to information and online literacy standards of practice, meeting a growing need (Long et al., 2016).

Summary

- CNLs can use their understanding of improvement science to advance roles as lateral integrators, advocates, information managers, lifelong learners, educators, and outcome managers.
- Knowing the intersection of critical appraisal of the research of improvement initiatives, the CNL uses this information about how an innovation may be implemented and evaluated to answer the question, "Does it work in a clinical microsystem?"
- Understanding forms of knowledge will guide implementation methods for EBP uptake in context of local care processes and patient outcomes.
- CNLs as clinical leaders in microsystem change are optimally positioned to bring teams together to sustain improvement.

Reflection Questions

1. Consider the impact of research priorities in implementation and improvement research. What microsystem change projects that you are currently engaged in fit into a particular priority area? Does an understanding of improvement science inform your project? How so?
2. Using the example of a change project from question 1, what improvement strategies best describe your approach to sustaining your innovation?

Learning Activities

1. What critical barriers to progress in improvement research, discussed in this chapter, have been noted when making a microsystem improvement change? Describe how you could overcome these barriers.
2. When critically appraising evidence to support your microsystems change, what have you noted regarding form of knowledge and strength of evidence? What lessons did you learn when critically appraising systematic reviews and clinical practice guidelines?
3. What implementation strategies have been demonstrated to have an impact on changing practice behavior? Do the strategies fit into the ideas for CNL projects?

References

Agency for Healthcare Research & Quality. (2008). *Health care innovations exchange.* http://innovations.ahrq.gov/

Altman, A. Butler, S., & Shern, L. (Eds.). (2016). *Assessing progress on the Institute of Medicine report The Future of Nursing.* National Academies Press.

American Association of Colleges of Nursing. (2011). *The essentials of master's education in nursing.* Author. http://www.aacn.nche.edu/educationresources/MastersEssentials11.pdf

American Association of Colleges of Nursing. (2013). *Competencies and curricular expectations for Clinical Nurse Leader education and practice.* Author. http://www.aacn.nche.edu/cnl/CNL-Competencies-October-2013.pdf

Brownson, R. C., Colditz, G. A., & Proctor, E. K. (Eds.). (2017). *Dissemination and implementation research in health: Translating science to practice* (2nd ed.). Oxford University Press.

Damschroder, L. J., Aron, D. C., Keith, R. E., Kirsh, S. R., Alexander, J. A., & Lowery, J. C. (2009). Fostering implementation of health services research findings into practice: A consolidated framework for advancing implementation science. *Implementation Science, 4*(1), 50.

Dolor, R. J., Proctor, E, Stevens, K. R., Boone, L. R., Meissner, P., & Baldwin, L. (2019). Dissemination and implementation science activities across the Clinical Translational Science Award (CTSA) Consortium: Report from a survey of CTSA leaders. *Journal of Clinical and Translational Science,* 1–7.

Dougherty D., & Conway, P. H. (2008). The "3T's" road map to transform US health care: The "how" of high quality care. *Journal of the American Medical Association, 299*(19), 2319–2321.

Glasgow, R. E., Harden, S. M., Gaglio, B., Rabin, B. A., Smith, M. L., Porter, G. C., Ory, M. G., & Estabrooks, P. A. (2019). RE-AIM planning and evaluation framework: Adapting to new science and practice with a twenty-year review. *Frontiers in Public Health, 7,* 64.

Glasziou, P., & Haynes, B. (2005). The paths from research to improved health outcomes. *ACP Journal Club, 142*(2), A8–A10.

Greenhalgh, T. (2018). *How to implement evidence-based healthcare.* Wiley Blackwell.

Grimshaw, J. M., Eccles, M. P., Lavis, J. N., Hill, S. J., & Squires, J. E. (2012). Knowledge translation of research findings. *Implementation Science, 7*(1), 50.

Grol, R., Baker, R., & Moss, F. (2004). *Quality improvement research: Understanding the science of change in health care.* BMJ Books.

Guirguis-Blake, J. M., Michael, Y. L., Perdue, L. A., Coppola, E. L., & Beil, T. L. (2018). Interventions to prevent falls in older adults: Updated evidence report and systematic review for the US Preventive Services Task Force. *JAMA, 319*(16), 1705–1716.

Harvey, G., & Kitson, A. (2015). PARIHS revisited: From heuristic to integrated framework for the successful implementation of knowledge into practice. *Implementation Science, 11*(1), 33.

Institute of Medicine. (1990). *Clinical practice guidelines: Directions for a new program.* National Academies Press.

Institute of Medicine. (1999). *To err is human: Building a safer health system.* National Academies Press. http://www.iom.edu/Reports/1999/To-Err-is-Human-Building-A-Safer-Health-System.aspx

Institute of Medicine. (2001). *Crossing the quality chasm: A new health system for the 21st century.* National Academies Press. http://www.iom.edu/Reports/2001/Crossing-the-Quality-Chasm-A -New-Health-System-for-the-21st-Century.aspx

Institute of Medicine. (2007). *The state of quality improvement and implementation research: Expert views. Workshop summary.* National Academies Press. http://www.iom.edu/Reports/2007/The -State-of-Quality-Improvement-and-Implementation-Research-Expert-Views-Workshop -Summary.aspx

Institute of Medicine. (2008a). *Creating a business case for quality improvement research: Expert views. Workshop summary.* National Academies Press. http://www.nap.edu/catalog.php?record_id=12137

Institute of Medicine. (2008b). *Knowing what works in health care: A roadmap for the nation.* National Academies Press. http://www.iom.edu/Reports/2008/Knowing-What-Works-in-Health-Care-A -Roadmap-for-the-Nation.aspx

Institute of Medicine. (2008c). *Training the workforce in quality improvement and quality improvement research.* IOM Forum Workshop. Washington, DC.

Institute of Medicine. (2011a). *Clinical guidelines we can trust.* National Academies Press. https:// www.nap.edu/catalog/13058/clinical- practice-guidelines-we-can-trust

Institute of Medicine. (2011b). *Finding what works in healthcare: Standards for systematic reviews.* https:// www.nap.edu/catalog/13059/finding-what-works-in-health-care-standards-for-systematic-reviews

Institute of Medicine. (2011c). *The future of nursing: Leading change, advancing health.* National Academies Press.

Kermaris N. C., Kanadaris N. K., Tziopis, G., Kontakis, G., & Giannoudis, P. V. (2008). Translational research: From bench to bedside. *Injury, 39*(6), 643–650.

Kilbourne, A. M., Goodrich, D. E., Miake-Lye, I., Braganza, M. Z., & Bowersox, N. W. (2019). Quality Enhancement Research Initiative Implementation Roadmap: Toward sustainability of evidence-based practices in a learning health system. *Medical Care, 57*(10 Suppl 3), S286.

King, C. R. (2013). Evidence-based practice. In C. R. King & G. S. O'Toole (Eds.), *Clinical nurse leader certification review.* Springer.

Leppin A. L., Mahoney J. E., Stevens, K. R,, Bartels, S. J., Baldwin, L. M, Dolor. R. J., Proctor. E. K., Scholl, L., Moore, J. B., Baumann, A. A., Rohweder, C. L., & Meissner, P. (2019). Situating dissemination and implementation sciences across the translational research spectrum. *Journal of Clinical and Translational Science, 4*(4), 371. https://doi.org/10.1017/cts.2019.392

Long, J. D., Gannaway, P., Ford, C., Doumit, R., Zeeni, N., Sukkarieh-Haraty, O., Milane, A., Byers, B., Harrison, N., Hatch, D., Brown, J., Proper, S., White, P., & Song, H. (2016). Effectiveness of a technology-based intervention to teach evidence-based practice: The EBR Tool. *Worldviews on Evidence-Based Nursing, 13*(1), 59–65.

Makary, M. A., & Daniel, M. (2016). Medical error—The third leading cause of death in the US. *BMJ, 353,* 2139.

McGlynn, E. A., Asch, S. M., Adams, J., Keesey, J., Hicks, J., DeCristofaro, A., & Kerr, E. A. (2003). The quality of health care delivered to adults in the United States. *New England Journal of Medicine, 348*(26), 2635–2645.

Mitchell, S. A., Fisher, C. A., Hastings, C. E., Silverman, L. B., & Wallen, G. R. (2010). A thematic analysis of theoretical models for translational science in nursing: Mapping the field. *Nursing Outlook, 58*(6), 287–300.

Moses, H., 3rd, Dorsey, E. R., Mattheson, D. H., & Thier, S. O. (2005). Financial anatomy of biomedical research. *Journal of the American Medical Association, 294*(11), 1333–1342.

Mulrow, C. D. (1994). Rationale for systematic reviews. *British Medical Journal (Clinical Research Edition), 309*(6954), 597–599.

National Institutes of Health. (2007). *Part II—Full text of announcement. Section I. Funding opportunity description. 1. Research objectives.* Institutional Clinical and Translational Science Award (U54). RFARM-07-007. http://grants.nih.gov grants/guide /rfa-files/rfa-rm-07-007.html#PartII

National Institutes of Health. (2019). Dissemination and implementation research in health. PAR 19-274. https://grants.nih.gov/grants/guide/pa-files/PAR-19-274.html

Nilsen, P. (2020). Making sense of implementation theories, models, and frameworks. In *Implementation Science 3.0* (pp. 53–79). Springer.

Ovretveit, J. (2017). Perspectives: Answering questions about quality improvement: Suggestions for investigators. *International Journal for Quality in Health Care, 29*(1), 137–142. http://doi.org/10.1093/intqhc/mzw136

Pawson, R., & Tilley, N. (1997). *Realistic evaluation.* Sage.

Pedersen, M. S., Landheim, A., Møller, M., & Lien, L. (2019). First-line managers' experience of the use of audit and feedback cycle in specialist mental health care: A qualitative case study. *Archives of Psychiatric Nursing, 33*(6), 103–109.

Powell, B. J., Fernandez, M. E., Williams, N. J., Aarons, G. A., Beidas, R. S., Lewis, C. C., McHugh, S., & Weiner, B. J. (2019). Enhancing the impact of implementation strategies in healthcare: A research agenda. *Frontiers in Public Health, 7,* 3.

Powell, B. J., Waltz, T. J., Chinman, M. J., Damschroder, L. J., Smith, J. L., Matthieu, M. M., Proctor, E. K., & Kirchner, J. E. (2015). A refined compilation of implementation strategies: Results from the Expert Recommendations for Implementing Change (ERIC) project. *Implementation Science, 10*(1), 21.

Proctor, E., Silmere, H., Raghavan, R., Hovmand, P., Aarons, G., Bunger, A., Griffey, R., & Hensley, M. (2011). Outcomes for implementation research: Conceptual distinctions, measurement challenges, and research agenda. *Administration and Policy in Mental Health and Mental Health Services Research, 38*(2), 65–76.

Proctor, E. K., Powell, B. J., & McMillen, J. C. (2013). Implementation strategies: Recommendations for specifying and reporting. *Implementation Science, 8*(1), 139.

Rogers, E. M. (2003). *Diffusion of innovations* (5th ed.). Free Press.

Rubio, D. M., Schoenbaum, E. E., Lee, L. S., Schteingart, D. E., Marantz, P. R., Anderson, K. E., Platt, L. D., Baez, A., & Esposito, K. (2010). Defining translational research: Implications for training. *Academic Medicine, 85*(3), 470–475.

Sackett, D. L., Rosenberg, W. M. C., Gray, J. A. M., Haynes, R. B., & Richardson, W. S. (1996). Evidence based medicine: What it is and what it isn't. *BMJ, 312*(7023), 71–72. https://doi.org/10.1136/bmj.312.7023.71

Sackett, D. L., Straus, S. E., Richardson, W. S., Rosenberg, W., & Haynes, R. B. (2000). *Evidence-based medicine: How to practice and teach EBM* (2nd ed.). Churchill Livingstone.

Saunders, H., Stevens, K. R., & Vehviläinen-Julkunen, K. (2016). Nurses' readiness for evidence-based practice at Finnish university hospitals: A national survey. *Journal of Advanced Nursing, 72*(8), 1863–1874.

Shojania, K. G., & Grimshaw, J. M. (2005). Evidence-based quality improvement: The state of the science. *Health Affairs (Millwood), 24*(1), 138–150.

Stevens, K. R. (2009). *Essential competencies for evidence-based practice in nursing* (2nd ed.). Academic Center for Evidence-Based Practice (ACE), University of Texas Health Science Center.

Stevens, K. R. (2013). The impact of evidence-based practice in nursing and the next big ideas. *The Online Journal of Issues in Nursing, 18*(2), 1–10.

Stevens, K. R. (2015). *Stevens Star Model of Knowledge Transformation.* Academic Center for Evidence-Based Practice. The University of Texas Health Science Center at San Antonio. https://www.uthscsa.edu/academics/nursing/star-model

Tabak, R. G., Khoong, E. C., Chambers, D. A., & Brownson, R. C. (2012). Bridging research and practice: models for dissemination and implementation research. *American Journal of Preventive Medicine, 43*(3), 337–350. https://doi.org/10.1016/j.amepre.2012.05.024

Stevens, K. R., & Ovretveit, J. (2013). Improvement research priorities: USA survey and expert consensus. *Nursing Research and Practice, 2013,* 695729. https://doi.org/10.1155/2013/695729

US Preventive Task Force. (2020). Home page. https://www.uspreventiveservicestaskforce.org/uspstf/

Weiner, B. J., Lewis, C. C., Stanick, C., Powell, B. J., Dorsey, C. N., Clary, A. S., Boynton, M. H., & Halko, H. (2017). Psychometric assessment of three newly developed implementation outcome measures. *Implementation Science, 12*(1), 108.

Wolk, C. B., Stewart, R. E., Eiraldi, R., Cronholm, P., Salas, E., & Mandell, D. S. (2019). The implementation of a team training intervention for school mental health: Lessons learned. *Psychotherapy, 56*(1), 83.

Zerhouni, E. A. (2005). Translational and clinical science—Time for a new vision. *New England Journal of Medicine, 353*(15), 1621–1623.

EXEMPLAR

Overcoming Resistance to Change with Complexity Change Theory

Gordana Dermody

Producing change in complex healthcare organizations requires new and innovative ways of attaining effective and sustainable change within microsystems such as hospital units (Harris et al., 2010). Complexity theory is based on mathematics and emerged in health and social sciences in the 80s in response to the recognition of the increasingly complex health systems and their challenges (Harris et al., 2010; Warren et al., 1998). The theory is classified as a nonlinear theory and assumes that systems changes occur over time in nonlinear ways. Linear change is based on a cause and effect relationship, in stark contrast to nonpredictable, chaotic change, also known as nonlinear change.

A high-acuity, high-traffic, stroke/telemetry unit caring for individuals with stroke and stroke-related diagnosis, isolation patients, and other medical patients was the setting. Insufficient promotion in patients with stroke and stroke-related diagnosis was the primary gap in care. As healthcare organizations are complex systems in which change is predominately rapid and unpredictable, complexity theory was used to initiate and sustain a nurse-driven mobility project in this setting. Complexity theory focuses on the process of change rather than an exclusive event. Any project must be adaptable to the complexities related to the frequently changing needs of the hospital unit such as changes in staffing levels and experience level of nurses and assistive personnel. Other unit-based factors that could impact the changes to be implemented include unit culture, workflow, and budget constraints (Paley, 2010).

Importantly the individuals that work within a given microsystem contribute to the unit-based culture and how change is viewed and adopted. The complex adaptive system has been defined by Plsek and Greenhalgh (2001) as "a collection of individual agents with freedom to act in ways that are not always totally predictable, and whose actions are interconnected so that one agent's actions changes the context for other agents" (p. 625). Examples of complex adaptive systems include microsystems such as this stroke unit and the individuals who are a part of the microsystem. The interactions between the members of the complex adaptive system is based on rules that have been internalized, which may include a specific mental attitude or model guiding the practice and behavior of medical professionals in the microsystem. While nurses working on this stroke unit were not providing sufficient mobility in patients, nurses held the inaccurate assumption that "someone" was promoting the mobility of the stroke patients. Nurses were not aware that the very few physical therapists were stretched thin and that they were not able to promote sufficient mobility. In addition, nurses did not perceive that providing early and frequent mobility to stroke patients as significantly beneficial or that it should be a nursing priority. The interactions between the members of the complex adaptive system show that the process of change depends on the system's beginning condition, in addition to intersystem interactions and feedback. This stroke unit was brought to the brink of change by providing evidenced-based clinical practice guidelines indicating the level of mobility patients with stroke diagnosis should have. In addition, comments from hospital-based satisfaction surveys were used to reveal the dissatisfaction of patients and their families with the lack of mobility during hospitalization. Last, an observation study was conducted on the unit to show nurses how perplexingly low the nurse-promoted mobility of patients was. This included the frequency and distance ambulated and the frequency of active/passive ROM and sitting up in the chair for meals. As nurses received the feedback, they began to interact with each other about this beginning condition of their practice and the unit.

Complex adaptive systems continually evolve and are influenced by other systems (Plsek & Greenhalgh, 2001). Boundaries within complex systems are fluid, enabling members to interact with others in their system and simultaneously be members of other systems. In addition, adaptive systems influence other systems, which produce irresolvable tension and paradoxical reactions. After bringing awareness to nurses, the resistance to change decreased significantly. Based on the changes desired by nurses, a unit-based stroke team was formed to develop and implement a nurse-promoted mobility protocol. The unit manager was very supportive but was resistant to purchasing the needed gait belts at the time of project implementation. However, through forming a trusting relationship and obtaining stakeholder buy-in by meeting the manager's unit goals, this resistance to change was overcome. The nursing staff was invited early on to participate in the change process. Initially showing nurses the CPG guidelines, coupled with the patient complaint of not receiving enough mobility after a stroke during their hospitalization allowed nurses to take ownership of a change that needed to take place on their unit—a certified stroke unit. In conclusion, resistance to change was overcome by involving the unit staff at every level of intervention and working alongside the staff.

Complexity theory can guide the CNL to focus on the processes of change rather than an exclusive event (Paley, 2010). Projects must be adaptable to the inherent unit-based complexities and the needs and goals of healthcare organizations. Promoting change is a journey and nursing staff and the interdisciplinary team need to be invited to be a part of this journey.

References

Harris, M. F., Chan, B. C., Daniel, C., Wan, Q., Zwar, N., & Davies, G. W. (2010). Development and early experiences from an intervention to facilitate teamwork between general practices and allied health providers: The Team-link group. *BMC Health Services Research, 10*(104), 1472.

Paley, J. (2010). The appropriation of complexity theory in health care. *Journal of Health Service Policy, 15*(1), 59–61.

Plsek, P. E., & Greenhalgh, T. (2001). Complexity science: The challenge of complexity in health care. *British Journal of Medicine, 323*, 625–628.

Warren, K., Franklin, C., & Streeter, C. L. (1998). New directions in systems theory: Chaos and complexity. *Social Work, 43*(4), 357–372.

CHAPTER 6

How Communication Improves Care and Builds Alliances

James L. Harris, Patricia L. Thomas, and Shanda Scott

LEARNING OBJECTIVES

1. Discuss how effective communication results in motivation, solutions, and success.
2. Explore how CNLs establish alliances with individuals, diverse groups, and consumers across the healthcare continuum.
3. Describe how group dynamics, process, and language affect communication.
4. Identify the link between decision support tools and communication.
5. Identify actions that CNLs can initiate to meet the triple and quadruple aims.

KEY TERMS

Active listening
Alliances
Assertiveness
Clinical support tools
Collaboration
Communication
Conflict management
Consumers
Crucial conversations
Culture
Decision support tools

Diversity
Group dynamics and process
Leadership
Motivation
Qualitative data
Quality improvement
Quantitative data
Stakeholders
Team coordination and synergy
Triple and quadruple aim
Value

CNL ROLES

Clinician
Communicator

Information manager
Leader

CNL PROFESSIONAL VALUES

Accountability
Acceptance
Empathy

Genuineness
Human dignity
Integrity

CNL CORE COMPETENCIES

Communicate information and
   technologies
Critical thinking
Design/Manage/Coordinate care

Ethics
Technology and resources
Therapeutic use of self

Introduction

Contemporary leaders engage in multiple conversations during presentations, e-mail, social conversations, and phone calls. Regardless of the medium, leaders must actively listen, persuade, and influence others to meet the demands imposed by regulations and challenges of healthcare reform. Open communication is a key component of growth in one's profession. "Many of the problems that occur in an organization are the direct result of people failing to communicate or communicating ineffectively" (Northcutt, 2009, p. 136).

While effective communication is important, it is not the primary objective. The objective is to achieve and foster understanding using effective communication as the tool (Fitzpatrick, 2010; Sanborn, 2006). CNLs have vast opportunities to effectively communicate with teams and patients across populations locally, nationally, and internationally. Understanding human interactions, diversity, problem-solving skills, conflict management, team coordination, and using a common language will foster success when communicating ideas and spreading evidence at the micro-, meso-, and macrosystem levels.

This chapter provides an overview of effective communication and techniques necessary to build alliances with diverse individuals, cultures, groups, and consumers of care. This chapter will discuss CNL's attributes in relation to effective communication aimed at building alliances and creating team synergy. The value of decision-support tools used to communicate plans and outcomes will also be discussed in meeting the triple and quadruple aims.

Effective Communication

Effective communication is fundamental in daily life and is defined as a two-way process where people take responsibility for their own part (Patterson et al., 2012). Communication is the instrument where information is exchanged to achieve trust and build lasting alliances (Chichirez & Purcarca, 2018). Communication is complex and includes numerous components that encompass verbal and nonverbal communication, participants, active listening, receptiveness, assertiveness, and conflict management that are unique to situations and individuals. The key is communicating in an effective and understandable way that clearly delineates the message being sent to the receiver. Maxwell (1999) described four essential qualities of effective communication:

1. *Keep it simple/convey a clear and simple message:* Communication extends beyond what is said and includes how a message is delivered. Keeping the message simple helps one connect with others.
2. *See the whole person:* Convey respect and belief in others. Use active listening skills.
3. *Demonstrate creditability/show the truth:* Display confidence and belief in what is said.
4. *Seek a response and validate that the correct message is communicated:* The goal of communication is action—give the receiver something to feel, think, remember, do, and motivate others.

In today's rapidly changing society, the vehicles of communication are typically a variety of technology versus face-to-face interactions. Technological advances allow patients to receive care through telehealth and other electronic devices, chat rooms, and blogs (Kaufman & Woodley, 2011). Regardless of the method, communication occurs at many levels and requires skills that facilitate understanding, create healthy relationships, impart cogent information, convey respect, and address both consumer and organizational needs. The impact of market forces, managing demands, changes in policy and reimbursement, and a diverse workforce will remain a challenge for CNLs (Nichols et al., 2015). While technology is typically viewed as a means of limiting face-to-face interactions and human components, a mutual understanding and respect is necessary for communication to be effective. Advances in technology are decreasing the less desirable aspects of technological interfaces, and CNLs are prepared to use multiple techniques to effectively communicate with patients, clinicians, teams, and groups. As more CNLs accept positions in telehealth, they will coordinate care in rural areas among diverse populations and communities facilitated by iPads, apps, and integrated EMR networks to address complex needs.

Intrinsically, CNLs are confronted daily with the challenges associated with interpreting verbal and nonverbal messages. Effective communication enables CNLs to realize the complexity of human interactions and form meaningful relationships with others. Intercultural competencies will therefore be required. When interacting with a patient, family, or colleagues, CNLs must use effective communication skills to convey clear messages, and in response to others when involved in collaborative quality improvement projects. Effective communication is persuasive, not abrasive, and requires one to be aware of emotions and tone of voice. These responses require self-control and are closely aligned to one's body language.

Understanding group dynamics enables the attainment of innovative improvement project goals in environments where consciousness-raising is solution-based (Crisp, 2014). What guides the success of a group can be determined by answering the following questions:

1. What is the group's alignment with organizational values, goals, and outcomes?
2. What decisions are required to ensure that group goals, implementation, timelines, and outcomes are consistent with the organization's goals, mission, and values?

3. What is the strategic plan to meet mutual goals?
4. How is the plan implemented across the health continuum?

As these questions are answered, the group can determine if they are moving in the right direction or if the goal needs to be revisited.

Many barriers, including the size of organizations, reporting structures, and the amount of information that is shared, affect all communication. As population needs and the demands of healthcare increase, organizations must ensure that providers are culturally competent in order to provide care and engage in improvements aimed at quality, safety, and patient satisfaction (Govere & Govere, 2016). To ensure effective communication, CNLs should organize strategies within the infrastructure that clearly delineates expectations to eliminate barriers. Understanding and integrating the mission, vision, and ensuring that feedback is available are critical factors in successful communication. Overcoming barriers requires one to manage crucial conversations. Patterson and colleagues (2012) define crucial conversations as those that address difficult issues and require positive outcomes when stakes are high. Managing crucial conversations requires one to frame dialogue in a constructive manner where other's perspective is understood and viewed as important (Gerzon, 2006). CNLs are prepared to manage such conversations based on skills and competencies mastered through formal education and lived experiences.

Building Alliances with Others

Responding to needs begins with trust, respect, openness, cultural sensitivity, and shared values. Throughout this process, alliances are created to achieve a specified goal. CNLs create alliances with patients as plans of care are developed. Alliances are also created as teams share the responsibility to meet the needs of patients, diversity in communities, and organizations. The ability to navigate and actively leverage differences among strengths, diverse styles of others, and cultural differences can be overshadowed if alliances are not managed. Openness to diverse ideas and thoughts create opportunities for actionable strategic outcomes within alliances and teams. Cultural differences contribute to team synergy and how the accumulation of behaviors and interactions guide the development of organizations to accept change in the current diverse, dispersed, and digital environment. Diversity in knowledge, experiences, norms, age, and gender are drivers for team success. A balanced team mix provides opportunities for creativity and innovation while limiting groupthink (Haas & Mortensen, 2016). The multifocal dimensions of communication and interpersonal relations are complex and are often associated with one's environment requiring attention by both CNLs and care teams (Sethi & Rani, 2017). As teams coexist and focus their consciousness on a particular patient issue and idea, it expands and a powerful momentum of knowledge and information evolves into a meaningful direction.

Implications for CNL practice are vast when one considers the number of alliances that are formed with diverse patient populations, communities, and healthcare teams that are sustainable for extended periods. When diversity is at the core of alliance building, inclusive environments become the norm. Culturally sensitive communication is valued and a new direction for healthcare policy, research, education, and practice alliances begin to evolve (Brooks et al., 2019; Iedema et al., 2019).

Hughes and Weiss (2007) identified five basic principles for managing alliances that include the following:

1. Develop the right working relationship. Successful alliances depend on the ability of individuals to reach consensus and share information about what relationship is desired, the roles of members, and desired outcomes.
2. Create means that foster alliance goals and progress. Instead of primarily focusing on the end results of an alliance, establish means that will foster the ultimate progress. Identifying the behaviors desired by all parties is a good indicator of the means of the alliance.
3. Embrace differences. Instead of attempting to eliminate differences, leverage them to create value. Diversity allows for a variety of experiences and opinions that motivate others and lead to innovation. There is much diversity in the environment such as age, gender, ethnicity, and religious differences. Embracing the differences will assist CNLs and teams to create opportunities for sustainable and measureable outcomes.
4. Enable collaboration. The need to cultivate collaborative behavior may seem obvious, but it is often unmet. Collaboration evolves over time and requires active involvement by individuals and a commitment to create opportunities from challenges.
5. Manage internal stakeholders. Remaining astute to the needs of internal stakeholders results in stronger alliances where trust is fostered and goals are attained.

While there is no prescribed formula for sustainable alliances and team effectiveness, the collective use of skills, data, collective thought, and the genius of detail arises as a goal is achieved. Alliances are therefore challenged to manage the alliance toward future success.

As previously stated, CNLs possess many positive attributes that foster effective communication, team building, and therefore generation of alliances that enhance their ability to lead, motivate, and inspire others. These attributes become the building blocks for successful communication and interpersonal relationships, as alliances are formed and mature. Each attribute promotes respect and person-centeredness, embraces strengths of others, maintains human dignity, respects differences, displays care and acceptance, and sustains healthy alliances. The six attributes include the following.

1. Therapeutic use of self. Quality is core to nursing. It engenders trust, acceptance, and a willingness to share similar experiences. This interactive process requires active listening, attentiveness to others, clear communication, and mutual respect. It positions the CNL to support, reassure, and gather data relevant to decision-making and efficient care delivery.
2. Genuineness. Refers to honesty and authenticity and infers openness and absence of defensiveness. It is the moral compass that underpins a CNL's genuineness.
3. Empathy. Capacity to identify with and vicariously experience another's situation, feelings, and motives without them becoming part of the self. Empathy enables the CNL to use objective approaches to evaluate and resolve highly emotionally charged situations.
4. Acceptance. Favorable reception, belief in or approval of others, and the value of differences. CNLs gain greater appreciation and acceptance of diverse

thoughts and a view that assists them in managing difficult situations and meeting care demands.

5. Self-awareness. Governed by behaviors that involve the acknowledgment and understanding of personal strengths, attributes, and vulnerabilities. A lack of self-awareness can result in defensiveness, personalization, and unwillingness to listen to others. CNLs who are more self-aware promote self through effective communication and establish coalitions throughout organizations.

6. Accountability. Responsible individuals account for what they do and how they perform. Accountability generates trust when there is a commitment to achieving an expected outcome. Being accountable is a way to build and sustain organizational trust and is a crucial leadership skill for CNLs in practice.

Using Clinical Decision Support Tools to Communicate Plans and Outcomes

Clinical decision support (CDS) tools are valuable assets when communicating plans, making clinical decisions, and documenting outcomes (AHRQ, 2015). More specifically, a number of benefits are gained from CDS tools that include:

- Increased quality of care and improved safe outcomes.
- Avoidance of adverse events and errors.
- Improved efficiency, resource management, and satisfaction of providers and patients.

CNLs use multiple decision-science tools, such as control charts and dashboard maps to communicate work outcomes and adapt projects. Both qualitative and quantitative methods are used to retrieve data in order to communicate with others.

Qualitative data provide rich information for communicating projects and their efficacy. Data are retrieved from focus groups, internet and social networking, and storytelling methods.

Measures of quantitative data include metrics from clinical databases, sociodemographic data, satisfaction reports, NDNQI, and marketing data specific to population and lifestyle practices. Metrics encompass the art and science of measuring value when they are comprehensive and action oriented.

Making decisions on what data to communicate, to what audience, and the frequency requires a thorough and deliberate process that will engender support from others and ignite patient and culturally diverse team engagement. CNLs have the responsibility to ensure projects are diverse and data are communicated in ways useful to all groups. While there is a paucity of studies related to managing the cultural competence of teams, CNLs must remain cognizant of managing such issues (Tormala et al., 2018). Mental models can be changed through data when based on different assumptions and comprehensive information.

Wahl (2013) identified ways that CNLs can unthink and be proactive, to embrace intuition, and spontaneously communicate. This holds the key to creative projects and the genius in one's ability to communicate facts and thoughts effectively to others.

Meeting the Triple and Quadruple Aims: The CNL's Contribution

Since the introduction of the triple aim, it has spread at an exponential rate across healthcare settings. Three basic dimensions of the triple aim include: improving the health of populations, enhancing the patient experience of care, and reducing the per capital cost of healthcare (Stiefel & Nolan, 2012). Using each of the three dimensions, CNLs can initiate purposeful actions toward meeting the intent of the dimensions when adopting a patient-centered care model.

Societal expectations for improved health in a timely and cost-efficient manner continue to rise. As expectations escalate, healthcare shortages are also increasing. Higher turnover rates and provider burnout are also increasing. Hence, there is a threat to patient-centeredness and meeting the triple aim (Bodenheimer & Sinsky, 2014).

Bodenheimer and Sinskey (2014) have proposed the fourth aim directed at improving the work life of clinicians and staff. CNLs are successfully initiating projects and assisting with designing structures to meet the fourth aim. Some examples of practice approaches include the following:

- Assisting nurses and interprofessional teams to develop coping skills to reduce and/or alleviate burnout.
- Developing documentation systems that assist all healthcare providers with documenting care delivery and outcomes of teamwork.
- Initiating previsit and appointment systems whereby elective surgery is a seamless process and more opportunities are available for patient education.
- Identifying what roles allow nurses and medical assistants/technicians to assume responsibility for preventive care.
- Standardizing processes that synchronize workflows that reduce wait times and appointment scheduling.
- Developing orientation programs that facilitate transition into practice whereby staff are prepared to assume new responsibilities that contribute to the health and the well-being of society.

Understanding how others engage in ways of work and life balances have become more common as the globalization of nursing and teams are accepted. This practice will assist organizations to meet the quadruple aim and a new opportunity for CNL practice (Bahreman & Seoboda, 2016; Street et al., 2007).

While the triple aim has provided a direction for meeting the demands of a dynamic healthcare environment, engagement by all professionals will result in meeting the fourth aim and meeting the needs for all care providers. CNLs are educationally and experimentally prepared to assist in this journey as they continuously develop valuable processes that reduce fragmented care toward a laterally integrated system.

Summary

- Understanding group dynamics is essential for communicating effectively with others and creating positive and sustainable outcomes.

- Alliances are created to meet needs of patients, communications, and organizations. The CNL plays an important role in alliance building at the microsystem level that can be extended throughout organizations.
- Diversity and cultural differences contribute to team synergy and effective communication for quality and safe practice.
- Attributes that foster alliances include the ability to lead and motivate others.
- Clinical decision-support tools are vital when communicating projects, outcomes, and managing data.
- CNLs are active partners in meeting the triple and quadruple aim through their actions.

Reflection Questions

1. What clinical experiences influence positive or negative group dynamics?
2. How can clinical support tools foster project development and the outcomes?
3. What primary action can a CNL initiate to meet the quadruple aim?

Learning Activities

1. Select a mentor and shadow them during an administrative or interprofessional team meeting.
2. Observe the group dynamics in an interprofessional team meeting and determine how team synergy and alliance building are formed.
3. Attend a new employee orientation session with a senior manager and observe the process for orienting employees to the culture of the organization. Identify the core values presented during the session and how they are actualized in the system.

References

Agency for Healthcare Research and Quality. (2015). *Clinical decision support.* http://www.ahrq.gov/professionals/prevention-chronic-care/decision/clinical/index.html

Bahreman, N. T., & Swoboda, S. M. (2016). Honoring diversity: Developing culturally competent communication skills through simulation. *Journal of Nursing Education, 55*(2), 105–108.

Bodenheimer, T., & Sinsky, C. (2014). From triple aim to quadruple aim: Care of the patient requires care of the provider. *The Annals of Family Medicine, 12*(6), 573–576.

Brooks, L. A., Manias, E., & Bloomer, M. J. (2019). Culturally sensitive communication in healthcare: A concept analysis. *Collegian, 26*(3), 383–391. https://doi.org.10.1016/j.colegn.2018.09.007

Chichirez, C. M., & Purcarea, V. L. (2018). Interpersonal communication in healthcare. *Journal of Medicine and Life, 11*(2), 119–122.

Crisp, N. (2014). Mutual learning and reverse innovation: Where next? *Crisp Globalization and Health, 10*(14), 1–4.

Fitzpatrick, V. (2010). *Effective communication leads to understanding.* The SANS Institute Management Laboratory.

Gerzon, M. (2006). *Moving beyond debate: Start a dialogue.* http://hbswk.hbs.edu/archive/5351.html

Govere, L., & Govere, E. M. (2016). How effective is cultural competence training of healthcare providers on improving patient satisfaction of minority groups? A systematic review of literature. *Worldview of Evidence Based Nursing, 13*(6), 402–410.

Haas, M., & Mortensen, M. (2016). *The secrets of great teamwork.* http://hbr.org/2016/06-the-secrets-of-great-teamwork

Hughes, J., & Weiss, J. (2007, November). *Simple rules for making alliances work.* https://hbr.org/2007/11/simple-rules-for-making-alliances-work

Kaufman, N. D., & Woodley, P. D. (2011). Self-management support interventions that are clinically linked and technology enabled: Can they successfully prevent and treat diabetes? *Journal of Diabetes Science and Technology, 5,* 798–803.

Iedema, R., Greenhalgh, T., Russell, J., Alexander, J., Amer-Sharif, K., Gardner, P., Juniper, M., Lauton, R., Mahajan, R. P., McGuire, P., Roberts, C., Robson, W., Timmons, S., & Wilkinson, L. (2019). Spoken communication and patient safety: A new direction for healthcare communication policy, research, education and practice? *BMJ Open Quality, 8,* e000742. https://doi.org/10.1136/bmjoq-2019-000742

Maxwell, J. C. (1999). *The 21 indispensable qualities of a leader.* Thomas Nelson.

Nichols, P., Horner, B., & Fyfe, K. (2015). Understanding and improving communication processes in an increasingly multicultural aged care environment. *Journal of Aging Studies, 32,* 23–31. https:// doi.org/10.1016/j.jaging.2014.12.00

Northcutt, S. (2009). *SANS Leadership and management competencies.* The SANS Institute.

Patterson, K., Grenny, J., McMillian, R., & Switzler, A. (2012). *Crucial conversations: Tools for talking when stakes are high* (2nd ed.). McGraw-Hill.

Sanborn, M. (2006). *How leaders communicate: Part I.* http://www.marksanborn.com/blog/how-leaders-communicate-part-1/

Sethi, D., & Rani, M. K. (2017). Communication barrier in health care setting as perceived by nurses and patient. *International Journal of Nursing Education, 9*(4), 30–35.

Stiefel, M., & Nolan, K. (2012). *A guide to measuring the triple aim: Population health, experience of care, and per capital cost.* Institute for Healthcare Improvement. http://www.ihi.org/resources/Pages/IHIWhitePapers/AGuidetoMeasuringTripleAim.aspx

Street, R. L., Gordon, H., & Haidet, P. (2007). Physicians' communication and perceptions of patients: Is it how they look, how they talk, or is it just the doctor? *Social Science & Medicine, 65,* 586–598. https://doi.org/10.1016/j.socscimedi.2007.03.036

Tormala, T. T., Patel, S. G., & Clarke, A. V. (2018). Developing measurable cultural competence humility: An application of the cultural formulation. *Training and Education in Professional Psychology, 12*(1), 54–61. https:// doi.org/10.1037/tep000183

Wahl, E. (2013). *Unthink: Rediscover your creative genius.* Random House.

Managing Conflict by Effective Communication

Samantha Gillam

Conflict can be a by-product of interaction. The conflict will most often follow miscommunication or demonstration of a lack of empathy for the opposing party. The best way to manage conflict is to avoid the negative interaction if possible. The use of therapeutic communication is often pivotal in by-passing a potentially conflictive situation. The therapeutic communication path involves use of self and asking relevant questions, which allows a person to feel heard, valued, and also offers opportunity for response, all of which can decrease the frustration that can lead to conflict.

To deflate an escalated communication transaction, there are some key communication elements that need to be invoked. Use of empathic listening is crucial to the de-escalation process. Being able to truly hear how something is being said will allow for greater understanding and therefore have the outcome of appropriate reactions, which in turn will decrease conflict. Taking both a nonverbal and verbal nonconfrontational stance can be extremely helpful when trying to manage conflict. Since confrontation breeds defensive responses in most, it is then important to relay a nonthreatening demeanor when interacting. The use of voice is also important for effective communication. Being able to present verbally in a calm, nonjudgmental manner can not only help to manage conflict but can also work to promote positive interactions. Positive communications build into a beneficial therapeutic relationship between clinician and client, which works to promote functioning and plan of care goal achievement.

EXEMPLAR

Value of Communication: The Elevator Speech of What Is a CNL?

Monique Swanson

The role of the CNL emerged from a call for change in the healthcare system as identified by the AACN, IOM, and multiple other stakeholders. The CNL was introduced in 2003 and was the first new nursing role in 40 years. Some, but not all, of the issues that assisted in the emergence of the CNL role were the increasing number of medical errors, need for evidence-based practices to be introduced at the bedside, and nurses as leaders and participants in quality and safety improvement projects. The CNL is a master's-prepared nurse who utilizes skills and evidence-based knowledge to coordinate care for a specified group of patients within a microsystem. While assuming responsibility for the specified group of patients, the CNL is responsible for healthcare outcomes and the utilization of available evidence to plan, implement, coordinate, review, and communicate patient outcomes (AACN, 2007). With evidence-based practice as a cornerstone, the CNL implements policy and practice changes to improve the overall functionality within a clinical microsystem. Through these practices there is increased quality of care provided and increased nurse and staff satisfaction. Looking through a quality and safety lens, the CNL conveys a different perspective to patient care that complements the functions of other nurses, managers, and treatment team members. Different "hats" may be worn by the CNL based on the needs of the microsystem including: clinician, outcomes manager, client advocate, educator, information manager, systems analyst, team manager, lifelong learner, and spreader of evidence.

Reference

American Association of Colleges of Nursing. (2007). *White paper on the education and role of the clinical nurse leader*. Author. http://www.cnlassociation.org/pdf/ClinicalNurseLeader.pdf

Communication and Conflict Management

Teresa Vanderford

CNLs can anticipate conflict as they lead improvement initiatives in the interdisciplinary healthcare team. Conflict is often a result of different goals, priorities, and values among the members of the team. An effective CNL must be competent at managing conflict.

Communication is key to conflict management. Emphasizing shared goals and priorities helps to promote communication and decrease resistance among team members. With this foundation, team members can engage in dialogue regarding current evidence and how evidence-based practice will help the team achieve its goals. In managing conflict, it is important to recognize one's emotions and not to be controlled by them. If emotions hinder a logical conversation it may be helpful to step away from the conflict and allow emotions to settle before resuming the conversation. This will facilitate a rational, objective conversation.

These principles were demonstrated in a conflict between providers regarding which patients were appropriate for discharge from the ED and which patients required observation in the hospital. The hospitalists felt the ED providers were placing patients in observation that could be discharged from the ED, while the ED providers felt the hospitalists resisted taking admissions.

The CNL student first emphasized the commitment to patient safety and guideline-driven care shared by all parties involved. With these priorities at the forefront, there was a discussion about current guidelines and evidence. When emotions were high, the CNL student took time to gather more data from the literature before responding. A consensus was reached regarding care pathways, and team members reaffirmed their commitment to evidence-based, guideline-driven care. The conflict required those involved evaluating current literature and evidence.

CNL Skill Set and the Pandemic

Beth Treizenberg and Rebecca Valko

The COVID-19 pandemic has been able to highlight some of the CNL's skill sets. The fact that the CNL specializes in organizational leadership, anticipating risk, process improvement, team communication, and collaboration makes this role a perfect choice in crisis. The CNL is an *advanced generalist*, which allows them to translate their skills to any setting or project.

At the start of the pandemic, our health system quickly realized the need to initiate N95 fit testing for all COVID-facing colleagues. The powered air-purifying respirators (PAPR) hoods, used for respiratory isolation for the past several years, were few in number and replacement supplies were not going to be available. The

CNLs were "tapped" by the command center to gather a team, create a process, and execute N95 fit testing within days of the first COVID patient admission.

Having already established trust and relationships within the organization allowed the CNLs to utilize their skill sets and execute within the accelerated timeline. Their knowledge of the organization allowed them to identify key stakeholders and quickly engage a team. Creativity, leadership, and risk anticipation skills were utilized to gather information and make swift decisions to develop processes. Initially multiple methods of communication were necessary, but within days they identified and implemented a communication plan to connect the command center, trainers, unit leaders, colleagues, supply chain, and employee health with the most up-to-date information on the process, supplies, and completion rates. In crisis and chaos, CNLs have the trust and grace to overcommunicate, anticipate needs, and implement a process that resulted in safe, effective, and efficient N95 fit testing.

CHAPTER 7

The Imperative for Collaboration and Interprofessional Team Improvement

James L. Harris and Charlene Myers

LEARNING OBJECTIVES

1. Describe tools, strategies, and methods used to create synergistic interprofessional teams.
2. Discuss the value of interprofessional team collaboration.
3. Identify the importance of interprofessional competency development and team effectiveness within healthcare systems.
4. Discuss what role emotional intelligence plays in interprofessional care delivery, coordination, and patient outcomes.

KEY TERMS

Accountability
Collaboration
Communication
Culture
Creativity
Emotional intelligence
Innovation
Interdisciplinary teams
Interprofessional teams

Language
Partnerships
Patient-centric
Quality
Safety
Team building
Team cohesion
Team synergy
Value

CNL ROLES

Clinician
Facilitator

Leader
Manager

CNL PROFESSIONAL VALUES

Accountability   Quality

CNL COMPETENCIES

Analysis   Emotional intelligence
Assessment   Evaluation
Communication   Innovation
Design   Leadership
Diversity   Management

Introduction

Achieving and sustaining optimal outcomes is a hallmark of any collaborative endeavor. As the healthcare industry has increasingly become more complex, collaboration among interprofessional teams is paramount. All health professionals are confronted with similar challenges as they respond to the myriad of mandates and needs of a globalized society. Joining forces and designing strategies for interprofessional teams to work together is predicated on new models of education and implementing various methods that are designed to transform effective and efficient care delivery. As healthcare professionals meet the challenges associated with the social determinants of health, more interdependencies will be created. An impetus to identify the complexity of interprofessional relations will emerge (D'Amour et al., 2009).

Effective and efficient care delivery will be driven by collaborative teams who complement and complete the care provided (Meleis, 2016). A workforce, working together, facilitates the engagement of patients, and the CNL is a key player in the process. CNLs identify gaps during microsystem assessments and as plans are developed for eliminating the gaps, interprofessional teams and patients are engaged to assist toward resolution. The engaged patient becomes the strategic imperative, and a culture of inclusivity emerges when teams are inspired. The odds for patient engagement are therefore increased. Knowledge will ensue as new ways occur that optimize patient pathways into the healthcare team (D'Amour et al., 2009; Stempniak, 2014; Vestergaard & Norgaard, 2017).

Finkelman and Kenner (2013) stated, "Collaboration is a cooperative effort that focuses on a win–win strategy. Collaboration depends on each individual recognizing the perspective of others who are involved and eventually reach a consensus of common goal(s)" (p. 353). Concepts that underpin the definition of collaboration include "sharing, partnership, power, interdependency, and process" (D'Amour et al., 2009, p. 116). A team that speaks a common language and understands the meaning of each term translates into measurable outcomes and team synergy. This knowledge mobilizes teams to collectively use different evidence-based tools and methods. Continuous communication, synergy, and consciousness raising toward innovative care delivery is then realized (Crisp, 2014). Rigorously aligning and integrating the needs and interests of individuals collectively creates a transformative connection. Ideas are shared and communicated toward a common goal. Being aware of how one manages and interacts with other team members is important.

Emotional intelligence plays an important role as teams are formed and collaborative projects are developed, implemented, and evaluated.

This chapter focuses on various tools, strategies, and methods used toward synergistic interprofessional team and competency development. The value of collaborative endeavors in meeting the demands toward a healthy society will be discussed. The role of emotional intelligence in effective team collaboration will also be explored.

To provide context for this chapter and throughout the text, it is important to distinguish between interprofessional teams and interdisciplinary teams given that both terms are used interchangeably. The terms have quite different meanings in the literature. Zaccagnini and White (2014) distinguish *interprofessional* as the inclusion of representatives from a discipline or knowledge branch with differing experiences, education, values, roles, and expectations. By comparison, *interdisciplinary* is more specific to a particular discipline. Generally, *interprofessional* is associated with a broader definition and context as related to projects, collaborative efforts, and their management.

Barriers to effective collaboration among interprofessional teams exist. Gaining an appreciation for what currently exists, the gaps, and new initiatives for collaborative endeavors must be leveraged in order to meet the challenges in contemporary healthcare settings.

Synergistic Interprofessional Teams

Today's workplace is extremely competitive. Individuals focus on surviving in a chaotic environment, where individualism is often the priority, and the reality of team synergy is often distant. In healthcare settings, personal accountability of health professionals often hinders team synergy. Teams often resort to managing the crisis of the moment without a coordinated effort that fosters effective team cohesion and long-range resolution of the issue (IOM, 2001). Opportunities are lost to analyze specific outcomes that are related to team synergy because the meaning or purpose focused on the crisis and quality work processes was absent (Porter-O'Grady & Malloch, 2015, 2017).

Shifting from an individual focus to an environment where individuals are free to grow relationships, seek and provide feedback, and gain insight from experiences is imperative for surviving in a turbulent healthcare environment. Attributes that contribute to synergy emerge as teams interact, actively listen, contribute, and motivate one another toward a common goal (Malloch & Porter-O'Grady, 2010). What starts as an unconscious process of individual actions transforms into collective creativity and innovation. Both positive and negative outcomes collectively self-correct and position the interprofessional team to capitalize on individual and the team's creative assets.

Leaders emerge in many situations, whether formal or informal. Leaders guide interprofessional teams toward a desired goal and outcomes where each team member is engaged in attainment of the goal, sharing a common language, and creating a synergistic environment that embraces inclusivity and differing perspectives. Leaders who effectively use a common language and actively listen contribute to how team members use imagination, life experiences, and foresight to meet a goal. Greater group interactions occur and open communication is appreciable

(Groysberg & Slind, 2012). Historically, there was the belief that individual actions and the accountability within the actions resulted in positive outcomes. As a result, silos were created, poor outcomes followed, and the absence of synergistic team efforts became the norm. The opportunity for the interactive dynamics of a team openly and actively collaborating toward meeting a common goal and emerging as a synergistic team was lost.

Dana (2013) posed six rules of synergy and team building that are foundational to interprofessional team effectiveness:

1. *Define a clear purpose:* Members are knowledgeable about the reason the team is forming, the goals, objectives, and team purpose.
2. *Actively listen:* Members must focus on others and actively listen to what is being stated without judgment.
3. *Maintain honesty:* Members must provide objective feedback and not have a sense of being belittled.
4. *Demonstrate compassion:* Members should listen in a caring manner.
5. *Commit to resolution of conflicts:* Members must agree to disagree as needed and work toward a common understanding and acceptance of the current issue.
6. *Be flexible:* Members must be open and flexible to other perspectives toward goal accomplishment.

Understanding the importance of the development and dynamics associated with an interprofessional team calls for reflection on the work by Bruce Tuckman (1965). Tuckman's model creates a framework for understanding group dynamic normalcy, discovering cohesiveness and synergy, producing measurable outcomes, dissolving, and moving toward other team goals. There are a series of phases that occur during this process to include:

Forming: Members define interpersonal boundaries and task behaviors.

Storming: Members resist others' influence or task requirements.

Norming: Resistance declines and cohesion emerges as expectations, ideas, and thoughts are freely shared.

Performing: Members are productive and work toward the common goal. Interpersonal relations become drivers of activities and results (Tuckman, 1965).

Adjourning: The team dissolves as the goal has been achieved (Tuckman & Jensen, 1977).

To ensure that interprofessional team collaboration and synergy are common denominators in healthcare environments, expectations and structures were created and supported by several organizations. Three examples are presented: TeamSTEPPS; situation, background, assessment, recommendations (SBAR) communication; and the Team Development Measure (TDM).

TeamSTEPPS is an evidence-based, systematic approach to improve and sustain a culture of safety by providing a curriculum, readiness assessments, and consultations to organizations that commit to implementation. Tools such as briefings, team huddles, and communication are foundational to the approach where fewer errors and improved outcomes emerge (AHRQ, n.d.).

SBAR communication is a technique aimed at improving communication by creating a structured support of critical thinking and setting expectations for consistency in information. The success of this tool has resulted in a standardized method for team and interdepartmental communication nationally (Malloch & Porter-O'Grady, 2010).

The TDM is used to promote quality improvement in team-based healthcare settings (Mahoney & Turkovich, 2008). The measure provides stakeholders an understanding of where they currently stand along dimensions of team functions at any phase of the team's life cycle, thereby providing opportunities for growth.

Each of the aforementioned tools can assist teams to achieve higher functioning and further engagement in managing complex situations that require interprofessional team interventions. Their value continues to be measured in the delivery of quality, safe, and value-based care by interprofessional teams across populations.

Value and Interprofessional Team Collaboration

Healthcare expenditures are expected to increase from 17 to 20% of the gross domestic product by 2020 (CMS, 2010). Regardless of the nation, all healthcare systems are challenged to identify processes aimed at gaining value. Strategically using existing resources fosters inter- and intradisciplinary collaboration achievement aimed toward patient safety, collaboration, and value. This requires interprofessional collaboration in order to develop empirical evidence on the relationship of collaboration, quality, safety, and value-based outcomes (Ma et al., 2018). Achieving high value is vital for survival in today's environment. Whatever the business, the value proposition, expressed mathematically as "Value = Quality/Cost," is applicable (Lighter, 2011). As value is achieved, stakeholders' benefits and the economic sustainability will increase (Porter, 2010).

Since value is expressed in terms of costs and efficiency, accountability is a shared responsibility for all individuals. This supports the notion that collaboration among interprofessional teams is a vital asset to the success where real-world experiences are the platform for value-based care (Tang et al., 2018).

Team collaboration can be viewed along a continuum from minimal to full engagement. Regardless of the engagement, interprofessional teams are effective innovators and are instruments to translate ideas and evidence into measurable improvements toward the well-being of society (Disis & Slattery, 2010).

More diverse teams increase the possibility of enhancing and accelerating innovation, discovery, and value increase. Combination of knowledge is more robust than that of a singular discipline. Sequential thinking by a single discipline can lead to unimaginative methods of problem solving with a shared mindset. Diverse interprofessional teams include extended networks and are associated with a higher likelihood of connective thinking where members make connections between multiple ideas. While team members may interpret goals differently, another member may have an idea that is the sum of input by all team members to substantially advance the idea (Disis & Slattery, 2010; Finkelman & Kenner, 2013; Post et al., 2009). The results are value-added innovations that others may replicate and further advance the innovative idea.

If a value-added team is innovative and functions to its full potential, the environment must be staged for the team and supported by leadership. While there are multiple determinants of successful collaboration within an organization (organizational determinants) and the environment (systemic determinants), their convergence will assist in the process and balance the value equation for sustainability (Martin-Rodriguez et al., 2005; Porter-O'Grady & Malloch 2015).

Four factors can assist in the previously mentioned process and include the following:

1. Instilling a culture of team collaboration, creativity, and staff accountability.
2. Connecting quality and financial data that supports decision-making (business intelligence).
3. Reducing variability and improving performance based on data.
4. Anticipating risks and managing care environments (Healthcare Financial Management Association, 2014).

To achieve a goal of value-added actions, interprofessional teams must be supported and an organizational culture that engenders value must persist. Progress from one success to a purposefully orchestrated common feature where outcomes are sustainable and spread to other healthcare systems will be required. Sustainable interprofessional team activity demands quality, safety, and value-based interventions in contemporary healthcare.

Interprofessional Competency Development and Team Effectiveness

Healthcare systems are challenged to respond to constant change while maintaining a sense of order. Responding to the challenge calls for creating environments that are sensitive to the needs, strengths, and diversity of interprofessional teams. Education and collaboration that is aligned to values, beliefs, and cultures often culminate in quality care and positive outcomes, which may be at the root of interprofessional collaboration and competency issues (Gunaldo et al., 2017; Hall, 2009; Suter et al., 2009). But the question arises, What is needed to ensure that interprofessional teams are effective and assist in responding to the myriad of demands imposed by 21st-century education, technologies, accreditation standards, and health reform mandates?

The Interprofessional Collaborative Practice Competencies (IPEC) panel proposed an answer in response to that question. The panel suggests the following steps to improve interprofessional team function and ongoing collaboration:

1. Create efforts across professions to ensure content is included in curricula.
2. Guide curricular development toward outcomes.
3. Provide foundations for a learning continuum across professions that embrace and engender lifelong learning.
4. Acknowledge that evaluation and empirical inquiry strengthen scholarship related to interprofessional competencies.
5. Prompt dialogue to identify goodness of fit between core competencies, practice, needs, and mandates (Interprofessional Education Collaboration Expert Panel, 2011, p. 7).

While the expected actions/competencies resemble a to-do list, significant outcomes are expected as the competencies are mastered. The actions/competencies include:

- Mutually respecting and sharing values.
- Collectively using knowledge to assess and address the needs of patients and populations.
- Openly communicating with others in a responsive manner that is supportive of team approaches to maintaining health and well-being of others.
- Applying relationship-building values and team dynamics that result in patient-centric care evidencing safety, timeliness, efficiency, effectiveness, and equality (Interprofessional Education Collaboration Expert Panel, 2011).

Emotional Intelligence and Interprofessional Teams

The emotional intelligence of interprofessional team members cannot be understated when considering the productivity of teams. Not considering how emotions can derail the most productive team is an error and can deter future actions of teams. According to Goleman (1988), emotional intelligence (EI) determines the potential for learning the practical skills of emotional competence and includes the following five areas:

1. *Self-awareness:* Ability to recognize and understand individual emotions, moods, and drives, as well as the effects on others.
2. *Self-regulation:* Ability to manage emotions to avoid ineffective team productivity.
3. *Motivation:* Desire to engage in work beyond individual or discipline-specific reasons.
4. *Empathy:* Ability to understand others' emotions.
5. *Social skill:* Skill in relationship management and network building to foster team rapport.

Effective team partnerships and collaboration evolve based on equity in relationships and equality in dialogue. EI fosters team intelligence as members learn, teach, communicate, reason, and think together toward a common goal (Gordon et al., 2012). As more emphasis focuses on the role of EI, interprofessional teams will use this knowledge to ensure that outcomes are measurable, replicable, and sustained.

Summary

- Healthcare systems are confronted with a myriad of issues where interprofessional teams can influence effective and sustainable change.
- CNLs are in pivotal positions to engage with teams toward patient-centric care delivery measured in quality, safety, and value-based outcomes.
- A common language that is understood among interprofessional team members is fundamental to team success.
- Synergy within interprofessional teams is a hallmark for success.
- Teams engagement and outcomes involve a series of actions whereby the common denominator is quality care and team collaboration.

- Interprofessional competency development is a cornerstone for responding to the dynamics of contemporary healthcare delivery.
- The IPEC panel suggests steps to improve interprofessional functions and interactions.
- Recognizing the value of emotional intelligence among team members will foster productivity.

Reflection Questions

1. As a member of an interprofessional improvement team, which attributes are essential for accomplishing the identified goal or aim based on the microsystem assessment?
2. What role does a common language and emotional intelligence play in effective interprofessional collaboration and team effectiveness?
3. What models/tools are available to foster interprofessional collaboration and team effectiveness? How can they guide CNLs toward effective interventions and team leadership?
4. What role does culture, values, social behavior, and customs play in fostering interprofessional team development?
5. How may CNLs use the value equation to measure quality outcomes across populations?

Learning Activities

1. Analyze the current culture in your organization and formulate an action plan to develop a culture of inclusiveness among interprofessional team members.
2. The value equation can provide multiple ways to measure quality outcomes. Using this information, develop a plan to measure quality and safety outcomes at the microsystem level.

References

Agency for Healthcare Research and Quality. (n.d.). *TeamSTEPPS: Strategies and tools to enhance performance and patient safety*. http://teamstepps.ahrq.gov

Centers for Medicare and Medicaid Services. (2010). *Affordable Care Act update: Improving Medicare cost savings*. http://www.cms.gov.apps/docs/aca-update

Crisp, N. (2014). Mutual learning and reverse innovation: Where next? *Crisp Globalization and Health, 10*(14), 1–4.

Dana, D. (2013). Organizational structure and analysis. In L. A. Roussel (Ed.), *Management and leadership for nurse administrators* (6th ed., pp. 213–307). Jones & Bartlett Learning.

D'Amour, D. D., Ferrada-Videla, M., Rodriguez, L. S. M., & Beaulieu, M. D. (2009). The conceptual basis for interprofessional collaboration: Core concepts and theoretical frameworks. *Journal of Interprofessional Care, 19*(Suppl 1), 116–131. https://doi.org/10.1080/13561820500082529

Disis, M. L., & Slattery, J. T. (2010). The road we must take: Multidisciplinary team science. *Science Translational Medicine, 2*(22), 1–4.

Finkelman, A. (2012). *Leadership and management for nurses: Core competencies for quality care.* Pearson Education.

Finkelman, A., & Kenner, C. (2013). Work in interprofessional teams. In A. Finkelman & C. Kenner (Eds.), *Professional nursing concepts: Competencies for quality leadership* (2nd ed., pp. 301–335). Jones & Bartlett Learning.

Goleman, D. (1998). *Working with emotional intelligence*. Bantam.

Gordon, S., Mendenhall, O., & O'Connor, B. B. (2012). *Beyond the checklist: What else health care can learn from aviation teamwork and safety*. Cornell University Press.

Groysberg, B., & Slind, M. (2012). Leadership is a conversation. *Harvard Business Review, 9*(6), 77–84.

Gunaldo, T. P., Brisolara, K. F., Davis. A. H., & Moore, R. Aligning interprofessional education collaborative sub-competencies to progressive learning. *Journal of Interprofessional Care, 31*(3), 394–396. https://doi.org/1080/13561820.2017.1285273

Hall, P. (2009). Interprofessional teamwork: Professional cultures as barriers. *Journal of Interprofessional Care, 23*(7), 188–196. https://doi.org/10.1080.13561820500081745

Healthcare Financial Management Association. (2014). *Learn, analyze, apply. The healthcare management association can change the world of healthcare finance.* https://www.hfma.org

Interprofessional Education Collaborative Expert Panel. (2011). *Core competencies for interprofessional collaborative practice: Report of an expert panel.* Interprofessional Education Collaborative.

Institute of Medicine. (2001). *Crossing the quality chasm.* National Academies Press.

Lighter, D. M. (2011). *Advanced performance improvement in health care.* Jones & Bartlett Learning.

Ma, C., Park, S. H., & Shange, J. (2018). Inter- and intra-disciplinary collaboration and patient safety outcomes in U.S. acute care hospital units: A cross-sectional study. *International Journal of Nursing Studies, 85,* 1–6. http://doi.org/10.1016/j.ijnurstu.2018.05.001

Mahoney, B., & Turkovich, C. (2008). *Team development measure.* http://www.peacehealth.org /about-peacehealth/medical-professionals/eugene-springfield-cottages-grove-team-measure /Pages/measure.aspx

Malloch, K., & Porter-O'Grady, T. (2010). *Introduction to evidence-based practice in nursing and health care.* Jones & Bartlett Learning.

Martin-Rodriguez, L. S., Beaulieu, M-R., D'Amour, D., & Ferrada-Videal, M. (2005). The determinants of successful collaboration: A review of theoretical and empirical studies. *Journal of Interprofessional Care, 19,* Suppl 1(1), 132–147. https://doi.org/10.1016.j.ijmedinf.2017.11.001

Meleis, A. I. (2016). Interprofessional education: A summary of reports and barriers to recommendations. *Journal of Nursing Scholarship, 48*(1), 106–112.

Porter, M. E. (2010). What is value in health care? *New England Journal of Medicine, 363,* 2477–2481.

Porter-O'Grady, T., & Malloch, K. (2015). *Quantum leadership: Building better partnerships for sustainable health* (4th ed.). Jones & Bartlett Learning.

Porter-O'Grady, T., & Malloch, K. (2017). *Quantum leadership: Creating sustainable value in health care* (5th ed.). Jones & Bartlett Learning.

Post, C., DeLia, N., DiTomasco, T., Tirpak, R., & Borwankar, R. (2009). Capitalizing on thought diversity for innovation. *Research Technology Management, 52,* 14–25.

Stempniak, M. (2014). *Your not-so-secret weapon to transform care.* https://www.hhnmag.com/display /HHN-news-article.dhtml?dcrPath=/templatedata/HF_Common/NewsArticle/data/HHN /Magazine/2014/Feb/fea-patient-engagement

Suter, E., Arndt, J., Arthu, N., Parboosingh, J., Taylor, E., & Deutschland, S. (2009). Role understanding and effective communication as core competencies for collaborative practice. *Journal of Interprofessional Care, 23*(1), 41–51. https://doi.org/10.1080/13561820802338579

Tang, T., Lim, M. E., Mansfield, E., McLachlan, A., & Quan, S. D. (2018). Clinical user involvement in the real world: Designing an electronic tool to improve interprofessional communication and collaboration in a hospital setting. *International Journal of Medical Informatics, 110,* 90–97. https://doi.org/10.1016/j.ijmedinf.2017.11.011

Tuckman, B. (1965). Developmental sequence in small groups. *Psychological Bulletin, 63,* 384–399.

Tuckman, B., & Jensen, M. (1977). Stages of small group development revisited. *Groups and Organizational Studies, 2,* 419–427.

Vestergaard, E., & Norgaard, B. (2017). Interprofessional collaboration: An exploration of possible prerequisites for successful implementation. *Journal of Interprofessional Care, 32*(2), 185–195. https://doi.org.1080/13561820.2017.1363725

Zaccagnini, M. E., & White, K. W. (2014). *The doctor of nursing practice essentials* (2nd ed.). Jones & Bartlett Learning.

The Use of a CNL as a Nurse Navigator to Decrease Length of Stay and Hospital Cost of Complex Trauma Tracheostomy Patients

Meridith Gombar

Trauma patients requiring tracheostomy have significant injuries that require substantial clinical knowledge and assessment skills, hospital resources, and high-level coordination. In 2013, the observed length of stay in this patient population in our Level 1 trauma center was higher than expected based on risk-adjusted modeling. As a result, Lean methodology was implemented to improve processes and minimize waste with the creation of a "Lean team" (LT), which was led by a CNL acting as a nurse navigator. The purpose of this study was to evaluate the effectiveness of the LT on length of stay and hospital costs in this complex patient population.

In 2014, the team developed a value stream map of the trauma tracheostomy patient, looking at people, processes, and the purpose. The multidisciplinary team, including physicians, nurses, respiratory care therapists, physical therapists, care managers, and a CNL identified barriers to optimal patient care. Three focus areas were identified to impact patient care: standardized rounding process, tracheostomy clinical pathway, and a navigator to guide the patient through the care delivery system. The initial implementation of a CNL as the nurse navigator showed improvements in length of stay and cost, but something more needed to be done. In 2015, the team completed a rapid improvement event consisting of an 11-week trial with a consistent multidisciplinary LT working collaboratively with this specific population across the continuum of care from admission to discharge. Demographics, care variables, and true cost (not charge) data was collected prospectively and compared with a historical control group of all the 2014 tracheostomy patients (CON).

During the trial period, 14 patients were followed by the LT from admission to discharge. The CON group consisted of 117 patients. Both groups were severely injured with median injury severity scores greater than 25 (LT: 30, CON: 26, $p = 0.97$). Continued work is currently being focused in the area of readmissions concerning this initiative but recent data reveals lower readmission results of the LT group as compared to the CON group. Additionally, the LT group resulted in a significant reduction in ventilator days (LT: 12, CON: 17, $p = 0.01$), overall length of stay (LT: 16, CON: 25, $p = 0.05$), and total costs (median LT: $57,894, median CON: $77,692, $p = 0.04$).

Utilizing Lean methodology resulted in a 36% reduction in length of stay and a 25% reduction in hospital costs for care of the trauma tracheostomy patient. Although there was an increase in the readmission rates of the LT group, through process evaluation and real-time action planning, recent data already reveals an improvement in this metric.

Successful implementation of an LT led by a CNL as a nurse navigator resulted in an annual savings of more than $2.3 million. This example highlights the added success any healthcare-related initiative or project is destined to have as a result of including a CNL.

Collaboration Impacts Patient Outcomes: An Exemplar Depicting How a CNL Advocates for a Client's Health via Interdisciplinary Collaboration and Partnership

Jessica Vaughn

A male patient in his 50s with leukemia has received several therapy regimens, all resulting in multiple disease relapses. He has traveled from his home state to an NCI-designated comprehensive cancer center to consider the option of receiving a clinical trial drug. On admission, he is chronically ill, febrile, and requires evaluation for possible pneumonia and empiric antibiotics.

In the following days after his admission, the CNL is alerted by the case manager that the patient's insurance will not cover his hospital stay. He has contacted his insurance provider several times concerning approval for the clinical trial, which is also expected to be denied. A week into his stay, the case manager reports that a compassionate care override for treatment has been denied by the cancer center medical director. The social worker states that he was informed by the social worker in his home state to seek treatment at the comprehensive cancer center within his home state, which will provide a similar clinical trial. The unit charge nurse is concerned that his respiratory status is declining, requiring increased levels of oxygen support. He is also having more fevers, and the medical team is concerned that he is experiencing disease progression.

The CNL acknowledges that the patient's health status is deteriorating with no long-term, alternate treatment plan for his progressive leukemia and advocates for an interdisciplinary team meeting to discuss the continuum of care on behalf of the patient. Representatives from the medical team, nursing team, case management, social work, patient advocacy, and ethics are requested to attend. On the day of the meeting, the patient cannot attend due to continuing decline in his respiratory status and is transferred to the ICU.

The CNL and unit charge nurse facilitate the interdisciplinary meeting, which results in the formation of a care plan that all care providers agree on. It is established that he needs immediate care at the current cancer center. Once medically stable and able to travel, he will return to his home state where he will seek out treatment at the cancer center covered by his insurance policy. The patient's attending physician agrees to contact his oncologist in his home state to determine which similar, if not same, clinical trial can be administered at the cancer center there. The nursing team agrees to continue to provide direct care and rehabilitation to prepare him for discharge and travel. Case management will continue to communicate with the patient's insurance company to anticipate any issues related to treatment in his home state. Social work agrees to investigate the option of air travel and ways to cover travel costs. Patient advocacy will continue to support the patient by responding to him regarding concerns related to this plan, and ethics recommends that he be informed of the estimated cost of the clinical trial to determine if this is feasible for him.

The patient returns to the inpatient leukemia unit three weeks later, requiring rescue treatment for progressive leukemia, continuing treatment for his confirmed pneumonia, and extensive rehabilitation for physical deconditioning related to acute illness. He was informed of the interdisciplinary conference while in intensive care, and he and his primary caregiver are in agreement with the plan. The CNL continues to collaborate with the previously mentioned disciplines, including representatives from additional consults such as nutrition, physical therapy, and occupational therapy. Within two months, his disease progression is controlled by standard therapy, his pneumonia has resolved, his physical status has improved, and he is cleared to travel. His primary caregiver has received confirmation that a similar clinical trial is available at a cancer center in his home state, and she will travel with him to help him enroll in the trial.

In this scenario, the CNL-facilitated collaboration among multiple disciplines designed and implemented a feasible care plan for this patient that addressed both short- and long-term needs. The CNL also acted as advocate, voicing the patient's concerns related to the uncertainties regarding his treatment plan. Through involvement in this care plan, the CNL was able to model both collaborator and advocate roles for nurses involved in this patient's care.

EXEMPLAR

Enhancing Continuity of Patient Care Through Improved Multidisciplinary Communication: A CNL Initiative in an Inpatient Oncology Unit Designed to Increase Participation by Interprofessional Teams in Weekly Care Conferences with the End Goal of Improving Continuity of Patient Care

Toby Meyers

The CNLs at an NCI-designated comprehensive cancer center observed that standing interdisciplinary care conferences (ICC) were poorly attended. The CNLs felt that coordination of patient care was suffering in part due to the lack of attendance at these regularly scheduled meetings among team members. The CNLs undertook an effort to improve attendance at the ICCs.

A work group of CNLs collaborated with interprofessional colleagues to identify barriers to attendance and developed a plan establishing consistent and regularly scheduled ICCs. The primary aim of this work group was to improve interprofessional attendance at the ICCs. A secondary aim was to improve communication, coordination, and collaboration among the team members to promote continuity and quality of patient care as a result of this collaboration.

Prior to practice change, the interprofessional work group reviewed the current unit process and required criteria for ICCs. According to the CMS guidelines, the meetings should at minimum involve representatives of two unique disciplines. To meet the group's aim and the CMS criteria, the CNLs proposed a more inclusive ICC that consists of case managers, social workers, nutritionists, chaplains, physical and occupational therapists, and registered nurses.

The CNLs met and discussed the proposal with the different disciplines to solicit their support in implementing the change. Additional changes discussed and approved included establishing a standard schedule for weekly ICCs, facilitating the ICCs for each of the three nursing pods on the unit, and utilizing a standardized form to document pertinent patient data after discussing patient care needs with the bedside RN in preparation for the ICC. The CNLs facilitated all ICCs to ensure consistency with the format.

After one year of participation in the new plan, attendance audits showed about 90% attendance from all disciplines. An informal survey of participants indicated that interdisciplinary team members find the new standardized ICCs improve communication and facilitate timely identification of needs and coordination of patient care. The CNLs monitored and trended Press Ganey and HCAHPS scores and observed a steady increase in patient-reported outcomes, specifically in the domains of discharge information and care transitions.

The ICC is a contributor to quality improvement, particularly in relation to developing individualized care planning for patients and timely, successful transitions of care. ICCs also reflect a core component of the CNL's role in coordinating interprofessional care at the microsystem level.

EXEMPLAR

Creating a Standardized Care Process for Incarcerated Patients: A CNL Initiative to Create a Standardized Care Process for Incarcerated Patients Receiving Stem Cell Transplants

Lihui Cao and Hilary Sullivan

In 2015, two CNLs assessed the needs for creating a standardized care process for incarcerated patients receiving stem cell transplants. The units have conducted SCT on four patients who were inmates of the state prison. Treating incarcerated patients with SCT in a civilian hospital posed significant challenges to the nursing, medical, and interprofessional teams. Particularly, the absence of forensic policy and guidelines of care, the knowledge gap for staff and correctional officers, and ensuring patient and employee safety was evident. Considering the average length of stay, acuity, and complications associated with SCT, education of key stakeholders and the development of a robust process were imperative.

The CNLs acting as a liaison, in collaboration with the unit leadership, formed a task force comprised of key stakeholders from both inpatient and outpatient SCT departments. The aim of the group was to develop a standardized care process and design a plan for information dissemination and staff education.

The task force held several meetings to review the SCT process flow, evaluate how to best integrate forensic care, and define roles and responsibilities. The SCT coordinators communicated referrals and provided updates accordingly, whereas the inpatient SCT leadership team scheduled interdisciplinary care conferences to address the inmate's special needs, medical and otherwise. Inpatient planning prior to anticipated admission date included room selection, special equipment procurement, nursing core team selection, and staff education (including correctional officers). During the inpatient admission, the CNLs organized and facilitated patient rounds and interdisciplinary care conferences to monitor patient progress, coordinate consults (e.g., physical therapy for limited mobility due to shackles), and plan discharge. The CNLs also served as the liaison between the medical/interdisciplinary teams and correctional officers to ensure a smooth transition throughout the SCT timeline: outpatient to inpatient, pretransplant chemotherapy to post-transplant recovery, and management of SCT-associated complications to discharge.

As a result of this collaborative effort, a standardized care process for incarcerated patients receiving SCT was developed, including communication and education tools, and the SCT forensic policy draft. The process flowchart shows the progression from inmate referral to initial clinic evaluation, interdisciplinary care conference to inpatient admission, and inpatient discharge to transfer of care back to referring facility. Some of the approved tools include an interdisciplinary care conference attendee list, patient admission teaching handout, admission and discharge checklists, tips for nursing care, and information packet for correctional officers. The SCT forensic policy is under final review and pending approval from the board.

During 2014–2015, a total of four prisoner patients received SCT. Three of the seven unit-based nursing teams provided care during this time. A four-point Likert scale survey was provided to the nurses, patient care partners (PCPs), and patient service coordinators (unit clerks) to elicit their feedback on interventions. Nursing staff and patient service coordinators overwhelmingly indicated that they felt supported in providing safe care to the prisoner patient throughout the continuum of care, while PCPs were less likely to have felt supported in providing safe care.

The CNL's leading role in coordinating this program bridged the gap between the different teams involved and ensured effective lateral communication to produce optimal healthcare outcomes for the incarcerated SCT patients.

EXEMPLAR

Improving Geriatric Patient Safety by Restricting Sleep Aids

Leslie Phillips

CNL observations of increased incidence of hospitalization-induced delirium in a geriatric population led to chart audits that reflected similarities between patients of advanced age, a history of dementia, and the use of sleep aids. The acute mental status changes displayed by these patients led to increased length of stay and diagnostic expenses. Complications also included emotional distress in patients and family members. Patient safety became compromised as patients often displayed the symptoms of hyperactive delirium. These behaviors demanded increased vigilance by the nursing staff to prevent injury. A review of the pharmacological evidence revealed the manufacturer's advice of restricted use in older adults, as the drug could induce increased confusion and motor dysfunction. When queried, the hospital pharmacist advised restricted use in geriatric patients. The unit medical director echoed this advice.

Collaboration among the unit nursing manager, medical director, CNL, and pharmacy led to the adoption of a new unit guideline restricting the use of sleep aids in patients 65 years of age and older. On the advice of the unit medical director, "new starts" of sleep aids were to be avoided as well. The CNL was responsible for educating the nursing staff, performing medication audits on newly admitted patients, and advocating for change with attending physicians. Nursing was challenged to promote sleep with alternative medications such as mild analgesics, sedating antidepressants and antipsychotics, warm drinks, and soothing music. With diligence, education, and patient advocacy, the incidence of medication-induced delirium decreased, thereby improving patient safety.

EXEMPLAR

Reducing Fall Rates Using an Interprofessional Team Approach

Bridget Graham

Falls are classified as a never event by CMS. Falls can result in devastating and debilitating injury for the hospitalized senior adult, leading to increased lengths of stay and increases in healthcare costs. The total number of falls for FY 2011 was 49. The fall rate for the 3 Lacks unit in FY 2011 was 5.52 per 1,000 patient days, compared to the national benchmark of 3.88 per 1,000 patient days. The goal on 3 Lacks was to eliminate patient falls with injury by the end of FY 2012 and to reduce the overall fall rate by 25%.

The CNL formed an interprofessional team that included RNs, PCAs, leadership, a CNL, and a pharmacist. Using the Lean process and a define, measure, analyze, improve, control (DMAIC) process improvement method, the group started by defining the problem and measuring the current state. The next steps included a root-cause analysis using the "6 Ms." The 6 Ms are materials, man, mother nature (environment), method, measurement, and machine. The RCA assisted the group in getting to the causes that were contributing to our increased fall rate. After the RCA was complete, the group proceeded to the improve phase and implemented several interventions:

1. Staff must do 1:1 education with family and patient and document.
2. Implement the following standards of care on 3 Lacks:
   a. Use bed alarms and chair alarms for anyone with a Morse Scale > 45.
   b. Educate staff on the use of gait belts (provided in each room).

    c. Use bedside commode if patient gait unstable.
    d. Staff stay with the patient while in the bathroom.
    e. RN/Physical therapist to complete whiteboards with specific plan such as up with 1 or 2, must use walker, etc.
    f. Create an individualized plan for each patient.
3. Pharmacist is reviewing medication lists daily of any patients with a Morse Scale > 45 to identify meds that may be contributing to fall risk. Pharmacist will discuss changes with the physician.
4. Discuss all falls in leadership group, getting to the cause of the falls. Super huddles completed immediately after a fall with all staff on the unit.
5. CNLs to monitor and ensure that daily Morse Scale is completed and safety actions are in place.
6. Hold staff accountable for lack of following standards/actions that put patients at risk.
7. Institute intentional hourly rounding.
8. Have targeted "lunch and learn" with PCAs specific to patient readiness for transfer, use of gait belts, etc.
9. Provide targeted education to student nurses.

Each intervention was assigned to someone and given a start and completion date. The group followed up on each intervention and its effectiveness.

In FY 2011, our fall rate on 3 Lacks was 5.52. At the end of FY 2012, our fall rate was 4.03. This is a 27% reduction in our fall rate. We had no falls with injury in FY 2012. The total number of falls in FY 2011 was 49, compared to 38 in FY 2012.

Our interdisciplinary falls team was able to positively impact our unit fall rate. A Lean process was utilized to help frame and direct the work group. As the group is now in the control phase of the project, we will continue to examine our compliance with the listed interventions; we are striving for the ultimate goal of zero patient falls.

EXEMPLAR

Collaborators of Care: Collaboration, Lateral Integration, Patient-Centered

Rebecca Valko

The role as a CNL is to strategically align the right people, at the right time, to create the best outcome for quality, safety, and experience for our patients and families. CNLs are facilitators of patient care, bringing members of the team together at the right time to achieve success in either: a discharge, a care plan, pain management, psychosocial challenges, an extreme length of stay, or an end-of-life decision. We keep the work going. We keep the entire team accountable, keep the story of the most complex, and advocate the best care for our most vulnerable and challenging cases. This happens *every day*.

A pivotal experience occurred recently, cementing the importance of lateral integration and our role as CNLs. It is no secret some physicians do not communicate with the team or with each other. We had a very complex patient with several months of repeated hospitalizations and declining health. The medicine team was supporting the patient and his family's wishes to begin hospice care. The specialist team was resistant to this, wanting to give him more time, which included an extensive surgery the patient did not want. These disagreements continued for about a week with different physicians asking the patient repeatedly if he wanted the surgery. As the CNL, I was the nexus to bring the physicians together to discuss the case instead of disagreeing in their respective progress notes. Advocating for the patient and his family was my priority—his voice needed to be heard with an emphasis on his quality of life. After enlisting palliative care, the patient finally transferred to hospice care and died 14 hours later. The family was so thankful for an advocate that was patient and family centered. The nursing staff was also thankful that I continued the discussion, keeping them out of the middle as they so often are in difficult cases. The nurses could give him compassionate care that he deserved.

EXEMPLAR

The CNL's Impact on Decreasing Nosocomial Infection Markers and Healthcare-Associated Infections Through Team Collaboration and Innovative Education Techniques

Courtney Edwards, Sharon Hayes, Sharon Mills, and Susan Blumstein

Introduction

According to the Centers for Disease Control and Prevention (CDC), healthcare-associated infections (HAIs), occur about 1 in every 25 patients and is linked to increased morbidity and mortality. Therefore, the purpose of this exemplar is to highlight the collaboration of an infection prevention team consisting of nurse managers, a director of nursing services, and a CNL in efforts to reduce the occurrence of nosocomial infection markers and HAIs at a 240-bed Baptist Health Hospital. The exemplar will also describe an innovative teaching strategy the CNL used to engage staff in purposeful learning, detail the technique used to reinforce performance and documentation of Foley/perineal care, implement best practices for central venous line management, and point out steps in collecting respiratory, urine, blood, and wound cultures.

Methods

The infection prevention team met biweekly to discuss current HAI and NIM results and review audits of patients who were positive for NIMs. An urgent need to address the education deficit and rising NIMs rate was identified through gap analysis.

Content was drafted to address respiratory, blood, wound, and urine nosocomial infection markers by the manager of infection control. The team reviewed the information biweekly to ensure correctness and alignment with the most current evidence. Once finalized, the team thought it important that distribution of the content not be presented in a computer-based learning module or in an on-site classroom. Prompted by the director of nursing services, the CNL was charged to devise a way that would engage staff as well as educate them on the content.

An impact story to detail the "why" behind the urgent need to prevent NIMs was developed by a charge nurse and fellow team member and presented during the educational roadshow followed by a storyboard that detailed the education content. An infection prevention tip sheet that was developed by the CNL was also distributed to each unit for display.

The educational roadshow was performed for one full week on both day and night shifts by the CNL and MICU nurse manager. There was much participation from staff, and many felt that it was a great way to get the information out. Followup was performed on the units one month after the initial education through NIMs Prevention Jeopardy where more tip sheets along with prizes were distributed.

Results

Prior to conducting the educational roadshow, the hospital NIMs rate was at its highest of 4.81. One month following educational rounds, the NIMs rate decreased from 4.81 in May to 2.81 by the end of June, and further decrease was noted in July at 1.94!

Conclusions

Nursing is a lifelong learning profession; one that is trusted to stay abreast on the latest evidence and best practice for patient care. As CNLs continue to be deployed throughout various healthcare settings, it is vital to utilize their skill set to develop innovative ways to deliver that information.

EXEMPLAR

CNL's Role in Leading and Building a Team in Decreasing CAUTI in the ICU

Toy Bartley

A CNL became aware of the increased CAUTI infection in the ICU. The CNL realized that she might be able to make a difference in decreasing the infection if she took the time to "go and see." She set out a date and time to make observations and photographed inappropriate practices of multidisciplinary caregivers that contributed to the infection, being mindful not to include patients in the photograph. The CNL compiled the photographs and created a poster of most common practices that contribute to CAUTI. The CNL analyzed the pictures taken and realized that all members of the caregiving team played a part in the cause of CAUTI; therefore, each member of the caregiver's team plays a role in decreasing CAUTI.

The CNL started fostering awareness among the interprofessional team consisting of physicians, nurses, patient care technicians, charge nurses, managers, transporters, environmental service staff, and respiratory therapists on the most common mistakes and practices that put patients at risk for CAUTI. A series of posters called "ICU CAUTI CAUTION," "No ladder in the bladder," and "It's good to have a flushing system" were posted by the huddle board, staff locker rooms, and staff lounge. In-services on universal precautions were provided in daily huddles and through e-mails.

Once a week during a huddle, a representative from each member of the interdisciplinary team reported back on observations of current practices in decreasing CAUTI. Gaps and opportunities for improvements were discussed to bring awareness to the whole team. Staff nurses were checked for competency on catheter insertion and perennial care.

The charge nurse performed daily room checks to assess whether patients with urinary catheters had the proper indications for use. If indications were not appropriate, staff were asked to use alternatives such as external catheter for males, incontinent pads, use of a bladder scan, and voiding schedule or intermittent catheterization.

During multidisciplinary rounds, physicians determined the appropriateness of the urinary catheter. Nurses were expected to report on the urinary catheter status—its indication, plan on discontinuing, or renewal of the order.

As part of the antimicrobial stewardship, physician residents were provided a "log book" to keep track of the patient antibiotic use. Elements tracked were specific to their patient's indication for antibiotics, number of days patients have been on antibiotics, and the treatment to escalate, de-escalate, or change course of antibiotic treatment based on microbiology results.

The nurse manager ordered extra supplies of urinary catheters and external catheter devices; nurses were able to take in an extra supply of urinary catheters during catheter insertion. If the first attempt to insert the catheter was not successful, the nurse had another one on hand. This prevented reinsertion of the previous catheter.

The CNL worked closely with the infection prevention team consisting of the medical director, epidemiologist, and microbiologist. The team reported to the CNL the incidences of CAUTI. The CNL investigated each incidence, prepared learning from a defects tool, and shared the information at huddles and via e-mails. Urgent huddles were performed when an incident of CAUTI was received.

Environmental service staff were educated and empowered to check on the placement of the urinary catheter (UC) in the bed. A corner spot in the bed became the designated area for hanging the UC bag.

Staff who made a big contribution were recognized for their efforts during the "Staff Appreciation Day." The unit experienced lower rates of CAUTI for 10 months, which paralleled lower usage of urinary catheters. The unit's 6 months of decreased use of urinary catheters were less than the national benchmark.

Many CAUTIs can be prevented by following the recommended and evidence-based prevention strategies. However, buy-in from all the stakeholders cannot be underestimated; each member of the multidisciplinary team has a role to play. Through consistent daily collaboration at the point of care with different members of the team on early urinary catheter removal, CAUTI was significantly decreased. In the comprehensive data for 2012 and 2013, CAUTI rates decreased in conjunction with decreased urinary catheter utilization rates.

The CNL initiated the creation of a nurse-driven protocol for urinary catheter discontinuation in collaboration with the infection prevention team, urology team, and nursing staff. The protocol is currently approved by the physician and nursing committees. This protocol will be implemented throughout all system hospitals.

EXEMPLAR

Embracing Innovation and Interprofessional Collaboration

Alex Nava

A CNL led a team on two acute care units partnered with the hospital's retail pharmacy in order to fill patients' prescriptions before discharge. The partnership became known as the pharmacy concierge service. The objective of the service was to decrease the risk of readmission among patients by ensuring they left the hospital with their medications and a pharmacist to speak to them to reinforce the rationale and side effects of the new prescriptions.

The CNL understood the importance of continual process improvement and the use of innovation to resolve issues. Complaints from patients and the staff were collected about the slow response of the pharmacy filling discharge prescriptions. A pareto chart indicated that waiting for filled prescriptions became a leading cause for the delay in discharges. The process was analyzed, and it was noted that the pharmacist relied on the staff nurse or CNL to inform them about discharge orders; hence, a delay occurred if the nursing staff did not communicate with the pharmacy.

The hospital utilized wireless communication devices to interact with interprofessional staff. The CNL and partner met with IT to discuss how we could use these devices to inform the pharmacy when the physician reconciled their patients' discharge medications. It was suggested that the communication device send a text message to users when a physician electronically ordered a discharge. IT stated they could implement this solution. The CNL then asked the pharmacy staff, charge nurse, and CNLs to receive these notifications. The text message notifications allowed the pharmacy staff to fill prescriptions in a timelier manner.

The pharmacy concierge service reduced the number of 30-day readmissions especially among our high-risk category patients and revealed an increase in patient experience. The hospital also recognized a new revenue source with filling additional prescriptions. Physicians were happy that their patients were leaving with their medications. An interventional cardiologist remarked that he was glad that his patients used the service because he was able to confirm they received their antiplatelet medication. The success of this service was disseminated through our hospital's evidence-based practice poster fair where it won first prize. The CNLs were instrumental with implementing this service.

This is another example of how CNLs use evidence to design and direct system improvements that address trends in safety and quality; implement quality improvement strategies based on current evidence, analytics, and risk anticipation; assume a leadership role of an interprofessional healthcare team with a focus on the delivery of patient-centered care and the evaluation of quality and cost-effectiveness across the healthcare continuum; and implement the use of technologies to coordinate and laterally integrate patient care within, across care settings, and among healthcare providers.

Improving Pain Scores in an Inpatient SCT Unit

Catherine Delanoix

Pain control is imperative in the provision of optimal patient care outcomes. In a 48-bed adult SCT unit in a comprehensive cancer hospital, the HCAHPS scores in the domain of pain well controlled were consistently below the 50th percentile rank when compared to other academic medical centers.

In February 2015, a CNL-led interprofessional work group was formed to analyze the primary source of pain on the inpatient STU unit and to implement a plan to improve HCAHPS scores in the domain of pain well controlled. Members of this work group included representatives from the departments of nursing, pharmacy, and pain services.

Acute oral mucositis occurs in nearly all patients undergoing an SCT. Despite routine use of cryotherapy as well as strict oral care regimens, acute mucositis pain was identified as the primary cause of uncontrolled pain in this patient population.

The CNL analyzed current practice and identified the following as limitations to adequate pain control:

- Delayed escalation of the pain control plan
- Poor communication between RN and physician when personal pain goal is not met
- Delay in writing/signing PCA orders
- Delay in initiation of PCA

The aim of this collaborative project was to improve the HCAHPS pain scores through the development of an algorithm designed to improve communication and to provide a standard for the appropriate escalation of the pain management regimen. The algorithm was meant to prompt nurses to notify physicians when specific qualifiers were met. The qualifiers included, but were not limited to, the number of "as needed" medications given during a defined period of time and the ratio of demand versus delivered patient-controlled analgesia (PCA) doses.

The CNL presented the completed pain algorithm to the SCT faculty in June 2015, and it was implemented on one 12-bed pod. Nursing feedback indicated a significant improvement in nursing autonomy and communication. This warranted unit-wide dissemination, which completed in September 2015. RNs received both written and verbal education provided by the CNL.

Analysis of HCAHPS scores indicates a significant increase in the domain of pain well controlled during the development phase and after implementation. To analyze the impact of the pain algorithm on nursing practice, an anonymous survey was sent to the staff. Using a four-point Likert scale, RNs were asked how they felt use of the algorithm affected pain management as well as their own practice and role in the pain management plan. Of the respondents, more than 78% believed the algorithm improved communication and understanding as well as improved the speed of PCA initiation, more than 70% of RNs believed the algorithm improved their pain assessment process, and finally, more than 60% of respondents indicated that use of the algorithm positively impacted their own professional practice and involvement in the pain management plan.

Increasing awareness of the barriers to pain management will significantly improve patient understanding, consequently improving overall pain scores. Further benefits include improved communication among the medical and nursing teams as well as with the patient/family and improved overall understanding of the efforts to control pain in the SCT population. The algorithm increased awareness of the role of nurses in providing optimal pain management and has empowered them to act as advocates for a better pain plan.

EXEMPLAR

The Impact of Collaboration Between Inpatient and Outpatient CNLs Navigating the Continuum of Care in Obstetrics

Leah Carnick Ledford and Sara Pratt

Care of the pregnant patient, if associated with chronic disease such as diabetes, hypertension, or obesity, involves several layers of care and many different facets of nursing, creating a strong need for synergy of all involved. CMC is a quaternary hospital that is part of the Carolinas HealthCare System located in Charlotte, North Carolina. In 2014, CMC delivered 6,649 babies, 2,869 (43%) of which were high risk. This number includes patients who are transferred from other facilities and/or are seeing multiple providers. To address this high-risk issue, CNLs took on the challenge of operating collaboratively within an inpatient and outpatient continuum of care with the intention of decreasing gaps in care, coordinating plans of care, and providing holistic education to complex, high-risk obstetric patients. The main goal of this initiative was to improve high-risk maternity care and provide evidence highlighting how CNLs working with obstetric patients could effect change across the continuum of care. Although similar research is currently being conducted with other patient populations as seen in the ample evidence related to the impact of healthcare navigators, CNLs at CMC are taking an innovative approach to clinical navigation by pairing an inpatient CNL and an outpatient CNL.

The high-risk obstetric (HROB) CNL collaboration began in 2014 when the observed to expected length of stay (LOS) for the women's division was identified as exceeding the target. The two CNLs working within the women's division at that time saw this as an opportunity to show the potential of the CNL role to impact quality of care and reduction in healthcare costs. The HROB CNLs created a plan focusing one CNL in the outpatient arena and one CNL within the inpatient arena in order to cover the entire continuum of care. Their goals were to help coordinate care, synchronize the interprofessional team, and identify potential barriers in the transition of care while decreasing length of stay and readmissions. These CNLs initially targeted high-risk diabetic and hypertensive obstetric patients for their focus because these patient types contributed significantly to the high readmission rates and extended LOS patients totals within the HROB population. The CNLs created clinical pathways for the patients and standardized a care-delivery process. The process includes the coordination of outpatient visits and home healthcare as needed, in-person patient education, daily collaboration with physicians, highly organized follow-up support for six weeks' postpartum, holistic care planning, resource obtainment, routine patient progress calls, and the encouragement of prenatal class and tour participation. This process centered on the objective of creating trusting relationships with patients and their families to improve outcomes. The CNLs review charts and/or interview all readmitted patients to identify opportunities for process improvement.

As of August 31, 2015, the HROB CNLs had cared for more than 53 patients since the initiation of this process in October 2014, and the number continues to increase. As of this date, 65% of the postpartum patients cared for by these CNLs have not had a readmission. The CNLs have noted an increase in one-week postpartum blood pressure checks as a direct result of their coordination of care and patient education. A larger percentage of the patients receive pregnancy care management referrals and TDAP vaccinations and are breastfeeding their babies. Although current work is being focused on teasing out the length of stay of patients seen by the CNLs, an improvement of patient outcomes and quality care is apparent with every exemplar they share with teammates. One example centers on a pregnant patient admitted with a diagnosis of uncontrolled type I diabetes mellitus and osteogenesis imperfecta. During a previous pregnancy, while not under the care of the HROB CNLs, the patient experienced nine readmissions during her pregnancy for uncontrolled blood glucose issues, recurrent UTIs, and hydronephrosis requiring two nephrostomy tubes. The patient's baby had to remain in the neonatal intensive care unit (NICU) for two weeks after delivery for continued medical care needs. When the HROB CNLS encountered this patient she was on her third pregnancy. The CNLs quickly enrolled her into their continuum of care process and followed their clinical pathway performing all of the aforementioned duties. As a direct reflection of the impact of CNL collaboration, the patient carried her baby for the full term and delivered via C-section, due to risks related to a vaginal birth. The patient was only admitted four times during this pregnancy, once for blood glucose control issues, once for shortness of breath, and once for pyelonephritis. The patient's baby was discharged with the mother, and an extended NICU stay was avoided.

In a second example, one of the HROB CNLs potentially prevented an HROB patient from harming herself and her baby. The CNL received a call from a patient informing the CNL that she had been feeling overwhelmed to the point that she sometimes felt like giving up. The patient reported no current thoughts of harming herself or others but was scared that she would soon get to that point if she did not get immediate help. The CNL further screened the patient and notified the HROB physician. The physician advised the CNL to have the patient call the behavioral health (BH) hotline to get immediate help. The CNL called the patient back and gave her the advice of the physician as well as the phone number to BH. The CNL asked the patient to call her back immediately after speaking with BH to provide an update. The patient soon called back and informed the CNL that someone from BH wanted to speak with her. The CNL called BH to find out that a referral from the doctor's office was needed in this patient's case instead of a self-referral. The CNL then called the HROB physician back and received the order for the referral. She sent this order to BH, and the patient was given an appointment the next day. The CNL notified the physician assistant who would be seeing the patient for her upcoming postpartum visit. She then comforted the patient and arranged to accompany the patient to her next postpartum visit. This is a prime example of the impact a CNL can have on a patient and family. Although the patient had family support in her home environment, the relationship she had built with the CNL was exactly what was necessary to protect her and her baby.

The HROB CNLs are currently working on an IRB-approved quasi-experimental study designed using a regression-discontinuity approach to quantify their impact on patient outcomes from 2014 to 2015. The study will compare pregnancy outcomes as well as results noted during the patient's six-week postpartum period.

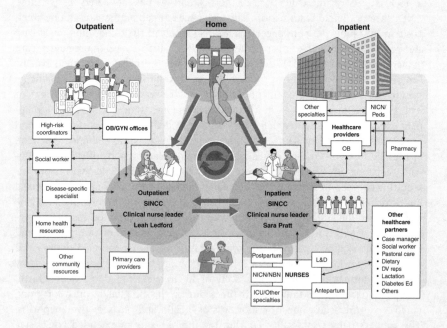

EXEMPLAR

The CNL's Role: Working Intra-collaboratively to Implement Safe Use of Bed Alarms to Reduce Falls in an Inpatient, Correctional Healthcare Setting

Kenia Latin and Jennifer Acklen

The Joint Commission publishes National Patient Safety Goals in order to improve patient safety. One of the goals for 2016 includes the effective and safe use of alarms on medical equipment (The Joint Commission, 2016). This goal can be directly tied to fall prevention initiatives to decrease patient falls by optimizing the hospital environment (AHRQ, 2013). Falls are reported as the most common adverse event in the acute care setting and frequently prolong a patient's hospital stay (AHRQ, 2016).

At this inpatient, correctional healthcare facility, bed safety alarms are used when a high-risk fall patient is identified. This is done as part of the fall precautions protocol. For security purposes, the inpatient acute care rooms are closed at all times. This prevented the bed safety alarm from being heard outside the room in the enclosed nurse's station. The CNLs met with the leadership team administrators, physicians, nurses, and security to devise a plan to ensure that the bed safety alarm was audible in the nurse's station. As part of the implementation, the CNLs met with the Fall Prevention Committee and bed vendor where it was learned that a cable was available that will attach to the existing bed safety alarm and allow the alarm to be heard in the nurse's station. After review, the leadership approved purchase of the cables, which are now available in all inpatient nurses' stations of the correctional hospital for use when a high-risk fall patient is identified. The CNLs participated in a hospital-wide campaign along with the nurse educator and nurse managers to provide didactic and direct hands on education of the bed and the cables to all the staff involved in direct patient care.

Since the implementation of this practice, the nursing leadership team meets regularly and makes frequent rounds on the units to obtain feedback from the staff on the use of the bed safety alarm features with the new cables. Developing, implementing, evaluating, and sustaining a fall-prevention culture that involves effectively and safely using medical equipment and alarms is an initiative that can positively impact patient outcomes in the area of fall prevention in which the role of the CNL is crucial for continued process improvement.

References

Agency for Healthcare Research and Quality. (2013). *Preventing falls in hospitals: A toolkit for improving quality of care*. http://www.ahrq.gov/professionals/systems/hospital/fallpxtoolkit/index.html

Agency for Healthcare Research and Quality. (2016). *Measure summary: Acute care prevention of falls: Rate of inpatient falls with injury per 1,000 patient days*. http://www.qualitymeasures.ahrq.gov/content.aspx?id=36945&search=falls

The Joint Commission. (2016). *Hospital: 2016 National patient safety goals*. https://www.jointcommission.org/hap_2016_npsgs/

A CNL's Approach to Sterile Processing, Quality, and Patient Safety

Dawn Stokley, Amy McRae, Amanda Johnson, and Kylia Parker

Introduction

CNLs manage care within clinical microsystems to improve patient outcomes by evaluating processes, designing, and implementing quality improvement initiatives that improve patient outcomes and safety (AACN, 2013). Traditionally, the CNL focused on specific patient cohorts and disease processes primarily at the bedside. The changing healthcare landscape, reimbursement guidelines, and a shift from in-patient to outpatient care has presented new opportunities for CNLs beyond the traditional microsystem. Guided by competencies, theories, and various frameworks, CNLs are evaluating processes, designing, and implementing innovative quality and safety improvement initiatives in a variety of microsystems such as sterile processing departments (SPD). This exemplar provides an example of a CNL student and graduate who initiated a project within an SPD and utilized the defining aspects of practice to include: risk anticipation; use of evidence-based guidelines; participation in leveraging human, environmental, and material resources; clinical decision-making; education; and facilitation of interdisciplinary and interprofessional collaboration to ensure safe and efficient sterile process outcomes.

Background

Surgical site infections are a leading cause of hospital readmissions, contributing to $10 billion in additional healthcare costs annually (Ames & Beauclair, 2019). The Joint Commission in 2018 reported noncompliance in cleaning medical equipment and surgical instruments as a contributing factor to infection rates in healthcare organizations (HCOs). Effective processing of equipment and instruments requires SPD technicians to acquire and maintain specific competencies based on policies, procedures, guidelines, and national standards (ECRI Institute, 2012). To ensure compliance and a competent staff, stakeholders within an HCO requested that a CNL student develop and offer educational sessions for SPD technicians based on an assessment of the department, staff competencies, current practice outcomes, and national guidelines.

The Improvement Initiative and Methods

As described by Roussel (2017), a microsystem assessment through the lens of the 5 Ps of quality improvement (purpose, patients, professionals, process, and patterns) is essential for a successful outcome. Based on the assessment and discussions with HCO administration, the purpose of all SPDs is to ensure safe materials are provided for patients and staff. This is consistent with TJC Resource Standard HR.01.06.01 (2014).

SPD staff must be valued to meet a monumental charge and duty toward patient care and safety. Staff in SPDs are often unrecognized for the contributions toward patient safety and quality outcomes (Brooks et al., 2019). Little or no compensation is offered for certification and is linked to poor motivation, limited voice, and lack of interest to excel beyond required daily workflow processes. Inconsistent training and competency validation also contribute to failures in job performance that result in unsafe sterilization and patient harm (Condon, 2012).

Following the microsystem assessment and input from staff using a survey, the PDSA approach to quality improvement guided the project. The method provided avenues for implementation changes and SPD staff input essential to a successful outcome. Using certification guidelines and standards, an educational format was developed that focused on cross contamination, accurate record keeping, infection control processes, cleaning procedures, required equipment, accreditation standards, and proper loading of sterilization case carts. Educational offerings were completed on each topic based on staff availability.

Initial Outcomes

While the project was not fully completed due to the time frame and unforeseen circumstances, initial steps were taken to introduced topics that were germane to work processes, opportunities for seeking certification as an SPD technician, and opportunities for fostering value of a dedicated workforce. Ongoing education was developed for future use and the need to recognize and advocate for the advancement and recognition of SPD staff.

Beyond the project activities, the CNL student realized the value of how competencies, frameworks, and evidence guide quality and safety projects that can be sustained and change practice. Making a difference as a CNL is an imperative in today's healthcare environment. CNLs are functioning in a variety of microsystems and contributing to sustainable and value-driven outcomes.

References

American Association of Colleges of Nursing. (2013). *Competencies and curricular expectations for clinical nurse leader education and practice*. https://www.aacnnursing.org/Portals/42/News/White-Papers/CNL-Competencies-October-2013.pdf

Ames, H., & Beauclair, S. (2019). The impact of sterile processing functions on hospital reimbursement. *Healthcare Purchasing News, 43*(3), 40–43. https://search-ebscohost-com.libproxy.usouthal.edu/login.aspx?direct=true&db=ccm&AN=135052842&site=ehos t-live

Brooks, J. V., Williams, J. A. R., & Gorbenko, K. (2019). The work of sterile processing departments: An exploratory study using qualitative interviews and a quantitative process database. *American Journal of Infection Control, 47*(7), 816–821.

Condon, L. (2012). Safe sterile processing supports safe patient care. *Biomedical Instrumentation & Technology, 46*, 20–23. https://doi.org/10.2345/0899-8205-12.1.20

ECRI Institute (2012). *Sterile processing department's role in patient safety*. https://www.ecri.org/components/PSOCore/Pages/PSONav0812.aspx?tab=2

The Joint Commission (2014). *Comprehensive accreditation manual for hospitals: The official handbook*. Author.

Roussel, L. (2017). The nature of the evidence: Microsystems, macrosystems, and mesosystems. In H. Hall & L. Roussel (Eds.), *Evidence-based practice: An integrative approach to research, administration and practice* (2nd ed., pp. 191–212). Jones & Bartlett Learning.

Improving Glycemic Control

Ann Eubanks

Problem Statement

Surgical site infections, and particularly sternal and mediastinal infections, have implications for significantly increasing both morbidity and mortality, as well as their associated costs in both man hours and dollars spent. Postoperative hyperglycemia is associated with the development of surgical site infections among cardiac surgery patients. Adequate glycemic control has been shown to decrease the incidence of deep sternal wound infection. According to Furnary and colleagues (2003), continuous insulin infusion protocols should be the standard care for glycometabolic control in all patients undergoing cardiac surgical procedures. Furthermore, the CMS publicly reports on postoperative glycemic control as part of the Surgical Care Improvement Project (SCIP). The goal of this project is to increase the percentage of cardiac surgery patients to at least 90%, meeting SCIP criteria for adequate glycemic control, with serum glucose levels less than 200 mg/dL on the first and second postoperative days.

Multidisciplinary Team

A multidisciplinary team was formed to address the design and implementation of updated glycemic control strategies to conform to current evidence-based practices. The team consisted of the nurse manager, staff nurses, diabetic educators, a clinical pharmacist, information systems analysts, and a cardiovascular surgeon. These individuals were chosen based on expertise in their respective disciplines. A retroactive chart review was performed to obtain baseline data; it revealed that glucose targets were only met in 40% of heart surgery patients.

Project Processes and Evaluation Methods

A microsystem assessment was performed in the cardiac recovery unit to determine knowledge levels regarding glycemic control and current methods of glucose management. Brainstorming and cause and effect analysis methods were used to determine possible causes of poor glycemic control. A literature review of best practices for postoperative glycemic control was undertaken by the team, and numerous evidence-based protocols were evaluated. A mutually agreed on continuous insulin infusion (CII) protocol was identified. Information systems analysts converted the protocol into an electronic form, which enabled bedside nurses to accurately titrate insulin infusion rates. The CII protocol was presented to the medical executive committee for approval as standing orders. The PDSA cycle was used to conduct tests of change using the agreed on protocol. Bedside nurses received comprehensive education on glycemic control and utilization of the new protocol prior to implementation.

Outcomes

Upon implementation of the new CII protocol, close supervision and clinical support was provided for all shifts. Data was monitored daily to ensure safety and to quickly identify problems. After the first quarter using the CII protocol, adequate glycemic control was achieved in 93% of patients. Through ongoing surveillance, the CII protocol has shown periodic decreases in surgical site infections and measurable improvements.

Reference

Furnary, A. P., Gao, G., Grunkemeier, G. L., Ying Xing, W., Zerr, K. J., Bookin, S. O., & Starr, A. (2003). Continuous insulin infusion reduces mortality in patients with diabetes undergoing coronary artery bypass grafting. *Journal of Thoracic Cardiovascular Surgery, 125,* 1007–1021.

CHAPTER 8

Networking and Community Advocacy

Linda A. Roussel and Lonnie K. Williams

LEARNING OBJECTIVES

1. Explore networking as a means of advocacy and influence.
2. Describe the CNL's roles as patient advocate and community leader.
3. Consider how the CNL makes connections and develops therapeutic relationships.
4. Evaluate tools and models used in discharge planning and assurance of continuity of care.
5. Outline creative tools for team building and collaboration.
6. Identify community outreach and networking opportunities for the CNL in a variety of community and ambulatory care settings.

KEY TERMS

Advocacy
Ambulatory care
Collaboration
Community outreach
Discharge planning
Influence

Population health
Networking
Social determinants of health
Social justice
Team building

CNL ROLES

Client advocate
Collaborator
Educator
Information manager

Lateral integrator
Outcomes manager
Systems analyst and risk anticipator
Team manager

CNL PROFESSIONAL VALUES

Accountability
Human dignity

Social justice

CNL CORE COMPETENCIES

Assessment	Human care systems and policy
Communication	Information and healthcare
Complexity and community networking	technologies
Disease prevention	Nursing technology
Ethics design/management/	Resource management
coordination of care	Risk reduction
Health promotion	

Introduction

Networking increases the ability to influence and advocate others. *Business Dictionary* defines "networking" as "creating a group of acquaintances and associates and keeping it active through regular communication for mutual benefit. Networking is based on the question, How can I help? and not with What can I get? This definition resonates with the CNL's role in its many facets as outcomes manager, systems analyst, and risk anticipator. Through actions and advocacy, the CNL increases capacity for building community, improving continuity and coordination of care throughout the system's leadership. Networking involves good communication and relationship-building skills. *Entrepreneur* identifies five steps to improving networking skills including: *mindset, the destination, the map, building a human connection*, and "*superconnecting.*" *Mindset* is taking the "work" out of networking, enjoying opportunities to extend self, and care for the other person. Being authentic increases credibility and defines the relationship being built in the connection. *Destination* refers to setting goals for reaching out, and extending self. What is the aim? How will you know that you have reached the goal in your networking opportunity? Is it to establish others from different disciplines and professions who might contribute to viewing one's work from a different lens? Is it finding opportunities for one to serve the community? What does one want to accomplish? Answering these questions, and thinking through actions provides guidance to the next step. *Map* provides the guide to follow for achievement of the aim and goals. Being as specific as possible, yet leaving room for serendipitous opportunities will help to ground efforts to extend reach and influence. *Building a human connection* puts communication skills to the test. Simply put, it is about asking insightful questions, asking better question to get better answers, and paying attention. Actively listening to what is being said, and being observant to the how of the interaction and engaging others will increase the ability to make connections. Listening and paying attention may be difficult as we are bombarded with multiple messages, competing demands, and daily distractions. Focusing on who is in front of you, being present, intentionally, and deliberately responding back are useful ways to connect. This is a skill that can be learned, and with practice becomes easier. *Superconnecting* extends one's reach when connecting with two or more people. *Entrepreneur* describes powerful ways to superconnect and include strategies such as: not keeping score, connecting with other superconnectors, interviewing others, and following up. CNLs are exquisitely poised to build capacity through networking. Cattelan (2016), a career and life coach, describes similar strategies, adding keeping it simple, building rapport, giving of self, and readily reciprocating. Mulligan (2016) builds on networking as an approach to achieve greater outcomes and includes connecting on social media, being prepared, and doing the research, supporting team and colleagues, staying in touch, seeing opportunities, and saying yes. Revisiting an elevator pitch is always important in preparation to "be out there," and seizing opportunities. While these strategies and techniques are not new to CNLs, they are not always included in preparing the CNL for clinical leadership, change management, and driving innovation. One cannot assume that this will occur easily, and stretching yourself out of a comfort zone through networking is an important skill set to learn.

The CNL, as the designer, manager, and coordinator of care, provides and assembles comprehensive care for clients—individuals, families, groups, and communities—in multiple and varied settings. According to the AACN (2007), "The CNL guides the patient through the health system using skills essential to this role. Such skills include communication, collaboration, negotiation, delegation, coordination, and evaluation of interdisciplinary work, and the application, design, and evaluation of outcome-based practice models" (pp. 25–26).

Preparation of the CNL

Preparing the CNL for community resource management and networking includes course work in leadership, interdisciplinary team building, organizational skills, information management, delegation, and cost-benefit analysis. The CNL considers the environment's readiness for change and the processes that are important to that end. Understanding organization and community culture and how decisions are made in translating best practices, as well as identifying key stakeholders, gives the CNL skill sets to accomplish these goals. The CNL does not work alone. Creating a vision for the stakeholders with those at the point of care (patients, family, staff, multidisciplinary teams, and community members) helps to spread and sustain quality and safe care. Patients' involvement in their care, working to facilitate decision making and self-management, is strengthened when interdisciplinary teams and community networks are involved.

Community Networks and Ambulatory Care

CNLs are positioned to facilitate community networking, which extends the reach to improve population-based care and address social determinants of health in ambulatory care settings. Networking and collaboration are essential to connecting partners and building meaningful, productive relationships. Ambulatory care settings are witnessing an increase in the volume of patients as the healthcare system transitions from a model of inpatient healthcare to a patient-centered system of care acknowledging the dominant role of outpatient and community-based care (American Academy of Ambulatory Care Nursing [AAACN], 2017; Roski & Gregory, 2001; Start et al., 2018). The Josiah Macy Jr. Foundation (2016) convened a group of national experts to address the need to transform primary care. This call to action identified the need to change the culture of healthcare and transform the practice environment. Specifically, the national experts recommended the development of primary care expertise among nursing faculty and subsequent education of nursing students in the role of the nurse in primary care. Their recommendations went further to advocate for the provision of support for the career development and opportunities for interprofessional education of nurses with a bachelor's degree in nursing (BSN). Furthermore, a report following the conference underscored the value of registered nurses (RNs) in primary care and their skill set to enhance their role in chronic disease management, care coordination, and preventive care (Berkowitz, 2017; Josiah Macy Jr. Foundation 2016; Start et al., 2018; Wojnar & Whalen, 2017). The CNL working in partnership with RNs and the interprofessional team can further advance services in the community as lateral integrators. Evident in Competency 2, Organizational and Systems Leadership, the CNL assumes a leadership role in an interprofessional healthcare team with a focus on quality and cost-effective patient-centered care across the healthcare continuum. The CNL advances outpatient and community-based care using systems theory in the assessment, design, delivery, and evaluation of healthcare within complex organizations (AACN, 2013).

According to the Bureau of Labor Statistics (2018), approximately one-fifth of the nearly three million RN workforce in the United States is employed in ambulatory care settings including primary care and other practice areas including home care. Also noteworthy is an expected 15% growth in employment of RNs in primary care by 2026 (Bureau of Labor Statistics, 2018). Berwick and colleagues (2008) imply that a strong infrastructure in ambulatory care service delivery is critical to reaching the triple aim, and RNs are the ideal team members to expand the capacity in primary care. Through the leadership of the CNL, working side-by-side, we as a nation can help further realize this goal because the impact of primary care has not been maximized (Josiah Macy Jr. Foundation, 2016; Start et al., 2018). Partnering with CNLs, RNs can advance competencies in care coordination and patient-centered care, making them uniquely poised to bridge gaps in the healthcare system (AAACN, 2017; IOM, 2010). Being able to reach this critical goal requires access to data, evaluation, and assessment skills to improve performance, and the promotion of value-based care for moving nursing forward in a purposeful way that will promote the creation of best practice.

Leadership and Interdisciplinary Team Building

As a horizontal leader, the CNL is pivotal to the healthcare team, serving as a critical navigator through the microsystem. The CNL knows the roles of the various team members and the value added to the transition of the patient into the community. The CNL understands concepts of team building and the skills necessary to build quality teams. Such skills include visioning, group dynamics, accountability, and the basics of conducting a meeting. For example, conducting a meeting involves establishing an agenda, staying focused on items to be covered at the meeting, and establishing follow-up actions. Complexity science advances concepts for the larger view of social systems and community networking, important knowledge for the CNL to possess. Strength-based leadership and emotional intelligence are critical skills to networking and advocating. There are several leadership and EI assessment tools that are useful to obtain baseline information concerning strengths, talents, capabilities, and opportunities to develop and grow as a leader and innovator

(Bradberry & Graves, 2009; Rath & Conchie, 2009). These assessments provide baseline information for the CNL student to develop a professional action plan for ongoing growth and development (Batool, 2013). The CNL, as an emerging leader of interprofessional teams, provides essential relationship-building and collaboration skills.

Complexity and Community Networking

Complexity theory provides new insights into the behavior and emergent properties of social systems. Complexity theory purports that the experience of community is both an outcome and the context of informal networking. A well-connected community is achieved when people feel part of a web of diverse and interlocking relationships. The networks sustain and shape an integrated and dynamic social and organizational environment, and support the familiar patterns of interaction and collective organization that characterize the voluntary and community sectors. Community development involves creating and managing opportunities for connection and communication across social identity and geographical boundaries. Termed *meta-networking*, it is a core function of the professional role. The community can be envisioned as part of the microsystem when the population of patients at the microsystem level is cared for within this system. Failing to take into consideration where patients are going (and coming from) and the neighborhood and community support available creates a fissure in the system. This failure underscores the silos that healthcare continues to reinforce, which are often related to reimbursement methods. Connecting resources and people maximizes capacity, impact, and influence. Grassroots efforts are important to the network process and can include several strategies such as hosting meetings, putting up posters, supporting a valued cause by providing financial support, facilitating letter writing, phone calling, and e-mailing campaigns.

The professional values of the CNL support active involvement with the community. When assuming responsibility for the comprehensive care of individuals, families, and population groups, the CNL participates in the care of the communities where clients live, work, and participate in recreational activities. The CNL advocates for the worth and value of all persons and individualizes a plan for continuity of care that reflects a commitment to the principle of social justice. Social justice is linked to the CNL's responsibility for fair, equitable care. Competency in providing healthcare to diverse populations and working with diversity are also integrated into social justice.

Tools and Models for the CNL's Role in Networking and Advocacy

Networking as previously described adds to the "tool kit" that the CNL continues to grow and expand their influence and reach, particularly across the continuum of care. Merriam-Webster defines *advocacy* as the act or process of supporting a cause or proposal. It is the act of advocating for others where we can achieve positive outcomes. Similar to networking, developing advocacy skills is also important to every aspect of the CNL's work. Learning how to advocate requires practice and builds on communication and relationship skills. As an advocate, it is important for the CNL to "know thyself," identify a style of leading, and manage change. Knowing one's strengths and talents can enhance advocacy capabilities. Just as with networking strategies, practice improves performance. Strategies the CNL can utilize to increase the ability to advocate include: presenting the issues in a way others can see them, being persistent, knowing facts and being able to present them in a credible and confident way, planning for small wins, being able to negotiate by looking for the good in others, staying the course, making issues local and relevant, getting broad-based support from the start, and working within the experience of your team. While there may be "lone" opportunities to advocate, there is strength in numbers; knowing the team members' strengths will be essential in aligning successful advocacy efforts (Community Tool Box, https://ctb.ku.edu/en).

Advocacy and networking can take many directions and represent a variety of strategies to that end. For example, applying advocacy and networking skills to the patient discharge process and care transitions can enhance the overall patient experience across the care continuum. Engaging the patient and caregiver in shared decision-making requires attention to expert communication, relationship-building skills, and interprofessional teamwork. Jurns (2019) identified that there are significant relationships and positive correlations between advocacy frequency and three variables: participant perceptions of speaking skills when communicating with a policy maker, understanding the organizational daily advocacy activities, and understanding policy creation.

The CNL uses networking, collaboration skills, and advocacy in various care coordination activities including discharge planning, care transitions, and interprofessional teamwork. The following sections provide specific skills and competencies that CNLs use when advocating for patients and providers.

Discharge Planning

Discharge planning is a process that has long been recognized as essential in the delivery of quality healthcare. The process advanced in healthcare management with the passage of legislation that mandated it as an essential service. Today, discharge planning is a critical process that requires interprofessional teamwork. The identification of cost-effective healthcare resources, as well as evaluation of these resources, is essential to the implementation of the CNL's role.

The key features of the discharge planning process are as follows:

- Planned and coordinated events in any patient care setting
- Contribution to the continuity of patient care services
- Promotion of health maintenance and safety of patients as they access and consume healthcare services
- Contribution to the cost-effectiveness of healthcare services
- An interprofessional process

Discharge planning begins during the first encounter with the patient. The individual patient assessment tools include information about the patient's diagnosis as well as living arrangements, family, and significant others. Each microsystem has standard tools for patient assessments. Information obtained in the patient's initial assessment directs the CNL to tools that will assist with the identification of discharge needs and community needs.

Transition Care Model

Transitions in care is defined by The Joint Commission (2014) as "the movement of patients between health care practitioners, settings, and home as their condition and care needs change" (p. 3). There are a number of evidence-based transitions of care models including Care Transitions Intervention (CTI), Transitional Care Model (TCM), Better Outcomes for Older Adults through Safe Transitions (BOOST), the Bridge Model, Guided Care, Geriatric Resources for Assessment and Care of Elders (GRACE), and Project Re-Engineered Discharge (RED; Bridge Model, 2012; Coleman, 2006; Counsell et al., 2006; Johns Hopkins Bloomberg School of Public Health, 2012; Naylor & Sochalski 2010; Society of Hospital Medicine, 2010). For example, the Care Transitions Program developed by Coleman (2007) refines the process of coordinated care and discharge planning by identifying specific goals for the process of moving patients between healthcare providers and healthcare settings. According to Coleman et al. (2006), the goals of transition care are to support patients and families, increase skills among healthcare providers, enhance the ability of health information technology to promote health information exchange across care settings, implement system level interventions to improve quality and safety, develop performance measures and public reporting mechanisms, and influence health policy at the national level. Coleman's model has great utility for any setting with providers prepared at varying levels.

Networking and Interprofessional Team Building

The CNL identifies the stakeholders in the clinical microsystem who contribute to the process. These individuals form the interprofessional team that becomes the patient and the community's source for direct care, primary prevention, and continued care and rehabilitation. The interprofessional team today reflects the expertise of providers from many disciplines: medicine, allied health, nursing, social services, clinical laboratory providers, and long-term care providers. In addition to these professionals, the family members and lay providers must be identified. The individuals provide essential support and validation for the patient. Networking skills can enhance team-building skills when working with interprofessionals. Understanding community health from a health promotion and illness prevention perspective provides foundational knowledge of epidemiological principles including the epidemiological triad and the natural history of disease model.

The Epidemiological Triad

Disease in humans is typically explained in terms of the epidemiological triad, which is a tool that is central to community diagnosis. The epidemiological triad describes the complex interaction of the human host with a disease-causing agent and the environment in which the interaction occurs. Host characteristics can be such factors as age, sex, race, religion, customs, occupation, previous disease, and immune status. Types of disease-causing agents may include biological, bacterial, viral, chemical, and nutritional. Temperature, humidity, altitude, crowding, food, water, air pollution, and noise are identified environmental factors that can cause an increased risk of human disease. It is the interaction of these factors (host, agent, and environment) that contributes to disease. Analysis of the host characteristics, possible agents, and environmental factors enable the CNL to identify risks that can contribute to the onset of disease and disability, which has implications for population health and social determinants of health. According to Gordis (2009), disease can be caused by biological, physical, and chemical factors. Psychosocial factors also contribute to disease occurrence but may not fit into the usual categorization of factors.

The Natural History of Disease Model

The natural history of disease model is a classic tool developed by Leavell and Clark (1965). The model describes the progression of disease, which has implications for population health. The CDC describes population health as an interdisciplinary, tailored approach that facilitates health departments' connection to practice and policy for change to happen at the local level. This approach uses nontraditional partnerships among different sectors of the community including public health, industry, academia, healthcare, and local government entities to achieve positive health outcomes. Specifically, population health is meant to assure that significant health concerns are brought into focus and addressed in ways that resources can be made available to overcome barriers that drive poor health outcomes in the population (CDC, n.d.).

There are two disease periods in the natural history of disease model: the pre-pathogenesis period and the pathogenesis period. The prepathogenesis period begins with the interaction of the host, agent, and environmental factors. As disease develops in a person, the model includes the phases of pathogenesis that the person experiences. The levels of prevention are correlated to the periods of prepathogenesis and pathogenesis (primary, secondary, and tertiary). Primary prevention focuses on the prepathogenesis period, whereas secondary and tertiary prevention focus on the pathogenesis period. Primary prevention considers health promotion and may include such interventions as health education; provision of adequate housing, recreation, and working conditions; and periodic selective examinations. Primary prevention can be related to specific protection against occupational hazards, accidents, and carcinogens; use of specific nutrients; and avoidance of allergens. Secondary prevention related to early diagnosis, prompt treatment, and disability limitation includes such interventions as case-finding measures, screening surveys, and adequate treatment to arrest the disease process and prevent further complications and contraindications. Tertiary prevention is included in the period of pathogenesis. Rehabilitation is central to tertiary prevention. Provision of hospital and community facilities for retraining and education for maximum use of remaining capacities describe important interventions in rehabilitation (tertiary prevention). Additional rehabilitation interventions may include education of the public and industry to employ the rehabilitated, selective work placement, and work therapy in hospitals. This model offers a blueprint for health promotion as well as disease management in individuals and at the community level. For example, the CNL who documents an increase in young males who are injured in motorcycle accidents will investigate primary prevention strategies for preventing accidents at the community level. A community diagnosis emerges when the absence of a needed service or the presence of an agent that contributes to disease is identified at the community level. Moving from basic epidemiological principles to reflective practices provides an integrated approach to community assessment. Tools such as mind maps and storytelling can enhance networking and advocacy capacity and the CNL's ability to influence and impact outcomes.

Mind Maps

Mind maps provide an excellent tool for leading teams through innovation. According to Buzan (2004), mind maps give depth and breadth of scope that a list of ideas cannot. (See **Figure 8-1** for an example of a mind map.) "By working from the center outwards, mind map encourages your thoughts to behave in the same way" (p. 8). The framework provides an illustrative view of ideas and their expansion and alternatives, radiating creative thinking. By using letters and numbers, colors and images, mind maps engage the left and the right sides of the brain. Starting from the center, working outwardly with ideas, symbols, colors, numbers, and other symbols, mind maps engage thinking power that increases synergistically. "Each side of the brain simultaneously feeds off and strengthens the other in a manner which provides limitless creative potential" (p. 9). Mind maps are useful for short- and long-term planning. Working with teams can be more efficient when employing mind maps. They can help a team focus on the way ahead and bring together a shared, creative, and imaginative vision. Techniques include incorporating equal time to listen and speak; showing interest in people and ideas; and having a clear idea of where the CNL, the team, and the organization are all headed.

For example, using mind maps, the CNL can focus the team on the core of their innovation; then, using brainstorming sessions, the team can work out specific strategies and ideas. Mind maps can be revisited as ideas are advanced or carried out, with new options surfacing with the changes. The mind map can serve as an agenda, a business plan, and the basis for developing project plans. Considering this nonlinear (complexity) way of thinking, mind maps offer a natural way to innovate.

Buzan also offers the trial, event, feedback, check, adjust, and success (TEFCAS) model as a successful mechanism for working with mind maps. Each aspect of TEFCAS identifies tools, a checklist, and strategies for applying a different way of thinking. TEFCAS helps to monitor and react to the outcome of project plans, focusing on goals and outcomes. This model reinforces project planning, adding new insights to ongoing processes.

The Use of Story: Messages to Innovate Team Collaboration

Loehr (2007) described the power of story as a means of changing one's destiny in business and in life. Narrative accounts or storytelling bring the voice and dynamic messaging often lost in quantitative data reporting. Hard data, graphs, and figures do provide critical information, however, may get lost in the overall purpose and mission of our innovations. Stories bring life to numbers, and can add a deeper level of understanding as a way of connecting all of our senses. Paying attention to what stories are messaging can enhance collaboration and sustained positive outcomes.

Bringing about ways to understand the CNL's story and that of an organization are critical to understanding the mission and goals to be accomplished. Knowing the CNL's own story (about success, challenges, and use of opportunities and challenges) is a good place to begin. Reflecting on values and beliefs, the "private

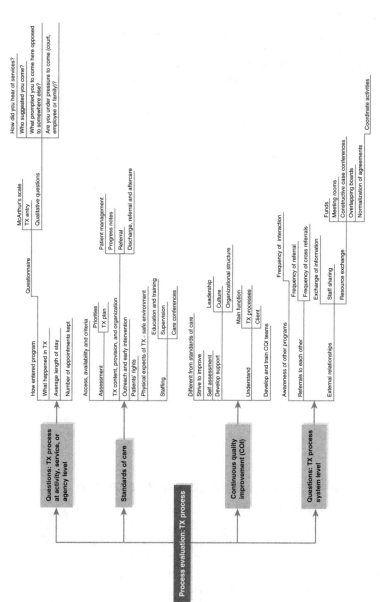

Figure 8-1 Process evaluation TX mind map

Note: Treatment (TX)

Permissioned by Margaret Moore-Nadler, DNP, RN, University of South Alabama, College of Nursing, 2020.

voice" in the CNL's head is part of self-awareness and self-reflection, qualities that are necessary for helping others to understand their stories and to mutually create one story for the team. Loehr identifies three rules of storytelling: purpose, truth, and action. *Purpose* considers the motives and overall intention of the story. What is the team striving for? What principle? What end? What goal? What does the team want to see at the end of the day or the year? Is the story taking the team where it wants to go? What is nonnegotiable? These are questions that can guide clarity of purpose (Loehr, 2007, p. 138). A shared vision through story can engage the head and heart.

Truth relates to the authenticity of the story. Being truthful gives credibility to leading innovation in patient-care delivery. *Action* relates to the purpose and the truthfulness of the story being told. "Does the story move others to action?" Knowing how explicit actions (plan) will be played out for desired outcomes can provide a dynamic template for the team. This action plan involves the stakeholders, their engagement in the process and outcomes, and how the story plays out.

Stories engage the heart and the mind. The CNL can use a story to bring alive what may seem like static processes, policies, and procedures that may be considered mechanistic and carried out in robotic fashion.

Prepared with knowledge and skills in discharge planning, community outreach, and creative collaboration, the CNL furthers the business case for safe, quality continuity of care. Effective discharge planning through a greater understanding of community outreach, networking, and tools such as mind maps and stories can improve financial, quality, safety, and satisfaction outcomes as teams come together.

Community Assessment

The CNL will demonstrate leadership, as well as creativity, in the provision of continuity of care. No skill better displays leadership qualities and the development of strategies for improving care for individuals, families, and communities than that of community assessment. Community assessment requires interprofessional communication and collaboration, along with the ability to prioritize. Community assessments identify resources and gaps in services in the community. Anderson and McFarlane (2000) identified eight elements of a comprehensive community assessment:

1. Physical environment
2. Recreation
3. Education
4. Economics
5. Communication
6. Health and social services
7. Politics and government
8. Safety and transportation

Box 8-1 provides an example of a community outreach assignment. Any service or resource considered for a patient needs to be evaluated. The questions in **Box 8-2** can serve as a guide to evaluating community resources. A case study in leadership and advocacy is also provided at the end of the chapter.

Box 8-1 Community Outreach Assignment

This assignment gives you the opportunity to evaluate community services, referrals, and other community resources that your patients/consumers access in your clinical microsystem. Consider patient discharge planning and how patients on your unit (in your microsystem) use community services (your major referral support services). In the same vein, where are patients being admitted from (in your community)? What patterns do you see regarding admissions and discharges? In other words, are patients coming from the same communities and settings (home, nursing homes, senior centers, etc.)? Are patients being discharged back to their same settings?

What have you learned from this assignment?

_____

_____

_____

Describe your microsystem's discharge plan considering referral and support sources. Do you observe any patterns? If so, what are the patterns?

_____

_____

_____

Outline primary sources and follow-up plans. Do you have contact with your patients after discharge? If so, describe the continuity of care and how this impacts the quality and safe delivery of services and patient satisfaction.

_____

_____

_____

Outline recommendations to improve community outreach and ongoing continuity of patient care in your microsystem. Yes or no?

_____

_____

_____

Assignment is in APA style, has a scholarly presentation, and uses reference citations liberally. Yes or no? _____

_____

_____

Box 8-2 Evaluating Community Resources

Is the agency an official or governmental agency?
Is the agency a private or voluntary agency?
What is the level of prevention addressed by the services of the agency?
What are the eligibility requirements for the services?
What are the costs of services, and what payment sources are accepted?
How are referrals made?
How are families and significant others included in the services provided?
What is the preparation and expertise of the service provider?

Summary

- Networking and advocacy skills enhance the community's health through strategies to increase communication, relationship building, and leadership.
- As reimbursement tightens and there are greater demands for efficient, effective care, discharge planning and community networking become more critical.
- The CNL—in the role of outcomes manager, client advocate, and team manager—provides an understanding of quality improvement data, using evidence-based practice methods to promote a smooth transition of care from setting to setting.
- As an educator, information manager, systems analyst, and risk anticipator, the CNL uses tools for discharge planning and community diagnosing, including the epidemiological triad and the natural history of disease model.
- Additional strategies include mind maps and story, which contribute to engaging staff and communicating and collaborating with teams.
- CNL core competencies—such as communication, assessment, nursing technology and resource management, health promotion, and risk reduction—are essential to the CNL's success in community outreach and participating in patient-centered care.
- Core competencies also include integrating disease prevention, information and healthcare technologies, ethics, and human care systems.

Reflection Questions

1. As a CNL, how do you determine the best strategies for networking with community partners?
2. As a CNL, what are some ways to best advocate for patients and community?
3. What are the best communication strategies for beginning a dialogue with community leaders and stakeholders?

Learning Activities

As a CNL on a fast-paced surgical orthopedic unit, suppose you have noted that after most of your patients are discharged into their community, they return just weeks later. You note that many of the patients require after-hospital care, including home health services, support groups, long-term care, and assisted-living services. Other services, such as Meals on Wheels, medication assistance programs, and assistance with durable medical equipment, are also important to your patients' discharge planning. You begin to see a pattern of inadequate resources within your community. You have also noted that your hospital has programs that may be useful to the community.

1. As an outcomes manager, what specific outcomes would be appropriate for you to address these issues?
2. What are the advocacy issues? As a client advocate, what are your responsibilities? How are these evaluated?
3. As an educator and information manager, how would you determine educational needs and how would you manage this information?

4. As a systems analyst/risk anticipator, how would complexity theory guide you in managing community resources?
5. Who would need to be at the "table" as you serve as a team manager?

References

American Academy of Ambulatory Care Nursing. (2017). American Academy of Ambulatory Care Nursing position paper: The role of the registered nurse in ambulatory care. *Nursing Economic$, 35*(1), 39–47.

American Association of Colleges of Nursing. (2007). *White paper on the education and role of the Clinical Nurse Leader (pp. 6–10). Author.* https://nursing.uiowa.edu/sites/default/files/documents/academic-programs/graduate/msn-cnl/CNL_White_Paper.pdf

Anderson, E. T., & McFarlane, J. M. (2000). *Community as partner: Theory and practice in nursing* (3rd ed.). Lippincott.

Batool, B. F. (2013). Emotional intelligence and effective leadership. *Journal of Business Studies Quarterly, 4*(2). http://jbsq.org/wp-content/uploads/2013/03/March_2013_8.pdf

Berkowitz, B. (2017). Registered nurses in primary care: A value proposition. *Nursing Outlook, 64,* 525–526.

Berwick, D. M., Nolan, T. W., & Whittington, J. (2008). The triple aim: Care, health, and cost. *Health Affairs, 27*(3), 759–769.

Bradberry, T., & Graves, J. (2009). *Emotional intelligence 2.0.* TalentSmart.

Bridge Model. (2012). *Illinois Transitional Care Consortium.* http://www.transitionalcare.org/the-bridge-model

Bureau of Labor Statistics. (2018). *Monthly labor review.* https://www.bls.gov/opub/mlr/2018/

Business Dictionary. (n.d.). *Networking.* http://www.businessdictionary.com/definition/networking.html#ixzz47XacOFj5

Buzan, T. (2004). *Mind maps at work: How to be the best at your job and still have time to play.* Penguin Group.

Cattelan, L. (2016). *Ten essential networking strategies.* http://www.humanresources.com/617/10-essential-networking-strategies/

Centers for Disease Control. (n.d.). *What is population health?* https://www.cdc.gov/pophealthtraining/whatis.html

Coleman, E. A. (2007). *Care transitions intervention.* http://www.caretransitions.org/definitions.asp

Coleman, E. A., Parry, C., Chalmers, S., & Min, S. J. (2006). The care transitions intervention: Results of a randomized controlled trial. *Archives of Internal Medicine, 166*(17), 1822–1828.

Community Tool Box. (2016). *Survival skills for advocates.* Chapter 30. http://ctb.ku.edu/en/table-of-contents/advocacy/advocacy-principles/survival-skills/main

Counsell, S. R., Callahan, C. M., Buttar, A. B., Clark, D. O., & Frank, D. I. (2006). Geriatric Resources for Assessment and Care of Elders (GRACE): A new model of primary care for low-income seniors. *Journal of the American Geriatrics Society, 54*(7), 1136–1141.

Entrepreneur. (May 14, 2015). 5 steps to seriously improve your networking skills. https://www.entrepreneur.com/article/245995

Gordis, L. (2009). *Epidemiology* (4th ed.). W. B. Saunders.

Johns Hopkins Bloomberg School of Public Health. (2012). *Guided care.* http://www.guidedcare.org (Accessed on May 2, 2016)

The Joint Commission. (2014). *Hot topics in health care: Transitions of care: The need for a more effective approach to continuing patient care.* http://www.jointcommission.org/assets /1/18/hot_topics_transitions_of_care.pdf

Josiah Macy Jr. Foundation. (2016). *Registered nurses: Partners in transforming primary care. Recommendations from the Macy Foundation Conference on preparing registered nurses for enhanced roles in primary care.* http://macyfoundation.org/docs/macy_pubs/2016_Conference_ Summary _FINAL.pdf

Jurns, C. (2019). Policy advocacy motivators and barriers: Research results and applications. *OJIN: The Online Journal of Issues in Nursing, 24*(3). https://doi.org/10.3912/OJIN.Vol24No03PPT63

Leavell, H. F., & Clark, E. G. (1965). *Preventive medicine for the doctor in his community: An epidemiologic approach.* McGraw-Hill.

Loehr, J. (2007). *The power of story.* Simon and Schuster.

Merriam-Webster. (n.d.). *Advocacy.* http://www.learnersdictionary.com/definition/advocacy

Mulligan, C. (2016). *Networking—10 tips to improve your networking skills.* http://claremulliganconsulting
.ie/networking-10-tips-to-improve-your-networking-skills/#sthash.4mupHX5P.dpuf

Naylor, M. D., & Sochalski, J. A. (2010). Scaling up: Bringing the transitional care model into the mainstream. *The Commonwealth Fund, 1453*(103), 1–12.

Rath, T., & Conchie, B. (2009). *Strengths-based leadership.* Gallup Press.

Roski, J., & Gregory, R. (2001). Performance measurement for ambulatory care: Moving towards a new agenda. *International Journal for Quality in Health Care, 13*(6), 447–453.

Society of Hospital Medicine. (2010). *Project BOOST—Better Outcomes for Older Adults through Safe Transitions. Implementation guide to improve care transitions.* http://tools.hospitalmedicine.org
/Implementation/Workbook_for_Improvement.pdf

Start, R., Matlock, A. M., Brown, D., Aronow, H., & Soban, L. (2018). Realizing momentum and synergy: Benchmarking meaningful ambulatory care nurse-sensitive indicators. *Nursing Economics, 36*(5), 246–251.

Wojnar D. M., & Whalen E. M. (2017). Preparing nursing students for enhanced roles in primary care: The current state of prelicensure and RN-to-BSN education. *Nursing Outlook, 65*, 222–232. https://doi.org/10.1016/j.outlook.2016.10.006

Tools of the Trade: Case Studies

Case Study 1: Individual Level

A 21-year-old pregnant woman who has a history of intravenous drug abuse is admitted through the emergency department. As the CNL on the labor and delivery unit, you admit the patient and begin the initial assessment and discharge planning. Consider the following questions as the discharge planning begins.

Who does the patient consider her family?

Where does the patient currently live, and where will she go when she leaves the hospital?

What personal, environmental, and safety concerns will the patient have when she leaves the hospital?

What health and medical follow-up care (including pre-/postnatal care) will be needed?

After considering these questions, use the natural history of disease model to identify primary, tertiary, and prevention interventions that might help the patient.

Case Study 2: Community Level

Examine the histories and assessment data of the patients on your unit or in your microsystem. Focus on the patients' demographic profiles. Do the patients come from one community or neighborhood? Are the patients referred by primary providers or by another agency, such as a nursing home or home care agency, or are they admitted through the emergency department? Are patients being discharged back to the same setting, or are they referred to another level of care?

Describe your microsystem's discharge process, and consider the referral and support resources used. Do you observe any patterns? If so, what are they?

Describe your microsystem's follow-up plan for patients. If the follow-up plan includes contact with the patients after discharge, describe that process.

How does your microsystem evaluate the discharge process and its effect on the patient and community? Is there a method for documenting outcomes?

Case Study 3: Leadership and Advocacy in the Community

Assessment of patient data, as well as the discharge planning process in your microsystem, reveals the following information.

A significant number of patients with type II diabetes have been admitted over the last year. The patients reside in the zip code where a new retirement community that provides housing for low-income persons over age 65 has just been established. The patients have different primary care providers. The neighborhood is on the public bus route that transports residents to a chain grocery and shopping center.

Who are the stakeholders in this neighborhood?
How would you go about initiating a diabetic management clinic for the retirement community?
What are the resources that will assist with the patients' care, and what is the first step you would take with each client?

EXEMPLAR

Community-Based Wound Care Integration

Ann Nguyen

Problem Statement

The current communication tools, patient education, and wound care network have not worked effectively within a healthcare system in San Francisco, California. Sending copies of current medication lists from skilled nursing facilities (SNFs) to wound care centers (WCCs) and faxing wound care orders from WCCs to SNFs do not provide nurses with adequate information about patients' conditions and comorbidities related to wound etiologies and treatment modalities. In addition, the lack of a networking system between the inpatient wound care team and the outpatient WCC delays the follow-up. Therefore, the number of wound care readmissions is high and the time of healing is prolonged.

Team Development

This project was developed by using Kotter's theory and Six Sigma methodology to achieve the positive goal of achieving effective and efficient wound-healing outcomes. This project had three parts:

1. Creating the status/condition/any laboratory result/new wound (SCAN) communication tool: collaboration between the wound care nurse and community-based setting nurse. The SCAN tool is included at the end of this exemplar.
2. Patient teaching handouts: patient centeredness.
3. Inpatient/outpatient wound care network: lateral integration.

Implementation

Providing the tools, continuing education, and presentation of materials to the WCC staff, five SNFs, five home health aides (HHAs), and case managers.

Working with community-setting partners for individual patients and every wound care visit through the SCAN communication book.

Collaborating with case managers and attending physicians on discharge plans for wound care patients.

Financial Impact and Outcomes

The SCAN communication tool saved $280,560 in four months for all WCCs, SNFs, and home health agencies and positively impacted patient/customer satisfaction.

The patient teaching handout saved $635 and $130 in four months for the WCC by reducing the length of treatment.

Wound care network implementation saved $56,700 in four months by reducing the readmission rate.

Wound Care "SCAN" Communication

PATIENT NAME: **DATE:**

PREVISIT NURSE: **PHONE:**

STATUS	Last FSBS/ Treatment		Last Dressing Change	On Coumadin	Others
				❑ YES ❑ NO *Dose:*	
CONDITION	**Fever (T°)**		**Loose Bowel Movement**		**Others**
	❑ YES	❑ NO	❑ YES *Treatment:*	❑ NO	
ANY LAB WORK	**Current Lab Result (Date)**			**Wound Culture**	**Others**
	CBC	Hemoglobin/ Hematocrit	Hb A1C	❑ YES	❑ NO
NEW WOUND	**Location**		**Date Identified**	**Current Treatment**	

POSTVISIT	NURSE/DATE:		PHONE:	
STATUS	Please refer to Nursing Assessment Sheets			
CONDITION	Stable		Others	
	❏ YES	❏ NO		
ANY LAB WORK	New Lab Order	Culture Result		Others
		❏ YES	❏ N/A	
NEW WOUND	Location	Diagnosis		Treatment
				Please refer to the Physician Order and Home Care Instruction

EXEMPLAR

Transferring Patient Care—Continuity between Organizations: The Psychiatric Patient Care Experience

Laurie A. Schwartz and Susan E. Koons

Pine Rest Christian Mental Health Services (PRCMHS) is a 150-bed freestanding psychiatric hospital located 10 miles from Saint Mary's Health Care (SMHC), a Trinity Health Organization. Psychiatric patients requiring medical assessment, treatment, or emergency services are frequently transferred to SMHC when medical situations arise. Following the ED evaluation, the patients are returned to PRCMHS or admitted to SMHC. The transfer process lacked standardization, causing communication gaps and prolonged patient ED stays, and was reflected in patient outcomes, unmet expectations, and increased staff dissatisfaction for both organizations. In response, the CNLs, at the direction of risk management and senior leadership at their respective facilities, partnered to lead a process improvement project.

Utilizing a Lean process improvement methodology, the CNLs directed a 15-member team of various disciplines from the two organizations through the project. Through deliberate collaboration, the team identified barriers, obstacles, and process gaps and developed and initiated a detailed action plan to improve the patient transfer experience to the ED.

Process flow improvements and tools were identified and developed at each organization. An improved patient transfer process flow, including collaborative design of a prearrival form (PAF) tool with telephone communication scripting and a patient transfer packet and checklist, improved the handoffs between the organizations. Internal process improvements at PRCMHS included an ambulance call system, psychiatric sitter guidelines, and an after-hour call tool for the psychiatric nurse communicating with the on-call medical team. At SMHC, whiteboards and hourly rounding with the psychiatric sitter have improved the communication flow and resulting communication to PRCMHS.

Initial outcome data, including staff surveys, indicate 100% completion and resulting satisfaction with the PAF, which alerts the ED to the incoming psychiatric patient. The after-hour general information to medical (GIM) tool, designed in an SBAR format, is a guideline to equip nurses in providing accurate, pertinent information to after-hour on-call medical providers. With the use of the GIM tool, during a three-month monitoring period, the average number of after-hour calls decreased by 55%. GIM tool usage increased from 5% to 90%. The average number of inappropriate, nonurgent, after-hour calls decreased by 50%. Patient length of stay in the ED and subsequent sitter time decreased by one hour for this patient population. Overall staff satisfaction improved by a rate of 50%, which was the stated outcome goal.

This collaborative effort was led by CNLs who have expertise in risk assessment and microsystem analyses in psychiatric and emergency nursing care. Implementation of this process improvement has generated additional system-wide awareness, produced an impetus for ongoing change processes, and generated transfer process revisions for programs and transfers to other facilities. Ultimately, it has improved relationships between two organizations, created an understanding of shared experiences, and improved the transfer process of a complex patient.

EXEMPLAR

Enhancing Palliative and End-of-Life Care

Vidette Todaro-Franceschi

The End-of-Life Nursing Education Consortium (ELNEC) core training is incorporated into our CNL graduate program, which consists of eight modules (introduction, pain management, symptom management, ethical and legal aspects, cultural aspects, communication, grief/loss, and final hours). One of the clinical objectives and concurrent written assignments for the students is to complete an assessment of end-of-life/palliative care practices in their microcosm and then create an action plan to address any deficiencies that they have identified.

The CNL program is in its infancy, with only 16 students thus far completing the assignment. However, the potential for change in this important area is notably tangible. Feedback from students who received ELNEC training has been positive, with the majority believing that end-of-life care pedagogy is a necessary component of CNL role development. Not only did the students realize that their own knowledge base and comfort level regarding dying and death had improved with ELNEC training, but many were then able to foster an increased awareness in staff as well.

One student who worked in an ICU, upon having an open discussion with staff and identifying that many had difficulty facing death, offered educational sessions to assist them in becoming more comfortable communicating with patients who are dying and their loved ones. Another, noting that there were frequent anticipated deaths on his unit, had a private room dedicated for patients in transition so that there would be a quiet space for staff and loved ones to be with the patient. Yet another student spoke with her practice council in the ED about end-of-life care, and they then recognized a need to address staff and patient concerns related to unanticipated deaths. The outcome was the creation of a bereavement packet for the loved ones of patients who die suddenly.

The student clinical logs also indicated a change in awareness as the students shared instances where they intervened on behalf of patients who were nearing the end of life. For example, one noted that she had spoken with a family at length about end-of-life care choices for their 94-year-old loved one who had been in and out of the ICU four times. After discussing concerns, the family decided that their loved one did not need to be in an ICU, and the patient was transitioned to comfort care. The student noted, "I would not have been able to have this discussion with the family had we not had classes on end-of-life care."

EXEMPLAR

Do We Always...?

Patricia Egan and Denise Bourassa

This project used methods designed to address health literacy and incorporate components of the teach-back method for patient education into a tool for nurses. With a focus on nursing indicators, the Do we always...? campaign was developed to elicit conversation between patients and staff regarding care delivery. Specifically designed for a 20-bed orthopedic unit, this campaign and teaching tool was developed for nurses to use with patients to achieve a better understanding of their medications.

A 5 Ps analysis was completed, which revealed several areas for improvement as well as an engaged and committed staff focused on excellence in practice and achieving good patient outcomes. A collaborative decision was made to focus the project on an initiative to enhance nurse communication with patients regarding medications and medication side effects. Recommendations from the IOM indicate that the use of common, everyday language to communicate with patients enhances patient understanding of their healthcare regimen. Requiring staff to use basic vernacular and the teach-back method are shown to be successful in achieving these goals.

A consistent, uniform, and standardized approach served to create staff fluency with the information and improved compliance with the guidelines. Another priority for this project was to create a tool that would be easy and efficient for the nursing staff to use—to have something handy at the bedside. This would eliminate the nurse having to make the extra effort to obtain and print out teaching information for the patient.

Inclusion of frontline staff was a priority in the development of this project. As this project involved a practice change for nurses, it was important to identify a few staff members to serve as the early adopters to the process and function as the change agents for their peers. Frontline staff working as change agents lends a measurement of credibility to a new initiative. This project could not have gotten off the ground and would not have been successful without the involvement of staff nurses. With the support of unit leadership, RNs were identified as champions and introduced to the Do we always…? concept to their colleagues. These champions provided information about their typical practice concerning medication teaching and were available for consultation and discussion during the development of the particulars of the teaching packets. These champions also supported the education effort and rollout of the project to their colleagues.

Patients and staff were surveyed prior to the initiative's rollout to set a baseline for what the nurses believed they were teaching their patients and what the patients understood. The disparities in the results were an eye-opener for the staff and reinforced the focus of the project.

The slogan for the project was Do we always . . .? This was designed with the idea that it would prompt conversation with patients, staff, and visitors. Lapel buttons and flyers were created with the message. Informational sessions were held for staff to introduce the project, explain the relevance to the surveys and patient outcomes and explain the health literacy concepts and to solicit feedback from the larger unit population on the content of the folders. One-to-one conversations with staff also contributed to the overall acceptance of the initiative. The expectations for rollout were explained, including that every staff member would wear the button, every patient would receive a folder, and that every nurse would use the medication fact sheet to communicate with patients each time they administered a medication.

The expectation was that the slogan Do we always…? would elicit questions from the patients and visitors of, "Do you always what?" The staff was instructed to answer, "Do we always talk to you about your medications in a way you understand?" "Do we always explain about medication side effects?"

An unanticipated and very positive outcome was the engagement of the nursing assistants. During the information sessions for staff, the CNAs were very vocal about what role they could play in this initiative. As all staff are required to wear the button, not just the RNs, the CNAs wanted to know how they should answer patients' questions, "Do you always what?" Upon discussion with several CNAs, it was realized that the concept of *always* is not limited to medications. The goal of this hospital is to always provide excellent care and the nursing assistants play a big role in this. They were encouraged to answer patients' questions by saying things like: "Do we always answer your call light in a timely manner?" "Do we always respect your privacy?" "Do we always explain things in a way you can understand and answer your questions?" It was heartening to know that the nursing assistants were engaged in this effort and wanted very much to be a part of it. High-quality care encompasses the entire patient experience, not just medications.

Another unanticipated result is the reception this project has had around the hospital. Staff from other areas and disciplines were curious about the buttons and asked to have them distributed in their areas. At the invitation of the vice president of patient care services, the project was presented at a meeting attended by the nurse managers, the corporate compliance officer, the director of patient experience, and a member of the board of directors. The project was received very well as a potential tool to be used to improve patient outcomes and, subsequently, patient satisfaction scores house-wide.

Four weeks after the initial rollout, the patients were surveyed again about their understanding of medications. The results indicated an improvement overall in nurse communication with patients about medications. The staff and unit leaders were made aware of these results and congratulated on their successes. Surveys of the nurses indicated they were focusing more on side effects while teaching about medications and report satisfaction with the ease of use of the teaching materials in the folders. A few nurses also reported that with the implementation of this project, they have a better understanding of how what they teach to their patients about medications has a significant impact on outcomes, which not only affects the patient but the hospital as well (with regards to the survey results and reimbursements).

A role of the CNL is to focus on patient outcomes and facilitate the incorporation of best practice into the daily workings of the nursing staff. Leaders should be supporting nurses in the care they deliver and ensure they have the right tools to succeed. Keeping all the initiatives focused on patient outcomes is what makes the most sense. It is imperative that leaders focus not only on the scores per se but on what the scores reflect—which is the overall patient experience. Interactions with nurses are the basis for the overall perception the patient has about their hospital experience.

One of the fundamental aspects of the CNL's role is advocacy for patients, communities, and the health professional team. This project embraces this essential aspect. Advocating for improved patient understanding of their medications to improve outcomes and reduce readmissions, the unanticipated outcome of engagement of CNA staff and others in the hospital to utilize the Do we always…? concept as a way of improving the overall patient experience and the creation of an easy to use teaching tool for nurses all demonstrate how the CNL can impact care delivery and improve patient outcomes.

EXEMPLAR

The CNL as a Patient and Family Advocate

John Sims

A. S. was a 91-year-old patient admitted with pneumonia. The patient did not respond well to treatment as evidenced by her declining labs and worsening mental status. The physician spoke with A. S.'s family and chose for the patient to be full code. Clinically, it was evident she would likely not survive this illness, and, therefore, it was prudent to readdress the patient's code status. The CNL student was able to speak personally and candidly with the patient's son regarding the patient's outcome. The CNL student explained the patient's diagnosis, prescribed treatments, and the potential consequences of continued treatments. The pneumonia was not clearing, kidney function was getting worse, and A. S. was becoming more lethargic. It appeared A. S. would succumb to this illness very soon. The CNL student answered the son's questions and provided emotional support. The son admitted he had not comprehended the gravity of A. S.'s condition, even after several discussions with physicians. The son expressed relief and thanked the CNL student for his candor. A. S. was made do not resuscitate (DNR) and transitioned to inpatient hospice a short time later. She died peacefully two days later.

Had the CNL student not intervened, A. S. would have coded, been intubated, and potentially had a poor prognosis. The time spent by the CNL student with this patient and her son proved to be the best possible outcome for A. S. as well as for the family. A thorough review of the plan of care, in a way the patient and family could understand, allows for end-of-life decision making on the patient's own terms.

The preceeding case example further illustrates the role of a student using the CNL competencies to enhance care and decisions. Specifically, the following competencies, while not all inclusive, are relevant: (1) demonstrate effective communication, collaboration, and interpersonal relationships with members of the care-delivery team across the continuum of care; (2) promote a culture of continuous quality improvement within a system; (3) ensure the inclusion of an ethical decision-making framework for quality improvement; and (4) advocate for patients within a healthcare delivery system to effect quality, safe, and value-based outcomes.

EXEMPLAR

CNL as Advocate in End-of-Life Care Delivery

Gladis Mundakal

Ms. B was a 55-year-old Caucasian female who went to a freestanding ED due to failed treatment for a urinary tract infection and back pain. The patient did not have health insurance but was established with a family physician for her healthcare needs on a self-pay basis. The patient did not have a known medical history, and she was not prescribed any medication before the recent back pain. This patient was employed as a hairdresser. She was single and had no children. Her mother was her next of kin and provided family support.

Within a few days of diagnostic testing, Ms. B was diagnosed with stage IV cancer. Her bilirubin continued to rise, thoracentesis was performed, and she was receiving Clinimix for nutrition. She was able to eat, but nutritional status was poor. The hospitalist consulted a gastroenterologist and an oncologist. She was not a candidate for chemotherapy and the oncologist recommended hospice. She was in complete denial, and she lost trust in the oncologist with that conversation. The patient transferred to the medical surgical unit without any further plans for discharge.

The CNL student visited the patient the next day after transfer to the medical surgical unit. Before much introduction of the CNL's role, she asked the CNL student, "I need to get out of bed. Can you help me?" The CNL student was knowledgeable of her situation and desires, but she did not know where to start the conversation. So, she took this as an excellent opportunity to talk with the patient about her diagnosis and plan of care. After she assisted Ms. B to the chair comfortably, she asked Ms. B to share what she knows about her health condition. The CNL was able to confirm that the patient had a clear understanding of her diagnosis. She said, "I need to get well, I need to get chemotherapy, and I am rescheduling my customers to next week." Now, the CNL student was in a shock, "How do I bring her into the reality?" The CNL student continued to visit with her every day and talked to her mother about the health status. The mother said, "I can't give up my daughter yet, help us to get some treatment." The mother had a recent loss of her partner due to cancer and was experienced with hospice care. The mother was financially able and was willing to help her daughter.

The patient requested to the hospitalist for the second opinion for cancer treatment. The care team attempted to transfer the patient to another hospital, but due to the patient's request and that she was not a candidate for chemotherapy per oncology, the transfer did not occur. Ms. B was adamant about getting the second opinion. In the discharge planning rounds with the team, the hospitalist said that if the CNL can find an oncologist for a second opinion as an outpatient, then a discharge will occur when the patient was medically stable. Meantime, the patient was titrated off Clinimix, and pain was controlled.

The CNL partnered with the hospital and coordinated an outpatient oncology appointment upon discharge and the social worker that was planning for discharge and home care. Home care was arranged and unfortunately a second opinion never occurred due to a cancellation by the oncologist prior to her death five days post-discharge.

This case illustration underscores the value of the CNL as an advocate who demonstrates interpersonal competency, collaboration, and active listening. CNLs use a variety of skills and techniques to ensure care is safe, address patients' desires, and provide and explain care transitions.

CHAPTER 9

Preparing Preceptors for CNL Immersions

Rebekah Barber, Kristen Noles, and Keaton Lloyd

LEARNING OBJECTIVES

1. Define preceptor and preceptee roles and identify core competencies for each.
2. Define the CNL's immersion in a clinical setting and requirements for a successful immersion experience.
3. Define and discuss the significance of a learning environment for a CNL's clinical experiences.
4. Identify steps in developing meaningful and sustainable clinical immersion projects.
5. Provide examples of clinical immersion projects and discuss the impact on the healthcare system.
6. Discuss the significance of academic-clinical partnerships.

KEY TERMS

Academic-clinical partnerships
Apprentice
Clinical immersion
Learning environments
Lifelong learning

Mentor
Preceptee
Preceptor
Professional development
Sustainable value

CNL ROLES

Educator
Lifelong learner

Member of a profession

CNL PROFESSIONAL VALUES

Advocacy   Human dignity
Altruism   Integrity

CNL CORE COMPETENCIES

Advocacy   Critical thinking
Communication   Outcomes management

Preceptor and Preceptee Roles and Core Competencies for Each

The clinical immersion experience consists of two central participants, the preceptor and the preceptee. In this relationship, the key participants incorporate the inter-professional team as essential key stakeholders in the work of the CNL's overall clinical experience. The preceptor must be knowledgeable of the CNL competencies to ensure that experiences are offered to meet each of them during the immersion experience. The preceptor will listen, direct, teach, and mentor the student, aligning competencies with clinical experiences and seeking what is most important to the preceptee during the clinical immersion. It is imperative to understand the precep-tee's passion as it relates to understanding certain systems in the healthcare setting and matching that passion with meaningful experiences.

The preceptee and preceptor must each enter the relationship with openness and commitment to creating a psychologically safe environment where both parties can communicate candidly, express ideas freely, ask questions, seek understanding, and plan objectives to ensure a positive experience. This optimizes the successful transformation of the student into a practicing CNL. The relationship between the two is crucial for success. Once a commitment is reached to precept a CNL student, it is important to meet prior to the clinical immersion experience and at regular intervals defined and agreed on by the preceptor and the preceptee. Open commu-nication is essential with the preceptor and preceptee relationship, as well as the relationship between the dyad with the instructor. This is often accomplished by telephone, in person, or through virtual classroom arrangements. The frequency of meetings should also be discussed with the academic course coordinator to ensure that they are in compliance with the requirements for the designated program.

The Preceptor

The preceptor provides individual attention to the novice student's learning needs by providing ongoing guidance and feedback regarding performance, making deci-sions, setting priorities, managing time, and offering insight into meaningful clinical experiences. A preceptor is a teacher, coach, tutor, instructor, professor, and other terms that identify "to instruct," and functions as an advocate for the advancement of the CNL's role in clinical practice. The preceptor functions as a change agent in environments, highlighting the CNL's skill set regardless of title and providing time to share with the preceptee clinical experiences that match the CNL's competencies.

The preceptor functions as the ambassador for the CNL in clinical practice to the preceptee and is the foundation for the clinical immersion experience.

The preceptor for the CNL student should be a CNL themselves, whenever possible (AACN, 2013). *Competencies and Curricular Expectations for Clinical Nurse Leader Education and Practice* (AACN, 2013) states, "An extended clinical experience, prior to graduation, mentored by an experienced Clinical Nurse Leader, is critical to the effective implementation of the role." The reality of obtaining an experienced CNL and pairing one with every student enrolled in a CNL program can be difficult due to nursing shortages and the lack of adoption of the CNL's role into clinical practice (Lillibridge, 2007). The newness of the role in healthcare and variations of the role in practice continues to create ambiguity; therefore, the partnership with a CNL and student is vital to establish the new role (Bender, 2016).

If a certified CNL is not available, using them as a consultant, even if they are not physically present, is advisable. If a CNL is not an option, faculty must take the time to familiarize the preceptor with the role of the CNL and expectations for the clinical experiences to optimize the immersion for the student. It is not unacceptable to assume that any preceptor who is not a CNL understands the role, nor do they understand the need of clinical experiences that support the success of the preceptee. If there are no available preceptors at the clinical site, faculty may also consider a team of preceptors to best facilitate the immersion experience. The nurse manager, assistant nurse manager, or coordinator may be the preceptor, with other department contacts (education, infection control, risk management, quality, and safety) available to widen the student's experiences (Moore et al., 2014). In settings such as freestanding skilled nursing and rehabilitation facilities, home care agencies, ambulatory settings and hospice programs, the director of clinical services may be the best main preceptor, with other interdisciplinary team members augmenting the overall clinical immersion experience. The student's instructor can guide the student to fulfill gaps to ensure that the student has an optimal immersion experience.

Identifying qualified individuals to function as mentors for CNL preceptees can be challenging for schools of nursing. One strategy used to maintain certified CNLs precepting students in the CNL program is to create and maintain a database of existing CNLs, graduates of the CNL program, and contacts at organizations in the area who have existing CNL roles. Another tactic is to develop a relationship with a former student who has excelled in the healthcare system to help match students with optimal preceptors. This individual can also assist with assigning immersion experiences that are aligned with strategic initiatives that have high visibility within the organization. If successful, this will provide visibility leading to additional advocacy for advancement of the role of the CNL in practice.

Preceptors who are actively involved in interprofessional teams and practice are desirable if the preceptee is to understand, engage in, and maximize the full learning experience (AACN, 2013). A preceptor should possess the same core competencies of the CNL, including advocate, member of a profession, team manager, information manager, lifelong learner, systems analyst, risk anticipator, clinician, outcomes manager, and educator (AACN, 2013). In the most beneficial preceptorship experiences, the preceptor acts as a role model, facilitates learning, supports socialization in the role, and encourages progressive independence (Payne et al., 2014).

The school of nursing must recognize and acknowledge the crucial role that dedicated preceptors assume to ensure the success of the CNL student, and must pursue individuals possessing such professional values as altruism, integrity, and respect. The initial meeting with the school faculty and the preceptor is important to ensure that the preceptor is an acceptable candidate to precept the student during the clinical immersion. This meeting is like an informal interview, but also is a touch point to establish expectations, share the need to achieve experiences related to all CNL competencies, and establish an open communication plan between the preceptor and the faculty member. At the conclusion of the initial meeting, it is vital that there is an understanding of the CNL's role, a commitment to the student's success, and openness to share experiences throughout the course(s). The support and backing that the preceptor offers to the preceptee, along with modeling successful interprofessional team relationships, is imperative for the student to reach full potential and thrive (Goode, 2012).

The Preceptee

The CNL preceptee is a student, but should also be recognized as a CNL emerging into clinical practice. The preceptee learns and develops under the direction and guidance of the preceptor, in much the same way an apprentice integrates knowledge learned from classroom instruction through on-the-job training. In the clinical immersion experience, the preceptee has the responsibility of assuming accountability for the learning process. Most schools of nursing, colleges, and universities have defined universal core competencies for students such as oral and written skills, information technology, and professional values. Core competencies that the CNL preceptee should possess, like that of the CNL preceptor, are an advocate and a member of a profession, dedicated to lifelong learning, and exhibiting a commitment to professional development. Acquiring and cultivating these key proficiencies determine the level of success during the clinical immersion experience. One of the best ways for the student to gain these behaviors is by observing and modeling the preceptor, highlighting the importance of the preceptor while being cognizant of individual behaviors and how they are exhibited to and perceived by the student (Akiyode, 2016).

The preceptee should have an honest perception of their personality and character, including strengths, weaknesses, beliefs, motivations, emotions, and biases prior to entering the immersion experience. It is important for them to perform a self-assessment prior to the clinical immersion to gain self-awareness and understand how they respond to others. The knowledge obtained by knowing oneself will assist the preceptee in navigating interactions with members of other professions as they work in collaboration with multiple disciplines to drive change.

There are additional behaviors the CNL preceptee can exhibit that will foster positive clinical immersion experiences, such as arriving prepared for clinical days, dressing professionally, communicating openly with the preceptor, asking questions, proactively seeking meaningful experiences, maintaining a positive attitude in all interactions, and marketing themself and the CNL's role. The preceptee should involve the preceptor in the didactic course of study and homework assignments so that they can follow along with the preceptee. They should also actively engage with and participate in the microsystem's interprofessional team structure by becoming a recognized team member, and not being an outsider merely doing a task to get a degree.

The preceptee must also remember to exercise patience and recognize that the preceptor will have additional job responsibilities that must be juggled throughout the CNL immersion. The preceptee should communicate openly with the preceptor about what is working well and what areas may need further attention. Important communication between the preceptor and preceptee for positive immersion experiences include establishing dedicated one-on-one time, establishing a mutual understanding of what both desire from the experience, and how and when those desires can be best supported. These one-on-one engagements are important to provide opportunities to reflect on clinical experiences, review lessons learned, provide support and guidance, and discuss alignment of the CNL competencies with what has been encountered. This prioritizes the student's time and allows for ongoing communication throughout the immersion experience.

The CNL Clinical Immersion and Requirements for a Successful Immersion Experience

The culminating educational experience for the preceptee is the CNL clinical immersion. This is a 300- to 400-hour concentrated practicum where the preceptee enters the healthcare environment and begins incorporating the knowledge and skill sets gained throughout the educational process, including previous didactic and clinical proficiencies. The CNL is accountable for patient-care outcomes through the translation of evidence-based information to design, implement, and evaluate patient care processes and models of care delivery, all fundamental aspects of CNL practice immersion. During the immersion, weekly opportunities to discuss experiences, ask questions, and reflect on events with other CNL students, faculty, or mentors should be made available (AACN, 2013). These can be in person or through virtual meetings.

Successful immersion begins long before the CNL preceptee enters the healthcare environment. It is imperative that a relationship is established between academic and clinical partners. This relationship establishes a foundation for an enriching clinical immersion through educating, having dialogue, interviewing, recruiting, and developing nurturing relationships. This is especially important to explain the history, framework, and competencies of the CNL's role for mutual understanding. Non-CNL preceptors should not be chosen regularly, but be the exception in areas where CNLs currently do not exist. In those circumstances, closer monitoring of both the preceptor and preceptee is essential. Candidates for preceptors should be made aware of and understand the level of commitment and guidance required before agreeing to function in this role. Schools of nursing should also assess and thoughtfully consider if potential preceptors are a good fit for meeting institutional goals. Once preceptors have accepted the responsibility and school of nursing faculty have deemed these preceptors a good fit, careful pairing of student to preceptor should occur. In these situations, it is essential that the academic partner educate, oversee, and support both the preceptor and the preceptee in preparation and throughout the clinical immersion experience.

Successful partnerships usually have common threads, such as clearly defined goals and purposes, awareness and understanding of each other's roles and responsibilities, and planned deliberate reviews of performance through ongoing observation, communication, and evaluation (Hunter & Perkins, 2012). Considering personality traits, strengths and weaknesses, and teaching and learning styles of both individuals also contributes to effective relationships. If personality conflicts exist, no matter how wonderful the individual preceptor or preceptee seems, extra challenges will resonate throughout the immersion, negatively impacting the student's experience.

Prior to the clinical immersion beginning and throughout the duration, regular and periodic meetings should be held between the schools of nursing, preceptors, and preceptees. These meetings are indispensable to ensure that a clear understanding of the CNL role is maintained, the core competencies are being achieved, and the student is progressing. There should never be any surprises. When possible, on-site visits should occur. If on-site visits are not practical for CNL programs that provide online distance learning, conference calls should be scheduled. This time should be used to evaluate progress toward and attainment of both short- and long-term goals, discuss and remove barriers, celebrate successes, and chart direction. The projected course curriculum, in-class assignments, and clinical opportunities should also be reviewed.

Successful immersions require the assistance and support of senior nursing leadership. A qualitative study of CNLs struggling to thrive in practice found a lack of organizational understanding of CNL competencies and how each is used to produce CNL workflow (Bender, 2016). Nurse administrators who reinforce and support the CNL's role and objectives increase the sustainability of the role (Moore & Leahy, 2012). Nurse managers also have a role in determining whether clinical immersion experiences are supported, as frontline leadership is pivotal to driving change at the microsystem level (Kujala et al., 2019). Because the focus of the CNL is the microsystem, the unit manager of the immersion microsystem must have an understanding of the CNL's competency objectives and project goals. Unit managers who are confident and secure in roles are more likely to welcome and support improvement projects and embrace change processes than unit managers who are insecure and more comfortable with the status quo.

The culture of the healthcare environment is vitally important, and should be assessed prior to assigning a student to a microsystem. If the environment is not conducive for an optimal clinical immersion experience, faculty should be proactive in finding a more conducive experience. Faculty should also take time to meet with microsystem leadership where the immersion is to occur to ensure there is understanding of the CNL's role and continue to affirm support throughout the student's immersion. Meeting with the unit leadership prior to confirming commitment to the microsystem allows faculty to evaluate possible challenges and decrease negativity toward the student that might impede a successful project plan implementation. If warranted, the faculty should be prepared to intervene and facilitate.

Clinical environments in which staff understand the skill set of the CNL in practice should be given priority for the student placement for the clinical immersion experience. Requisites for ensuring successful immersions between schools of nursing and healthcare settings include education about the role, thoughtful planning and pairing of the preceptor and preceptee, and support of the CNL's role by nurse administrators and nurse managers. Senior leaders can strategically partner CNL students with certified CNL preceptors to focus on key areas in need of improvement. When support, oversight, and commitment to the student are given, the immersion has the potential to have an outcome that is meaningful to others in the organization, thus resulting in potential replication and sustainability of the intervention. If formalized more frequently, senior nurse leaders can optimize the impact of the immersion experience for value-based gains.

The following example offers how aligning an organizational need with a student's improvement project resulted in ED throughput. The purpose of the project was to examine how having an area designated on treating mid-acuity patients could decrease the average length-of-stay (LOS) time and the left-without-being-seen (LWBS) rate in the ED. Emergency Screening Index (ESI) level 3 patients make up a majority of the arrivals at the ED on any given day. How quickly the patients are seen, treated, and discharged is one of the primary factors influencing LOS and LWBS metrics. Research demonstrates the physician-in-triage can help with these metrics; however, in the ED the physician-in-triage only focuses on low-acuity patients (Santistevan et al., 2020). Between the physician-in-triage focusing primarily on the lowest-acuity patients and the remainder of the ED tending to the sickest patients, the mid-acuity patients can wait multiple hours in the waiting room to be seen. This interventional process used a triage screening as well as a physician-in-triage to evaluate the patient before placing the patient in the dedicated mid-track location. The dedicated location was a semiprivate room with recliner chairs for patients to receive treatment. Once the patient arrived to mid-track, they were followed by a nurse practitioner until the patient's disposition was determined. The use of the mid-track process resulted in a decrease LOS for ESI level 3 patients by an average of 50 minutes and slightly reduced the LWBS rate by 0.1%. There was an average of 571 boarders per month, with the average increasing over a four-month period to 845 per month. This cycle for improvement was completed during the month with the highest numbers of boarding patients at 931. As the number of boarders increased, so did the LOS and LWBS averages, except for during the mid-track trial. It was considered that the number of arrivals was the main factor affecting the metrics; however, these metrics were dependent on how well patients moved through the department (throughput). Despite record boarding rates during the month of the trial, implementing a mid-track process focused on mid-acuity patients decreased LOS averages and LWBS rates. These results conclude that creating a process for mid-acuity, or ESI level 3 patients, to be seen in a dedicated area greatly improves the LWBS rates and LOS averages, optimizing ED throughput.

Learning Environment and Lifelong Learning

Schools of nursing should partner with healthcare organizations committed to learning environments for the CNL's clinical immersion. In such an environment, educators and clinicians work collaboratively to create an atmosphere where all members have a concentrated focus on teaching and learning (Fourie & McClelland, 2011). Factors contributing to satisfying and successful student learning experiences include the quality of planning, welcome and orientation of the student to the unit, peer encouragement and teamwork, cooperation of the unit manager and charge nurses, and support of clinical and faculty preceptors (Fourie & McClelland, 2011). When students are in environments that allow them to flourish, they can practice innovation at the bedside, eliminating workarounds that are often developed by staff and optimizing care from the bedside up, instead of the usual way from administration downward (Noles et al., 2019).

When preceptees begin the clinical immersion journey, it is often with anxiety and trepidation. "How will I be received? Will the nurses on the unit welcome me? How can I earn the respect of staff and management?" In learning environments where staff and management routinely work with CNL students, staff is acclimated to a student role, and the student perceives that careful and thoughtful planning of this immersion was completed in preparation for the immersion experience. Benefits of such clinical environments include clear and identifiable learning objectives, anticipated trajectories, assistance with the development and acquisition of CNL core competencies, and a final CNL project plan.

Time should be allocated early in the immersion experience for the CNL student to orient with charge nurses and staff nurses, unit secretaries, patient care associates, the unit manager, and the medical director to learn each member's role and how this role contributes to the overall function and purpose of the unit. Time spent orienting with individual team members helps create and establish relationships that enable the CNL student to work freely in the work environment, become part of the "team," and assume accountability and responsibility for unit performance, opportunities, outcomes, and culture. This engagement and evolution of becoming a team member is beneficial to the student experience and critical for the overall success of the immersion, as well as the project plan implementation and sustainability.

Data about unit performance should be accessible and shared freely with the CNL student. It is crucial that the CNL student understands the definition of data points and can match the data to each workflow. Data integrity frequently delays the acquisition of relative information to perform a thorough microsystem assessment (Vimalachandran et al., 2016). Because data integrity is a challenge, it is important that the CNL has a good understanding of the data. A CNL preceptor should search and advocate for truth in the data shared. A clear understanding and validation of the integrity of the data is imperative to the CNL as a leader in practice. Real change can only be planned once the current state is fully understood.

Transparency is the hallmark of a high-reliability organization, and any attempt to avoid weaknesses within the system can hinder effective and meaningful project plans. Unfortunately, healthcare is not a high-reliability industry like commercial aviation and nuclear power (Chassin & Loeb, 2013). To become a high-reliability organization, transparency is the first step. Transparency includes a responsibility on the part of the student and faculty to ensure that any sensitive information that could be disparaging to the institution remains confidential. Agreements between schools of nursing and healthcare organizations where CNL preceptees complete clinical immersions should be obtained prior to the clinical experience to ensure confidentiality. Organizations that are not willing to share necessary information and data prevent the CNL preceptee from achieving maximum results, creating a culture of distrust and futility. Carefully selecting and maintaining partnerships with institutions and providing ongoing education promotes an environment of trust, clarity, and openness.

Developing Meaningful and Sustainable Clinical Immersion Projects

The clinical immersion project is the pinnacle of the preceptee's educational experience. Completion of a process or quality improvement project provides the student with a means to demonstrate all objectives, course work, and competencies acquired throughout the CNL program of study. The project is scheduled at the end of the learning experience, after the required experiential learning in order to complete such a challenge. Diligently checking off the CNL's competencies day-by-day offers the CNL student with the skill set and knowledge essential for implementing a successful project. Conducting the microsystem assessment and performing a gap analysis easily identifies inconsistencies. These are opportunities within the microsystem that can be potential project plan ideas, moving toward the ideal future state for the microsystem.

Common mistakes made among CNL students are attempting to identify a project plan too early in the clinical immersion experience, allowing the preceptor to dictate the project prior to completion of the microsystem assessment, or selecting a project that is so broad that there is not sufficient time or resources to allow for adequate preparation, implementation, and measurement. Sequenced steps, which if followed, can ensure successful project plan implementation. Identifying and selecting the appropriate project plan, setting measurable and attainable goals, developing a realistic step-by-step time line for implementation and evaluation, and summarizing events are key factors for accomplishing desired project goals. If a student can clearly identify the current state of the microsystem, focus on one aspect, and map it out, identify the gaps of opportunity, and implement an intervention to improve, the student is successful. If the intervention fails to improve the identified problem, all will learn from the experience. If the metric the project is driving matters, the team can learn from failure and perform another iterative cycle of improvement after the student has completed the experience. The focus on what matters and celebrating failure in a psychologically safe environment will lead to clinical practice transformation.

Identifying and Selecting a Project Plan

Identification and selection of a project plan is the most important step in implementing a successful process or quality improvement. It is also the most difficult step of the endeavor. Many times, preceptors or unit leaders have projects for the student to complete prior to the student's completion of the microsystem assessment. Many students also enter the healthcare setting with individual ideas and agendas for what the project plan will be and how it will be implemented before becoming familiar with the culture or goals of the organization and microsystem. Both are missteps and usually result in failure. Seven steps that safeguard effective project plan selection include: (1) completing an overview of the organization, (2) recognizing the importance and value of the introductions and orientations to the facility, (3) listening, (4) conducting thorough literature research, (5) seeking feedback, (6) obtaining buy-in, and (7) aligning with organizational priorities.

Step 1

Complete an overview of the designated healthcare organization prior to entering the clinical immersion setting. Formulate an impression by talking to people, asking questions, being present, and observing. Go to the cafeteria, waiting room, or coffee shop, and observe and listen. Conduct online searches to determine the history, purpose, development, and progress of the institution. Learn the mission, vision, and values of the organization and discern if those values line up with your own.

If not, be aware entering and be prepared for situations that may prove challenging during the immersion experience. Commit the mission, vision, and values to memory or save them to a location where they can be reviewed throughout the year. Assess periodically if the organization "walks the walk" of the vision. Do the executives know the mission? Do they live the mission? When observed, are the mission, vision, and values consistently exemplified with the decisions made by middle management? It is important that the student know who they are and understand personal values. There are several self-evaluations that can be completed to see how one can potentially impact the organization. This self-assessment will also guide the student to assess if the values of the organization are aligned with personal values. Students who complete some degree of background homework first are usually able to begin contemplating project plan ideas sooner and experience a less stressful transition into the clinical setting.

Step 2

Acknowledge the value and importance of introductions and orientation to the clinical immersion setting and microsystem. Introductions to personnel during the orientation period is the time when the CNL student learns the who, what, where, and how of obtaining information and support, and serves as the formative time for establishing the underpinnings necessary for building and developing interdepartmental relationships. Being visible to key stakeholders in the hall, cafeteria, at the nurses' station, and in other key gathering places is important for the student's experience. Spend time shadowing individuals of various roles in the microsystem to gain insight and mutual respect from team members. Sit at the unit secretary's desk, talk, look, and listen. Orientation with team members in the microsystem helps form alliances and bonds that will be instrumental as the time for project plan identification and implementation approach. Spending time with and learning the roles of key personnel in other departments and roles enables the CNL student to identify the "go-to" people and resources readily available. This will also provide staff the reality that you respect various roles on the team and value opinions.

Inquire about regularly scheduled meetings, either in person or virtually, and ask for all opportunities to participate in any meetings as an additional invite. Do not be afraid of the virtual world. Although it is new for many in healthcare, it is an opportunity that eliminates wasted time moving from location to location. The virtual world allows for all to be seen and share. Attending larger organizational meetings, as well as meetings within the microsystem, provides a plethora of information pertaining to goals and objectives for future reference for project ideas.

Step 3

The most important undertaking for developing meaningful and sustainable clinical immersion projects is to be present, listening and seeking clarity from the preceptor if not understanding. If there are common themes that are discussed at all levels of the organization, write them down. The CNL must have an understanding of data and the story behind it; this is key in executing an intervention and sustaining the effort. Spend time reflecting on all experiences during the immersion. Which themes touch your heart? Which themes do you have a personal passion to improve? By listening and observing, you can identify the aims of the organization, pinpoint objectives of the chief nurse officer and director of nursing, see how all roles in the microsystem function as a team, understand the challenges of the providers, and ascertain the goals and aspirations of the unit manager, CNL, and the interprofessional team at the microsystem level.

Once immersed, begin a list of possible project plan ideas, and continually add to this list as the clinical immersion progresses. Ensure that someone is talking about some aspect of the project to ensure that your plan for improvement matters. What you choose to pursue must matter to someone or it is not worth attempting. Take in everything. Listen to everyone and, above all, do not try to establish the project plan too early. Be patient. Allow the course work and immersion time to provide insight and focus, giving project plan ideas time to emerge.

Step 4

Conduct literature reviews and research the recurring themes that have been identified to seek understanding. Determine if studies have already been completed in this area, and if there are any evidenced-based best practice standards that have been successful in improving outcomes. It is important to not focus solely on the reported intervention, but also pay attention to the studied patient population, the size and type of the organization where the study was conducted, as well as if the improvement was sustained. Review as much literature as necessary until the point of saturation occurs. The project plans found in the literature must offer sustainable value.

Consider the costs involved and determine if the project plan requires capital, workforce, supplies, or resources. Consider the return on investment for the organization. How much does the current outcome cost the organization? Ensure that the scope of the project is not so large that it cannot be implemented or evaluated within the time constraints of the immersion. Determine if the project plan creates or reduces work for members of the interprofessional team and associate a dollar amount to this if able. Ascertain if the manager, CNL, or members of the team have an interest in this idea. If the project produces positive results, how will it be sustained? Once the research has been completed and thoughtful contemplation given to all contributing factors, eliminate those ideas that are not feasible, and retain the ideas that remain possibilities.

Step 5

Share the results of the microsystem assessment conducted and seek feedback from a variety of members of the interprofessional team. Data gathered should be discussed or posted on bulletin boards on the unit level, with graphs highlighting areas of focus and concern. Discuss project plan ideas, how they were identified, and the results of the literature review with the designated preceptor. Identify the goals and expected outcomes of each project plan idea, as well as limitations, anticipated obstacles, potential barriers, and roadblocks together. Be flexible and open-minded. Trust the preceptor and foster open communication so that both preceptor and preceptee can talk through whether the microsystem is ready for and open to the change process. Allot time for interactive discussion, questions, dialogue, and careful and deliberate consideration. Allow time after the initial conversation for all parties to consider thoughts and views expressed and make an appointment to revisit these project plan ideas later. Time spent away from the discussions for processing thoughts and exploring new ideas can produce innovative and insightful results.

Step 6

Determine buy-in. The most excellent project plan ideas can crumble and deteriorate if buy-in is not obtained prior to implementation. While it would be unrealistic to expect support and backing from the entire team within the microsystem, it is essential that buy-in exist among key stakeholders. The unit manager, preceptor, appointed and informal leaders within the unit, and the CNL student should all believe in the project plan selected and share in the development and implementation of the identified goals. Even though the student will be leading the project, for it to be sustained, ownership of the team must be established. This cannot be a top-down approach, or in this case a student "push" approach. Seeking team members who believe in the effort and are excited about the initiative should be included in the planning phase. If kept engaged and included, these champions who are part of the microsystem team will own the effort when the immersion is completed.

Step 7

Carefully consider and then clearly communicate which organizational-, departmental-, and unit-level goals the project aligns with and supports. Alignment with these goals is essential to make a project impactful. If a project is not meaningful to the organization, then the immersion experience is just a checkbox for completion of the objectives. The immersion experience and student project can have a huge impact on transforming care delivery at the microsystem level. If possible, the student should provide the financial impact for the organization and not primarily focus on the metric itself, equating a dollar amount to the impact of the change, as finances get the most attention from administrators. It is very difficult for them to reject or discount actions that will positively impact finances and improve desired areas of focus.

Set Measurable and Attainable Goals

Setting measurable and attainable goals is essential for implementing a successful project or quality improvement initiative. It is important to be realistic in what one can hope to accomplish. A time line for gathering baseline data, implementation, and reviewing post-implementation data should be established. It is important to know when data is routinely collected by the organization and what period one is reviewing. Although data may be collected electronically, it may only be reported quarterly or have a lag time of a month. Timeliness of data reporting will help guide the data collection as well as establish realistic measurable goals within a time frame. Change is slow, and sustained change requires a conscious effort from others to practice a task or behavior differently than how previously practiced. Establishing a baseline period for education and implementation and a due date for measuring results allows the CNL preceptee to assess the degree of improvement and success.

Selection of the baseline data is critical and requires careful thought and realistic planning. For example, a project aim statement from a preceptee on a med-surg unit *to reduce ED boarding time by 50% over a two-month period as compared with the previous year* may not be practical if the ED had an average of 10 hours of boarding last year. First, a two-month period of measurement should not be compared to a year's worth of data. Instead, when selecting a baseline, consider the amount of time you have for project implementation and measurement. If you are lucky enough to have an entire quarter of a year (three months) for project implementation, then select a quarter of data from a previous period as the baseline. If you only have one month to implement a project and measure results, include the last three to six months prior to establish a trend and set a goal to reduce or improve performance by a realistic percentage of that number. The prior example of reducing boarding hours identified many factors related to boarding hours that would be outside the scope of the project. The student preceptee should focus on a more manageable improvement within their microsystem that affects the larger goal of reducing ED boarding. Perhaps a better project goal would be to *reduce time from discharge orders being placed on Med-Surg Unit 4 to patients being discharged from a room*. Since ED boarding is impacted by no available rooms to send admitted patients to from the ED, discharging patients timelier from a unit reduces the boarding time in the ED.

Selection of attainable goals must also be considered. There is a tendency for CNL students to set sights high and aspire to lofty goals that usually cannot be reached within the designated time for immersion completion. Avoid the tendency to "conquer the world" and instead, set goals on improving one small piece. Change is more easily accomplished when it is simple, entailing one or two steps that do not require additional work and extraneous efforts or tasks. Do not avoid any project idea that creates additional time for a nurse to function as a nurse, decreases steps in any workflow, or helps to improve an overall goal, even if the project is a small step in the change process. The simplicity of a project plan optimizes the chance for ownership by the interprofessional team, ensuring successful sustainability leading to transformative clinical practice.

Develop a Step-by-Step Time Line

Developing a realistic step-by-step time line is imperative. Be smart and think through everything occurring throughout the clinical immersion experience. Create a calendar and include every day of the week, including weekends, throughout the clinical immersion. Include test dates and assignment due dates for classwork, any events required outside of clinical time, clinical days, and workdays. Divide readings so that there is approximately the same amount of material to read daily. Change the scenery where the reading and time spent on the computer occurs, and enter these locations in a calendar. This will support your mental well-being.

Social well-being is equally important. Add important personal events such as birthdays, holidays, and children's events, if you are a parent. Do not forget the importance of your physical well-being. Schedule time to walk, plan meals, and maintain regular exercise habits. Until a clear picture emerges delineating the expected time and obligations required to meet and fulfill deadlines, do not stress. Simply write in your calendar the time needed to support physical, social, and mental well-being throughout the finality of the program. Remember to include some downtime and strive to maintain some type of balance among work, home, and school. Remind yourself that while completely "free" time will be minimal, it is only temporary.

Once the calendar is completed, plan an outline with an accompanying period for project plan goals. Ask the preceptor to assist you with planning. Often students create time lines for projects without considering other projects, mandatory education, or activities already planned by unit leadership for staff. Coordinating a project time line with the preceptor who is knowledgeable of the other priorities being pushed to the staff will aide you during implementation. Work backward for project plan due dates. Determine the period desired to collect and analyze all concluding data and add this to the calendar. Determine how long the project plan or process change needs to be in effect after education is provided and mark that time. Consider the time required to educate teams about the project plan, and remember to factor in various schedule patterns, which may require up to two weeks of education before implementation to ensure all staff are aware. Once all dates are added to a master calendar, you will be able to identify a due date for project plan selection.

Implementation and evaluation of the project plan is usually the time when the difficult mental work ceases and the oversight and reinforcement begins. Observing daily for compliance, reinforcing objectives, and collecting and logging data as often as possible becomes the focus of the remaining clinical days. Meetings with the preceptor should occur regularly, and findings, deviations, barriers, and successes should be discussed. Open communication between the preceptor and preceptee is imperative. Do not be afraid to adjust the project plan if unforeseen obstacles occur that hinder project goal attainment, with recognition that the adaptation of the original plan is another cycle for improvement. It is important to document each effort to improve.

Summarize Findings and Results

Summarize findings and results of the project plan. Return to the baseline data and demonstrate progress made toward goal attainment with trends noted. Do not forget to include unforeseen barriers that presented roadblocks along the project's course. Consider using graphs, run charts, or line charts. Brief summaries with picture boards and educational material developed to promote project plan goals are interesting to the reviewers and should be included in the summary.

Examples of Clinical Immersion Projects and Impact on the Healthcare System

Exemplars of CNL clinical immersion projects can be in various books and textbooks written for the CNL, poster presentations from previous CNL summits, Clinical Nurse Leader Association (CNLA) regional conferences, CNLA chapter meetings, other CNL conferences via the internet, and from the CNLA website. Ongoing monthly continuing education units (CEUs) provided by the CNLA offer a variety of CNL topics, including projects CNLs or former CNL students have completed or are presently working on within organizations. The book *Project Planning and Management: A Guide for CNLs, DNPs, and Nurse Executives* (Harris et al., 2015) is an excellent resource for guiding the CNL student through project plan selection and implementation. Networking with other CNL students and certified CNLs can also provide ideas for meaningful and sustainable clinical immersion projects. Several venues to network have been created through schools of nursing or CNLA chapter development. Some organizations that employ several CNLs have weekly or monthly meetings to discuss current projects. Students should ask the faculty and preceptor about networking opportunities within the clinical setting.

On a 20-bed medical surgical unit, a CNL student noted that discharges before 1 p.m. were only at 21%, with most discharges from the unit occurring after 4 p.m. The inquiry of the student was to better understand why discharges were not happening earlier in the day. The ED was on diversion during the week from Monday through Thursday quite frequently. Why is the hospital turning away patients, if in fact we could move patients from the ED more efficiently? The CNL met with the lead team, which was an established accountable care team (ACT) for the unit. As the data were presented, the team decided to address improving discharge times before 1 p.m. as a focus. The team initially decided to create a flyer that was posted in every patient's room that communicated the expectation was to discharge before noon. The coordinator developed scripting and education for the interprofessional staff to consistently communicate the expectation beginning on admission. This education took two weeks to hardwire. Patient whiteboards were used to identify the day of discharge, and were audited daily with follow-up coaching from leadership. This unit team owned the CNL student's project and became very competitive and focused to achieve 50% of all discharges to be completed by 1 p.m. This goal was communicated at shift huddles, among the entire team, and the goal was posted at the nurses' station and in the break room. Initially, after two weeks, the team had achieved 35% of all discharges by 1 p.m. At one-month post-implementation, the team had achieved 47%. The second, third, and fourth months post-implementation, the student's project was completely owned by the team, with the unit achieving 61% of all discharges being discharged by 1 p.m. This has been sustained and the unit continues to carry the hospital medicine group for their total discharge before 1 p.m. metric.

Summary

- The preceptor and preceptee are the two key players in the CNL's clinical immersion experience. Both have core competencies that facilitate the mutual success of one another. This relationship is vital to a successful experience for both parties.
- Clinical immersion sites that partner with academia and understand the CNL's role foster an enriching learning environment. A clinical setting that employs CNLs is optimal to further pave the way for future CNL immersions.
- Learning environments where CNL preceptees are welcomed and routinely complete clinical rotations instill lifelong learning trajectories shaping ongoing professional development. Meaningful and sustainable CNL immersion projects can be identified, implemented, and sustained.
- Identifying and selecting the appropriate project plan, setting measurable and attainable goals, developing a realistic step-by-step time line for implementation and evaluation, and summarizing events are key to project plan success. For sustainability to be achieved, it is important to create ownership early on by engaging unit champions.
- Examples of former successful CNL projects can be located through CNL books, textbooks, websites, organizations, and networking. Hard work is rewarded with success.

Reflection Questions

1. How are core competencies of the CNL preceptor and the CNL preceptee alike? How are they different?
2. What requisites are important to you for achieving success in the clinical immersion experience?
3. What barriers could prevent you from achieving success in the clinical immersion experience?
4. Why is it important for a CNL to understand the data? What is the importance of equating a financial amount to the data?
5. What do you feel constitutes meaningful and sustainable clinical immersion projects?
6. What is the most important element needed to determine the clinical immersion project?

Learning Activities

1. Complete a self-evaluation to determine your preferred methods of communication and feedback and be prepared to discuss these methods with your preceptor. Ask your preceptor about their preferred method of communication and ascertain what type of feedback they need to maintain open lines of communication and exchange of ideas. Work together to establish means and frequency of communication acceptable to both parties. This relationship is vital for the clinical immersion experience.
2. Identify your strengths and weaknesses in your roles as student, preceptee, nurse, and a member of a profession. In one column, list strengths and in the other column list weaknesses. Identify ahead of time strategies for handling weaknesses that are part of your individual makeup prior to the clinical immersion experience, acknowledging that these weaknesses will be magnified during peak times of stress, fatigue, and weariness.
3. Assess your values and biases that you may have prior to going into the immersion. How will you react if your values are not aligned with the organization? Are you aware of your nonverbal communication cues? It is important to have complete self-awareness prior to the immersion to be prepared in any situation or discussion.
4. Assess your ability to organize and prioritize events in your life. Pinpoint events and triggers that cause you to go astray and lose focus. Research ways to minimize these triggers. Think of events in your past that made you want to give up and quit, and analyze those events to identify the mitigating factors that caused these feelings and/or actions. Develop an action plan to recognize when these situations are threatening and how to prevent and halt their progression.
5. Are you committed to complete the CNL immersion? The CNL track is a time commitment. Have you talked through the commitment with your family, your boss, and your friends? It is important to be transparent with those whom you care about related to the time commitment of the program. This will allow each of them to provide additional support along the way.

References

Akiyode, O. (2016). Teaching professionalism: A faculty's perspective. *Currents in Pharmacy Teaching and Learning, 8*(4), 584–586.

American Association of Colleges of Nursing. (2013). *Competencies and curricular expectations for clinical nurse leader education and practice*. Author. https://www.aacnnursing.org/News-Information /Position-Statements-White-Papers/CNL

Bender, M. (2016). Clinical nurse leader integration into practice: Developing theory to guide best practice. *Journal of Professional Nursing, 32*(1), 32–40.

Chassin, M., & Loeb, J. (2013). High reliability healthcare: Getting there from here. *The Milbank Quarterly, 91*(3), 459–490.

Fourie, W., & McClelland, B. (2011). *Enhancing nursing education through dedicated education units*. The National Centre for Tertiary Teaching Excellence. http://akoaotearoa.ac.nz/download/ng /file/group-1658/enhancing-nursing-education-hrough-dedicated-education-units.pdf

Goode, M. L. (2012). The role of the mentor: A critical analysis. *Journal of Community Nursing, 26*(3), 33–35.

Harris, J. L., Roussel, L., Dearman, C., & Thomas, P. (2015). *Project planning and management: A guide for CNLs, DNPs, and nurse executives* (2nd ed.). Jones & Bartlett Learning.

Hunter, D., & Perkins, N. (2012). Partnership working in public health: The implications for governance of a systems approach. *Journal of Health Services Research & Policy, 17*(Supp.), 45–52.

Kujala, S., Horhamer, I., Heponiemie, T., & Josefsson, K. (2019). The role of frontline leaders in building health professional support for a new patient portal: Survey study. *Journal of Medical Internet Research, 21*(3), e11413.

Lillibridge, J. (2007). Using clinical nurses as preceptors to teach leadership and management to senior nursing students: A qualitative descriptive study. *Nurse Education in Practice, 7*(1), 44–52.

Moore, L. W., & Leahy, C. (2012). Implementing the new clinical nurse leader role while gleaning insights from the past. *Journal of Professional Nursing, 28*(3), 139–146.

Moore, P., Schmidt, D., & Howington, L. (2014). Interdisciplinary preceptor teams to improve the clinical nurse leader student experience. *Journal of Professional Nursing, 30*(3), 190–195.

Noles, K., Barber, R., James, D., & Wingo, N. (2019). Driving innovation in health care: Clinical Nurse Leader role. *Journal of nursing care quality, 34*(4), 307–311.

Payne, C., Heye, M. L., & Farrell, K. (2014). Securing preceptors for advanced practice students. *Journal of Nursing Education and Practice, 4*(3), 167.

Santistevan, J., Lee, A., & Hamedani, A. (2020). CareSTART: A physician in triage front-end model improves patient safety and ED efficiency. *American College of Emergency Physicians, quality improvement & patient safety*. https://www.acep.org/how-we-serve/sections/quality -improvement--patient-safety/newsletters/july-2017/carestart-a-physician-in-triage-frontend- model-improves-patient-safety-and-ed-efficiency

Vimalachandran, P., Wang, H., Zhang, Y., Heyward, B., & Whittaker, F. (2016). Ensuring data integrity in electronic health records: A quality health care implication. *2016 International Conference on Orange Technologies (ICOT)*, pp. 20–27. IEEE.

EXEMPLAR

Follow the (Clinical Nurse) Leader

Keaton Lloyd

The preceptorship was a formative experience. Paring with a CNL allowed me to see what that role looked like in action. I was able to take those experiences and build on them by collaborating with different teams. With guidance from my preceptor, I began to think and perform like a CNL. I was transformed from the observing student to the apprentice. By the end of the preceptorship, I was able to successfully gather a multidisciplinary team for a quality improvement project and help drive change with evidence and purpose. Ultimately, I was able to gain a more comprehensive perspective for healthcare systems that has helped me even in the role I am in today. I learned how to press into the *why*—Why do we really do the things we do? Why does it really matter? Why does it matter to others? This education has been invaluable to understanding and relating to others. The CNL preceptorship helped transform my thought process and give me the skills to put things in action.

EXEMPLAR

Less Is Not Always More

Nick Hall

In December 2018, a major academic medical center completed its full conversion from intravenous (IV) Brand 1 catheters to IV Brand 2 catheters in an effort aimed at reducing hospital-wide costs by an estimated $20,000 per year. The IV Brand 2 catheters were trialed throughout the hospital system beginning in summer 2018, and a complete systemwide conversion was made to the IV 2 products beginning in December 2018. The CNL student collected data for tracking IV Brand 2 catheter use beginning in December 2018 through February 2019 and compared that data to IV Brand 1 catheter use from December 2017 through February 2018.

After compiling usage data, the CNL student could clearly show that the number of IV Brand 2 catheters being utilized exceeded that of the IV Brand 1 catheters during the comparative time frame, even though the number of patients being seen during these evaluation times were relatively equal. According to the initial review of data, IV Brand 2 product usage translated to an increased expense of $2,000 per month, contradicting the projected cost savings the conversion anticipated. In addition to increased costs, patient and nurse satisfaction has been reduced related to the increased number of sticks required to obtain sufficient intravenous access since conversion to the IV Brand 2 product.

EXEMPLAR

The CNL and CNS: Partners in Quality Care

Donna M. Meador

Although the National League of Nursing (NLN) first advocated the CNS in the 1940s, it took many years to advance the role. With the advent of the CNL, many concerns have been raised among healthcare leaders regarding overlapping of duties between these two roles. In an effort to clarify the roles, the AACN published *Working Statement Comparing the Clinical Nurse Leader and Clinical Nurse Specialist Roles: Similarities, Differences and Complementarities* in 2004. One major difference between these specialties is that the CNL is educated as a generalist and the CNS as an expert (AACN, 2004). In addition, the CNS has the ability to practice as an APRN (AACN, 2004). The CNL is not eligible to board as an APRN.

While the CNS and CNL roles are unique, in many cases their objectives are similar. Both coordinate care for patients, advocate for quality, and serve as a mentor to staff. They are partners in providing safe, high-quality care and can augment each other in this endeavor. For example, the CNL may identify a gap in a microsystem. The CNL can then enlist the assistance of the CNS to translate evidence-based practices, formulate a plan, and advocate for change in a clinical specialty. The CNL and CNS would then work together to test the modifications and share the knowledge at the unit level. Another example includes the identification of a knowledge deficit among staff on a medical unit regarding new insulin preparations and dosages. The CNL consults with a CNS who specializes in diabetes management who provides an evidence-based in-service to staff.

Ongoing collaborative efforts by all team members will continuously foster quality and safe care for patients. The complimentary actions by CNLs and CNSs are no exception. Embracing the partnership and recognizing the contributions of the CNL and CNS results in positive outcomes in an era of constant change within healthcare systems.

Reference

American Association of Colleges of Nursing. (2004). *Working statement comparing the Clinical Nurse Leader and Clinical Nurse Specialist roles: Similarities, differences and complementarities*. Author.

EXEMPLAR

The CNL as a Mentor

Bridget Graham

In February 2011, our hospital opened a 32-bed acuity-adaptable senior adult unit (3 Lacks). Staff members who had a passion for working with senior adults were hired for the unit. The majority of staff that was hired was competent in medical-surgical nursing but did not have any intermediate experience. Fewer than 12% of the staff members were intermediate competent. CNLs and the unit's CNS teamed up to develop and execute RN intermediate education in order to provide the professional development, education, and coaching required to ensure safe and excellent patient care.

Our first objective was to determine the minimum competencies for an RN to be considered intermediate trained. The criteria were as follows:

RNs must understand, verbalize, and demonstrate the use, effects, and monitoring requirements for the vasoactive drips used on our unit.

RNs will understand, verbalize, and demonstrate the use of hemodynamic monitoring.

RNs will recognize the signs/symptoms of and care for patients with respiratory and cardiac failure.

RNs will understand, verbalize, and demonstrate continuing assessment and reassessment of the intermediate patient.

RNs will verbalize and demonstrate the knowledge and ability to access additional resources during their shift (e.g., rapid responder, e-library, unit literature, CNLs, and CNS).

RNs will complete 3 Lack's specific intermediate competency checklist.

All non-intermediate RNs will have telemetry/EKG classes and four hours of didactic intermediate training.

A unit-specific intermediate competency tool was developed, which was to be completed by the end of training. This served as a record of completion. Charge nurses were the priority group to receive intermediate training. All RNs were paired with a CNL or the CNS for three 8-hour shifts. We worked one on one at the bedside to ensure education and monitor progress. The CNLs and the CNS worked the schedule of the nurse, whether it was days or nights. After three shifts, the RN and/or the CNL and CNS could determine the need for continued education. Training would continue if the RN required additional education. Intermediate education binders were also placed on the unit as a resource for staff.

When we began our training and mentoring, only 11.76% of our RN staff members were intermediate trained. Currently, 76% of our RN staff members are intermediate trained. The CNLs and the CNS continue to mentor staff. We have increased the level of trust between staff and the CNLs/CNS. RNs who have completed intermediate training verbalize that they feel empowered to teach new RNs on the unit intermediate skills.

By training our staff to care for the intermediate patient, we have prevented transfers to a higher level of care. Handoffs to RNs on a higher level of care were decreased by 32%.

The financial impact of training the nurses was minimal. One-on-one training and mentoring with CNLs or the CNS came at no additional cost to the unit. We paired with staff on their already budgeted shifts and therefore incurred no cost.

The CNLs on 3 Lacks played an instrumental role in the mentoring and training of intermediate RNs for the new unit. Through collaboration, education, evidence-based practice for seniors, and application of clinical skills, the CNLs impacted patient safety on the unit and helped to ensure a higher standard for the level of care expected. Working closely with the RNs fostered the growth of knowledge and skills for the bedside nurse.

EXEMPLAR

CNL Preceptor Role Satisfaction on a Dedicated Education Unit

Sherry Webb and Tommie Norris

Aim: To describe CNL preceptor role satisfaction

The role of the preceptor is critical to the achievement of the end-of-program competencies for Model C master's entry-level CNL students. Preceptor role satisfaction ensures preceptor continuity for students in adult health, pediatrics, acute care, leadership, target population diagnosis, and clinical leadership practicum courses.

Expert staff nurses on the dedicated education unit (DEU) were selected by the nurse manager, trained by the faculty at the university, and evaluated as DEU preceptors by students and faculty. Surveys of the DEU preceptors indicated overwhelming satisfaction with their role in working with CNL students, and preceptors expressed interest in serving in future courses. They believed that they provided realistic clinical opportunities, which helped students achieve their course outcomes, and they were proud of their students' successes. The DEU preceptors valued the relationships that they formed with their students and faculty and believed that the DEU partnership bridged the gap between academia and practice. They reported that they learned about quality, safety, risk reduction, and evidence-based practice from the students, which made them interested in returning to college to advance their education. Faculty served as ambassadors of the college and provided letters of recommendation for the CNL program. In addition, the DEU preceptors became more interested in pursuing achievement in the hospital's clinical ladder program for advancement. DEU preceptors received recognition from their colleagues, nursing leadership, hospital staff, patients, and families through verbal feedback, hospital newsletters, performance appraisals, and site visits by other organizations. Six clinical teachers received the preceptor of the year award presented during the College of Nursing Alumni Day awards celebration. DEU preceptor satisfaction is critical to the success of CNL student education.

EXEMPLAR

Preceptors' Use of Portfolios for Career Advancement

Tommie Norris and Sherry Webb

Aim: To prepare preceptors on dedicated education units

Portfolios can be organized to showcase achievement of career advancement criteria. Preceptors working with CNL students assigned to DEUs were impressed by the portfolios prepared by their students. Faculty were interested in facilitating the development of the preceptors' portfolios as one way to express gratitude to the preceptors for sharing their expertise and role-modeling professional nursing. Faculty worked with preceptors to develop portfolios that would demonstrate achievement of specialized skills and career advancement criteria established by the employer. In an informal survey, DEU preceptors reported that their portfolios helped them to feel prepared for their annual evaluations, impressed their supervisors, and provided evidence of meeting advancement criteria. Preceptors also reported that portfolios proved to be a great vehicle for retaining records of continuing education needed for certification renewal. All portfolios developed by preceptors contained an updated résumé. Faculty provided a template that enabled preceptors to "click and insert" demographic information, work experience, education, and honors/awards. The portfolios were individualized and contained various sections such as evidence of achieving certification including basic CPR, advanced cardiac life support, and/or pediatric advanced life support. Continuing education (CE) hours earned in pursuit of lifelong learning or as a requirement for employment (such as fire safety or HIPAA) were included. Membership in professional organizations and leadership positions was incorporated. Nurses returning to college to advance their education included transcripts of completed coursework, and many included examples of assignments such as quality improvement projects. Development of educational tools and patient pamphlets were included as examples of innovative practice. An agency always strives for patient satisfaction, and preceptors were encouraged to include "thank-you" letters/notes from patients and peers providing evidence of patient-centered care or teamwork.

CHAPTER 10

Creative and Meaningful Clinical Immersions

Patricia L. Thomas, James L. Harris, and Linda A. Roussel

LEARNING OBJECTIVES

1. Describe the purpose of the clinical immersion and the key elements.
2. Apply the business model to CNL clinical immersions and projects.
3. Discuss how using data assists in identifying needs and developing meaningful immersions and clinical projects.
4. Identify the importance portfolios and their value to CNL success.
5. Discuss the value of performance contracts toward achieving measurable goals.
6. Explore ways the clinical immersion can serve as a springboard for role success and integration of the CNL's role into operational practice models.

KEY TERMS

Business principles
Collaboration
Gap analysis
Metrics

Needs assessment
Portfolio
Planning

CNL ROLES

Clinician
Coordinator of care
Information manager
Lifelong learner

Member of a profession
Outcomes manager
Systems analyst/risk anticipator
Team manager

CNL PROFSSIONAL VALUES

Accountability
Evidence-based practice

Fiscal stewardship
Integrity

Interdisciplinary teams
Outcome measurement

Quality improvement
Quality patient care and safety

CNL CORE COMPETENCIES

Assessment
Communication
Designer/Manager/Coordination of care
Environment of care management
Horizontal leadership

Information and healthcare
   technologies
Membership in a profession
Team leader

Introduction: Intention of the Immersion—Value Added for the Organization

An imperative for educating future generations is a philosophical and programmatic transformation that is aligned with the changing healthcare delivery system and reform legislation (Jukkula et al., 2013). Meaningful and innovative clinical immersions are imperative for CNL students to develop the skills to respond to the changing care environment. Immersions are the culmination of the academic and clinical experiences in a CNL program. As such, the usefulness can be limited when faculty, clinical partners, and students do not mutually identify needs and create developmental opportunities within a microsystem. Clinical immersions for the CNL student should be based on identifying and assessing gaps and needs within an organization focused on improving the health of a population of patients within a given microsystem. This critical point cannot be overstated. Without thoughtful planning that is detailed and deliberate, the clinical immersion experience can be misaligned and opportunities for successful launching into the CNL role can be missed.

Nelson and colleagues (2007) identified the importance of discovering the microsystem by studying its 5 Ps—purpose, patients, professionals, processes, and patterns—and the ways each of the parts interacts with one another. Even the smallest measurable details should be analyzed, and iterative work redesign and learning cycles should be developed that result in changing work processes and developing database and feedback systems at the microsystem level. Thus, gaps between the unit and organizational levels are closed, improvement in the usefulness of information occurs, and a management focus that corresponds with the real work is created. The unit of work is therefore aligned with the unit of analysis and unit of intervention (Gerard et al., 2012; Nelson et al., 2007; Thomas, 2018).

A meaningful clinical immersion is established when CNL students are able to integrate their coursework into valued clinical work through the enactment of the CNL's role. The clinical immersion experience is intended to provide the platform to support transformative learning, initially for the CNL student and the microsystem, and eventually for the organization. Transformative learning is the culmination of past experiences and perspectives, joined with new learning, to support resocialization. Resocialization involves critical reflection on past and present perspectives in an effort to understand the learner's essential self and thinking processes. Beliefs and old ways of thinking are examined, and critical reflection is triggered, leading to alternative ways of thinking and acting. Within a clinical immersion experience, students are encouraged and supported in changing their worldviews and roles, as well as in internalizing new ways of thinking, communicating, and behaving. They are supported by a precepted clinical immersion experience in a microsystem (Bombard et al., 2010; Fletcher & Meyer, 2016; Hayes & Graham, 2019; Mezirow, 1997; Morris & Faulk, 2007). Fundamental to early outcomes, clinical partners and students need to question assumptions, beliefs, and values and consider multiple points of view while seeking to verify the rationale for the clinical immersion experience (Bouchard & Steel, 1980; Fletcher & Meyer, 2016; Jukkula et al., 2013; Mezirow, 1997; Mezirow & Associates, 2000; Stanley et al., 2007).

Because the CNL role is relatively new and has been implemented in a variety of ways, many CNL students and organizations struggle with the development of an appropriate immersion experience. Organizations have no or few CNL-prepared preceptors and are therefore challenged by identifying people in the organization to guide CNL students through the immersion period. CNL faculty and nurse leaders experiment to create structured immersions using CNL competencies and existing organizational roles. The overarching goal is to establish a tapestry of experiences that allows the novice CNL to use knowledge and skills that validate competence and that also address organizational needs within a microsystem.

To a great extent, the ability to define the scope of a CNL project determines success. Key factors in the scoping process:

1. Definition of a problem or project in a microsystem
2. Establishment of a clearly defined problem statement
3. Clarity in leading, lagging, and outcome measures
4. Documenting cost-benefit or cost-effectiveness expectations
5. Identification of key stakeholders and executive sponsors

Once the project is scoped, using a defined project and quality improvement framework that documents each aspect of the work is a necessity so sustainability and replication can occur.

Using Data and Resources to Identify Needs to Craft Meaningful Clinical Immersions

A variety of data and resources that correspond to the learning objectives of the CNL student are available for analysis at the microsystem level. Examples include balanced scorecards, quality markers, performance and target measures, satisfaction indices, key performance indicators, and actions to reduce or eliminate inefficient practices. The identified microsystem gaps can be transformed into meaningful clinical immersion experiences and projects that develop CNL student skills and ability, create additional examples of outcomes for portfolios, and benefit the overall function of the microsystem. In examining unit or microsystem data, CNL students can identify an area of interest to bring innovative approaches in how to address an issue that is easily recognized in the microsystem. **Table 10-1** provides examples of clinical project data and sources.

Table 10-1 Unit Clinical Project Data and Source

Type of Data	Source of Data/Data Collection Method	Target Compliance Percentage	Actual Compliance Percentage
Troponin level returned to provider for review and action within 60 minutes of order	Acute coronary syndrome performance measure **Balanced scorecard**	100	90
Percentage of patients who received smoking cessation at least once during inpatient admission	Smoking cessation performance measure; inpatient **Inpatient education tracking**	80	50
Percentage of inpatients diagnosed with heart failure who received all five components of the discharge instructions	Heart failure discharge instructions; inpatient **Balanced scorecard**	100	15
Percentage of patient readmissions with heart failure within 30 days	Patient education on admission, during hospitalization, and telephone contact within 1 week of discharge **Balanced scorecard**	100	85
Percentage of skin assessment completion on admission and daily during hospitalization	Admission and daily skin documentation **Inpatient skin assessment form**	100	92
Percentage of overall patient satisfaction scores with admission and discharge processes	Patient satisfaction metrics **Press Ganey survey scores, patient satisfaction**	5*	4.2*

*Based on 5-point Likert scale where 1 = very poor, and 5 = very good.

The planning process commences after scoping a project wherein the CNL student, the CNL faculty member, and the nurse leaders in the organization come together to craft a deliberate and detailed plan for success. Outcome data can point the CNL student and faculty to areas that require change, but a critical success factor for the CNL is the ability to apply new tools and knowledge to "old problems." A potential pitfall for the clinical immersion experience is addressing a current situation with past problem-solving strategies and practices. Key to a successful immersion experience are the use of a framework for planned change, innovative and creative thinking, documentation and use of proven quality and process and improvement tools, and analysis and synthesis of evidence-based interventions from the literature (Bombard et al., 2010; Gerard et al., 2012).

The AACN's White Paper on the Role of the Clinical Nurse Leader (2007), CNL Job Analysis Study (AACN, 2011), and Competencies and Curricular Expectations for the Clinical Nurse Leader Education and Practice (2013) offer distinct expectations and strategic reviews expected of CNL role enactment. These guiding documents offer current organizational role competencies found in nursing and ancillary departments that are key to the development of the clinical immersion experience. Often, no single person or department holds responsibility for measurement, leadership, and integration of practices. With support from CNL faculty and nurse leaders, the CNL student in an immersion experience has an opportunity to establish new relationships, new dialogue, new teams, and new ways to approach microsystem concerns. Detailed review and documentation of current process and practices and identification of points of coordination and competence position CNL students in immersion environments to deal with complexities, organizational culture, and norms.

A thorough gap analysis is the starting point for CNL work during the immersion experience and after graduation. Once gaps are identified, the CNL student can organize a clinical immersion project that meets the objectives in the clinical immersion course while simultaneously addressing important concerns in the microsystem. Linking a microsystem issue or concern to the planning of the immersion project then benefits both the student and the organization. Using the unit assessment tools provided in didactic courses offers the CNL a framework for analyzing opportunities in the microsystem. Different tools are used but commonly follow the 5 P approach (purpose, patients, professionals, processes, and patterns) or the Dartmouth Institute's clinical microsystems assessment (Dartmouth Institute, 2003; Nelson et al., 2007). Irrespective of the tool used, the assessment framework provided highlights the most pressing concerns and provides a springboard for specific problem identification. This leads to quality improvement methodologies, team engagement, and team leader opportunities, as well as specific measures and metrics to demonstrate outcomes. This also creates additional examples of outcomes for the CNL student's portfolio, benefits patient care delivery and patient outcomes, and ultimately creates a system transformation that builds a continuous improvement culture (Bombard et al., 2010; Gerard et al., 2012).

When establishing a project status summary, attention needs to be placed on the process and patterns that the student observes in terms of collaboration with the interdisciplinary team members, inclusion of staff in quality improvement initiatives, relationships established with departments or project champions in the organization, and the responses of patients, family, and staff. Because CNLs are expected to serve as the team or project leader, insights are gained as students reflect on their interactions and leadership skills are expanded. CNL students can use tools from their didactic learning or incorporate the sponsoring organization's tools so that future replication and organizational learning can occur. For team and project leaders, leadership skills are requisite as projects and supporting structures and processes that then foster collaboration and redesign of care delivery within a given microsystem evolve (Cebel et al., 2006; Porter-O'Grady et al., 2010; Rankin, 2015). **Figure 10-1** is an example format for a clinical summary project.

Summary of Project:		
Problems Encountered:	**Actions Taken:**	**Milestone Achievements:**
1.	1.	1.
2.	2.	2.

Figure 10-1 Clinical project status summary

Applying the Business Model to CNL Clinical Immersions

The often uncontrollable issues in clinical settings can interfere with the development of innovative approaches to problem resolution and work redesign. Staff members find themselves performing multiple tasks, getting trapped in existent business models and processes that are ineffective and obsolete. Without awareness and insight to this, the CNL student's clinical immersion experiences can be plagued by organizational memory and may be less than meaningful, and lack the innovation to demonstrate the incorporation and integration of advances of new technologies and methods (Gerard et al., 2012; Hwang & Christensen, 2008; Welton & Harper, 2015). This raises the question of how to use the elements of a business model to guide a CNL clinical immersion experience.

Business models consist of three components: a value proposition, resources and processes, and a profit formula. The value proposition is the service (quality and safe patient care) that assists an individual in accomplishing desired goals and objectives (Hwang & Christensen, 2008; Pourabdollahian & Copani, 2014). For the clinical immersion experience to be successful, resources must be dedicated, including expert and knowledgeable staff, engagement of academic partners, and the equipment necessary to provide care. Processes are identified to ensure activities and actions that result in desired outcomes are developed and initiated and are framed for data capture and future trending. The final component is the profit formula, where any organization determines the costs and benefits that can be sustained over time. Organizations can use this model as other services are envisioned and ultimately offered. With changing reimbursement structures found in at-risk contracts, value-based purchasing, and bundled payment models, efficiency and effectiveness are key to organizational success, coupled with evolving cross-continuum care models, the opportunity to define value through lower cost is emerging (Hwang & Christensen, 2008; Welton & Harper, 2015). The evolving payment models provide CNL students and assigned preceptors an opportunity to call forward this model as a road map to develop the clinical immersion experience. While once considered optional, today this is a necessity as awareness of organizational resource consumption for any change is reviewed and prioritized based on improving care costs as part of a wider framework of quality improvement, population health, and costs derived from the triple aim.

The CNL student can work with clinicians and managers to develop a cost-benefit analysis in concert with course objectives. This project can continue

Table 10-2 Clinical Immersion Project: Medical/Psychiatric Unit

Value Proposition	Resources and Processes	Profit Formula
Medical/Psychiatric unit dedicated to comprehensive care for patients requiring acute and chronic medical and psychiatric interventions by an interdisciplinary team skilled in medical and psychiatric care	Unit design and construction, staff development, equipment purchase and staff training, and marketing strategies that include patient education materials	Cost-benefit analysis that includes all start-up costs and savings of a comprehensive unit that eliminates transfer of psychiatric patients with acute and chronic medical problems off a medical unit that historically required 1:1 sitters

throughout the entire clinical immersion. While once a unique attribute of CNL impact and value, establishing the cost of a practice change or the financial benefit to implementing a change is now an expected metric in organizations as part of resource management and prioritization of work. Clear statements of cost impact have become an expected proposition prior to implementing a practice change that involves interprofessional team members and organizational resources. An example of a clinical immersion experience for a CNL student that incorporates each of the three components of the business model is illustrated in **Table 10-2**.

The Usefulness of Portfolios

The dynamic nature of the healthcare environment and the changing market with greater focus on value-based care requires educators to use innovative methods to measure learning outcomes. A professional portfolio is one such method. The portfolio is a summary and history of collected documents that showcases accomplishments and documents continuous improvement. It demonstrates how various elements of a professional's role functions are related, highlighting competence and the development of a role over time (Billings & Kowalski, 2008; Cope & Murray, 2018; Green et al., 2014; Sherrod, 2005; Wassef et al., 2012).

Portfolio content, whether compiled of paper documents or stored electronically, can serve as a vehicle to demonstrate developmental milestones, assessment, or showcasing of accomplishments. Developmental portfolios demonstrate progress students have made during a specified time period to demonstrate ownership and engagement in learning. Assessment portfolios are used to demonstrate competence or mastery of programmatic standards. Showcase portfolios house student examples of exemplary work at the end of a program that can be shared with potential employers. Often, portfolios contain developmental, assessment, and showcase documents (Cope & Murray, 2018; Wassef et al., 2012). Recently, options to incorporate technology within an e-portfolio has extended the medium by which students can share their work. Electronic platforms allow sharing of documents, videos, and audio recordings, enhancing the professional and personal elements to be shared with others (Cope & Murray, 2018; Green et al., 2014; Willmarth-Stec & Beery, 2015).

Right from the beginning of their coursework in a CNL program, students should start collecting documents from assigned classroom activities and save examples of their writing and accomplishments. The examples become a tool kit that can be shared with prospective employers to demonstrate accomplishments shared on a résumé. The examples become the vehicle to communicate to a prospective employer that academic knowledge has been translated into meaningful actions and interventions that can be used to improve a microsystem. Upon graduation, the portfolio can be used to persuade an employer or supervisor that the CNL can enact AACN's CNL end-of-program competencies and CNL practice experiences (AACN, 2006, 2013) as evidence to support what is claimed on his or her résumé.

The portfolio presented at the fruition of a clinical immersion experience chronicles successful completion of the capstone project. The portfolio document for the clinical immersion includes a detailed plan that identifies the microsystem problem to be addressed, project objectives, deliverables, time lines, implementation of structured quality and process improvement tools, data, and measurement metrics. Less evident to an untrained eye are the redesign efforts undertaken to improve clinical outcomes of care for the population of the microsystem and the leadership efforts required to guide an interdisciplinary team to success.

Aside from the information related to the CNL's education, licensure, work experience, and certifications, additional tips for creating an effective paper portfolio design includes:

1. Creating a well-designed cover
2. Placing information behind tabs to organize the content
3. Using colorful charts or graphics to demonstrate impact or outcomes achieved
4. Examples that illustrate cost savings and innovations (Cope & Murray, 2018; Elbow & Belanoff, 1997; Green et al., 2014).

Performance Contracts

As CNLs graduate and accept positions, the performance contract is a common mechanism used to define the role expectations and markers of impact and success. The portfolio documentation serves as a quick reference to prospective employers about past performance—evidence that CNL performance has been demonstrated in the past and can be expected in the future. An example of a performance contract is shown in **Figure 10-2**.

Measurement of CNL Success

The challenge for the CNL student and those in practice is to design methods that measure impact and clinical outcomes that are sustainable. Nelson and colleagues (2007) stated that measurement is forward progress, and clinical leaders functioning within a microsystem must engage all staff to be innovative and creative and to participate in the improvement of healthcare delivery. Didactic coursework and clinical immersions must prepare the CNL student to understand and collaboratively develop measurement tools that are applicable to the practice environment. Within all microsystems are numerous data points waiting to be mined, analyzed,

Rating Period: _____ – _____

Name: _____ **Unit Assigned:** _____

Measure	Target	Comments from Quarterly Review
Infectious disease: Blood cultures collected before administration of first antibiotic	93%	
Immunizations: Patients received immunization during flu season (_____ – _____)	90%	
Evidence of satisfied inpatients during each stay	95% (6 months' post-introduction of the CNL)	

_____ / _____

Clinical Nurse Leader/Supervisor Signatures Date

Figure 10-2 CNL performance contract

and displayed. Creating an area to display data as a "data board" allows the CNL to visually demonstrate each metric for the members of the microsystem to observe. This is a key role for the CNL. One commonly cited barrier of CNLs is the lack of consistent and uninterrupted time to appraise literature and analyze data. When negotiating CNL roles and positions, persistent and deliberate attention must be paid to the generation and distribution of data to microsystem staff as a way to bring awareness to issues and visualize team success. Data should represent the current value or target and the impacts over a period of time. This information can drive clinical and quality improvements and identify other improvement projects that are necessary to meet organizational goals, regulatory requirements, and specific microsystem improvements that ultimately enhance quality and delivery of care.

But how does the CNL identify appropriate metrics? A starting point is to review unit goals, the population served, and the services provided. For example, a CNL assigned to a long-term care area may focus on increasing residents' functional status by measuring involvement in daily activities offered by staff. The CNL assigned to an ambulatory surgery unit can measure the number of cancellations and the financial impacts incurred by each cancellation. This can be further measured and trended by service or product. The information can then be used by the project improvement team to develop strategies and tactics to improve efficacy and efficiency. These are only two examples of the many projects CNLs can measure and have an impact on to enhance both financial and quality outcomes within a microsystem.

Summary

- CNL clinical experiences must be creatively developed, meaningful to the student, and add value for the organization.
- Multiple data and other resources are readily available for CNL students to access when developing a clinical immersion project.
- The business case for a CNL project must be supported by outcomes and evidence-based data.
- Portfolios of CNL projects can be of value to healthcare facilities for displaying quality outcomes and partnerships with academic affiliates, and to the CNL for applying for positions.
- A performance contact is a useful method for the CNL and the organization to track successes and identify opportunities for improvement.

Reflection Questions

1. What part of the clinical immersion project do you feel most prepared for? What part do you feel least prepared for?
2. What are the critical elements of a clinical immersion project?
3. What resources do you have to assist you in completing the clinical immersion?
4. What documents do you have that demonstrate your skills and accomplishments in the CNL role?

Learning Activities

1. Gather documents to create a professional portfolio. Consider how you will organize the information. Share your ideas and documents with a classmate and ask him or her to perform a peer review.
2. Form a group with two or three other students and brainstorm about assignments that have been completed that would be appropriate for inclusion in your portfolios.
3. Bring a project plan that you have completed for a past project to class. The project plan should include a time line with detailed action steps, contact persons/responsible parties, and deliverables. Describe how a project plan for your clinical immersion would be different from this previous project plan.

References

American Association of Colleges of Nursing. (2006, May). *End-of-program competencies & required clinical experiences for the Clinical Nurse Leader*. http://apps.aacn.nche.edu/CNL/pdf/EndCompsgrid.pdf

American Association of Colleges of Nursing. (2007). *White paper on the role of the clinical nurse leader*. http://www.aacn.nche.edu/publications/white-papers/cnl

American Association of Colleges of Nursing. (2011). *CNL job analysis study*. http://www.aacn.nche.edu/cnl/publications-resources/job-analysis-study

American Association of Colleges of Nursing. (2013). *Competencies and curricular expectations for Clinical Nurse Leader education and practice*. http://www.aacn.nche.edu/cnl/CNL-Competencies-October-2013.pdf

Billings, D., & Kowalski, K. (2008). Developing your career as a nurse educator: The professional portfolio. *Journal of Continuing Education in Nursing, 39*(12), 532–533.

Bombard, E., Chapman, K., Doyle, M., Wright, D., Shipee-Rice, R,. & Kasik., D. (2010). Answering the question, "What is a Clinical Nurse Leader?": Transition experience of four direct-entry master's students. *Journal of Professional Nursing, 26*(6), 332–340.

Bouchard, J., & Steel, M. (1980). Contract learning. *Canadian Nurse, 76*(1), 44–48.

Cebel, R., Rebitzer, J., & Taylor, R. (2006). Organizational fragmentation and care quality in the US health care system. *Journal of Economic Perspectives, 22*, 93–111.

Cope, V., & Murray, M. (2018). Use of professional portfolios in nursing. *Nursing Standard, 32*(30), 55. https://doi.org/10.7748/ns.2018.e10985

Dartmouth Institute. (2003). *Clinical microsystems assessment tool.* https://clinicalmicrosystem.org/uploads/documents/microsystem_assessment.pdf

Elbow, P., & Belanoff, P. (1997). Reflections on an explosion: Portfolios in the 90's and beyond. In K. Yancey & I. Weiser (Eds.), *Situating portfolios: Four perspectives* (pp. 21–33). Utah University Press.

Fletcher, K., & Meyer, M. (2016). Coaching model + clinical playbook = transformative learning, *Journal of Professional Nursing, 32*(2), 122–129. https://doi.org/10.1016/j.profnurs.2015.09.0001

Gerard, S., Grossman, S., & Godfrey, M. (2012). Course strategies for Clinical Nurse Leader development. *Journal of Professional Nursing, 28*(3), 147–155.

Green, J., Wyllie, A., & Jackson, D. (2014). Electronic portfolios in nursing education: A review of the literature. *Nurse Education in Practice, 14*(1), 4–8.

Hayes, C., & Graham, Y. (2019). Understanding the building of professional identities with the LEGO® SERIOUS PLAY® method using situational mapping and analysis. *Higher Education, Skills and Work-Based Learning, 9*(1), 99–112. https://doi.org/10.1108/heswbl-05-2019-0069

Hwang, J., & Christensen, C. M. (2008). Technology: New technologies demand new business models. In *Futurescan: Healthcare trends and implications 2008–2013.* Health Administration Press.

Jukkula, A., Greenwood, R., Mote, T., & Block, V. (2013). Creating innovative Clinical Nurse Leader practicum experiences through academic and practice partnerships, *Nursing Education Perspectives, 34*(2), 186–191.

Mezirow, J. (1997). Transformative learning: Theory to practice. *New Directions for Adult and Continuing Education, 74,* 5–12.

Mezirow, J. & Associates. (2000). *Learning as transformation: Critical perspectives on a theory in progress.* Jossey-Bass.

Morris, A. H., & Faulk, D. (2007). Perspective transformation: Enhancing the development of professionalism in the RN-to-BSN students. *Journal of Nursing Education, 46*(10), 445–461.

Nelson, E. C., Batalden, P. B., & Godfrey, M. M. (2007). *Quality by design. A clinical microsystems approach.* Jossey-Bass.

Porter-O'Grady, T., Clark, J. S., & Wiggins, M. (2010). The case for clinical nurse leaders: Guiding nursing practice into the 21st century. *Nurse Leader, 8,* 37–41.

Pourabdollahian, G. & Copani, G. (2014). Proposal of an innovative business model for customized production in healthcare. *Modern Economy, 5*(13), 1147–1160.

Rankin, V. (2015). Clinical Nurse Leader: A role for the 21st century. *Med-Surg Nursing, 24*(3), 198–201.

Sherrod, D. (2005). The professional portfolio: A snapshot of your career, Nursing Management, 36(9), 74–75

Stanley, J., Holing, J., Burton, D., Harris, J., & Norman, L. (2007). Implementing innovation through education practice partnerships. *Nursing Outlook, 55*(2), 67–73.

Thomas, P. (2018). Developing metrics that support project plans, interventions, and programs. In J. Harris, L. Roussel, C. Dearman, & P. Thomas, *Project planning and management: A guide for nurses and interprofessional teams* (3rd ed., pp. 193–220). Jones & Bartlett Learning.

Wassef, M., Riza, M., Maciag, T., & Delaney A. (2012). Implementing a competency-based electronic portfolio in a graduate nursing program. *Computers, Informatics, Nursing, 30*(5), 242–246.

Welton, J., & Harper, E. (2015). Nursing care value-based financial models. *Nursing Economics, 33*(1), 14–19, 25.

Willmarth-Stec, M., & Beery, T. (2015). Operationalizing the student electronic portfolio for doctoral nursing education. *Nurse Educator, 40*(5), 263–265.

EXEMPLAR

Identifying a Meaningful Immersion Project

David C. Mulkey

The most important decision for a CNL student is choosing an innovative and valuable immersion project. Successfully executing an immersion project begins with discovering a quality project idea that supports the organization's philosophy and vision. The first step in isolating a perfect project idea begins with a detailed and methodical needs assessment and gap analysis. Weekly meetings with senior leadership allow opportunities to discuss the findings from the assessment and gap analysis. For example, data revealed that first year turnover rate was severely greater for new graduate nurses. Asking the fundamental five *whys* in a root-cause analysis can reveal gaps in the current clinical orientation process for new graduate nurses, who need a structured orientation model that provides direction. Goal setting is used to provide the direction that new graduate nurses need to succeed. The CNL creates a sense of urgency with stakeholders to market the project idea. This sense of urgency is supported by project outcomes and evidence-based data. The project idea increases confidence and readiness for practice in the clinical setting. The project idea fosters a developed and meaningful experience for the CNL student while adding value to the organization.

EXEMPLAR

Selling Your Idea for a Clinical Project: The Steps and Process

David C. Mulkey

A challenging task for the CNL to accomplish is to gain buy-in from stakeholders on goal-directed clinical orientation for new graduate nurses. The CNL student should communicate the vision and use persuasion styles to gain staff engagement and satisfaction. To receive buy-in from stakeholders, the CNL student uses four simple steps in the art of effective persuasion: (a) survey the situation, (b) remove barriers, (c) make a pitch, and (d) secure commitments (Shell & Moussa, 2007). These steps allow stakeholders to have a clear understanding of the project idea, background, and gaps that were determined in a gap analysis of clinical orientation for new graduate nurses. To remove barriers, face-to-face meetings will build trusting relationships with stakeholders, instead of communicating via email or other electronic methods. The CNL student can make an extra effort to be friendly to those involved. During these meetings, a pitch for the project idea is made using data points for staff satisfaction, staff retention, and first-year turnover. These pressure points speak clearly to stakeholders that change is necessary. Last, before allowing stakeholders to leave, commitments should be established to support the change of clinical orientation. Following these steps successfully persuades stakeholders that change is necessary.

Reference

Shell, R., & Moussa, M. (2007). *The art of woo*. Penguin.

CHAPTER 11

Using Evidence to Guide CNL Project and Clinical Outcomes

Clista C. Clanton, Linda A. Roussel, and Patricia L. Thomas

LEARNING OBJECTIVES

1. Describe the CNL's role as an information and outcomes manager.
2. Identify the CNL's use of information systems and the technology and skills needed to synthesize data, information, and knowledge in evaluating and improving patient outcomes.
3. Discuss some of the core competencies that have been identified for the master's-prepared nurse for evidence-based practice.
4. Describe critical appraisal tools for evaluating quantitative and qualitative research evidence.
5. Discuss reference management software programs that are useful in the collection and organization of information sources and the formatting of in-text citations and bibliographies.

KEY TERMS

Core competencies for evidence-based practice
Critical appraisal tools

Evidence-based practice
Information management
Reference management

CNL ROLES

Client advocate
Clinician
Educator
Information manager

Lifelong learner
Member of a profession
Outcomes manager

CNL PROFESSIONAL VALUES

Accountability   Integrity
Genuineness

CNL CORE COMPETENCIES

Critical thinking   Nursing technology and resource
Information and healthcare   management
  technologies

Introduction

The first definition of EBM involved the integration of individual clinical expertise with the best available external clinical evidence from systematic research (Sackett et al., 1996), with later definitions including patient preference as part of the triad utilized in the decisions made regarding patient care. As EBM spread and was adopted by other healthcare disciplines, several notable EBP models, such as the ACE Star Model of Knowledge Transformation (Stevens, 2015), the Iowa Model-Revised (Iowa Model Collaborative, 2017), and the Johns Hopkins Nursing Evidence-Based Practice Model (Dang & Dearholt, 2017) evolved in nursing to help guide practice. Regardless of the model or approach used to implement research in practice, certain skills are necessary to locate, appraise, and use information. The CNL has been tasked with both an information management and outcomes manager role that requires using information systems and technology and synthesizing data and other evidence in order to evaluate and improve patient care processes and models of delivery (AACN, 2013). Developed by the AACN in 2000, the newness of the CNL role means that the number of published accounts of how CNLs approach or use evidence in their practice is limited. One doctor of nursing practice project did report that recent CNL program graduates with less than five years of nursing experience continued to use their CNL competencies as they gained experience in a clinical environment (Klich-Heartt, 2010). Encouragingly, over two-thirds ($n = 35$) of the survey respondents reported that they were able to assimilate research-based evidence to improve their unit outcomes. While there are several studies that emphasize the importance that CNLs place on their role in the implementation of evidence in their practice setting as well as studies that indicate improved quality outcomes after the introduction of the CNL in microsystems, there is still little known about the structures and processes that influence successful CNL integration or the components that facilitate or hinder successful CNL effectiveness and sustainability (Bender, 2014).

Given the limited published data on CNLs in practice when it comes to their role as information managers and evidence-based practitioners, we can also look at RNs, those in other advanced practice nursing roles, and hospitals with Magnet designation for examples of how nurses are adopting and using EBP. The picture that emerges from published studies is one of both individual and organizational barriers that hinder the effective adoption of EBP in clinical settings. Lack of time to conduct searches remains one of the most frequently cited individual barriers, followed by limited searching skills and problems with access to appropriate resources (Sadoughi et al., 2017). A large sample from 19 different hospitals or healthcare systems in the United States found that the nurses surveyed did not believe they were meeting established EBP competencies, and although nurses with advanced practice degrees rated themselves somewhat higher, they did not rate themselves as competent in any of the 24 competencies. There was also no difference in EBP competency ratings between nurses who worked in Magnet vs. non-Magnet hospitals in this study (Melnyk et al., 2018).

CNSs access written evidence from a variety of sources, most often using literature tailored to their specialty or clinical practice, clinical practice guidelines, internet use at work, nursing literature, and medical literature. However, at least one study showed that they "never to rarely" conducted their own computerized literature searches using databases. They also "never to rarely" used search services or librarians, nor did they use the affiliated libraries at their university, college, or health institution. Information is sought frequently from people-based evidence sources and include personal experience, what has worked for years, physicians, clinical experience on a previous or current unit, or other nurses working in their clinical setting (Profetto-McGrath et al., 2010).

Another study conducted in a critical care setting showed that nurses preferred information from colleagues over text and electronic information sources to support clinical decisions (Marshall et al., 2011). Relying on evidence from the research literature to support decisions in clinical practice was viewed as problematic by both the bedside and senior nurse clinicians. Reasons for this included the volume of available information and the expertise needed to locate and critically appraise research articles—classic obstacles that have been cited by health professionals for as long as implementing evidence into practice has been emphasized in healthcare (Cook et al., 1997; Sackett, 1997; Shorten & Wallace, 1997).

Nurses with the highest level of capability beliefs reported that they used research findings in clinical practice more than twice as often as those with lower levels of capability beliefs. They also participated in the implementation of evidence seven times more often (Wallin et al., 2012). Originating out of the social cognitive psychology field, capability beliefs are also known as self-efficacy beliefs; they have been defined as a person's belief in their ability to succeed in specific situations (Bandura, 1997). Self-efficacy is also linked to competency, as opposed to being an intrinsic individual characteristic. Given that EBP can be used as an approach to solving problems, a familiarity with and competence in the steps necessary to form clinical questions, searching for and appraising clinical evidence, and applying that evidence in the CNL's practice domain should reinforce feelings of self-efficacy and strengthen capability beliefs.

There are multiple core competencies that have been identified for both RNs and advanced practice nurses for evidence-based practice (Melnyk et al., 2018), and aspects of those that are integral to the CNL's information and outcomes manager roles include:

- Conduct searches for locating primary research studies in multiple databases
- From multiple sources, locate evidence summary reports for practice implications in the context of EBP
- Using existing standards, critically appraise evidence summaries for practice implications in the context of EBP

- Assemble evidence resources from multiple sources on selected topics into reference management software
- Assemble clinical practice guidelines from various sources

Given that one of the reasons for creating the CNL role was to promote patient safety, here is a core competency developed for patient safety research that elegantly summarizes some of the key elements of the EBP core competencies:

Able to find, appraise and synthesize the evidence, to translate research findings into concrete changes, to communicate effectively to a variety of audiences, to employ change management techniques, and to take a leadership role in promoting patient safety within an organization (Andermann et al., 2011).

EBP Core Competency: Systematically Conducts an Exhaustive Search for External Evidence to Answer Clinical Questions

There are many different information sources that can be used in EBP. The sheer volume can lead to a sense of frustration and uncertainty about which resource to use or an overdependence on resources that are familiar but not always appropriate. To efficiently retrieve high-quality evidence to support decisions, it is important to know what resource to use with different questions. A useful classification model for information sources is the 6S model, which arranges evidence sources into a six-layer pyramid (DiCenso et al., 2009). In the 6S model, the goal is to start with the highest level of information resources and work downward to locate evidence to answer questions. Higher-level databases consist of resources that have some type of value-added process included, such as critically appraised synopses of research by diseases or condition. These type of resources are designed to save time and help with the difficulty in accessing and assimilating large amounts of research findings from the primary journal literature, which are commonly cited obstacles to implementing EBP (Cook et al., 1997; Sackett, 1997). See **Figure 11-1** for a visual representation of the 6S model.

The lowest level of the 6S pyramid contains original studies from the journal literature, which are indexed in databases such as PubMed, Ovid MEDLINE, CINAHL, Scopus, and PsycINFO. These databases provide a way to do topic searches; each database has its own search interface, indexing or classification system, and ways to limit search results. Although search engines like Google are not listed in the 6S hierarchy of resources, it is naïve to think that Google or other internet search engines are not being used by health professionals when information is needed. Google does index PubMed, so it is possible to bring up pertinent health science–related articles when doing a topic search. Using Google Scholar (https://scholar.google.com/) is a better option for EBP information, as it weeds out nonscholarly content such as blogs, personal websites, and advertisements. If you do not know the URL for Google Scholar, the easiest way to locate it is to google it, as direct links to the Scholar version are not prominent among the Google suite of links for its products. A Google search for "clinical nurse leader evidence-based practice microsystem implementation" returned 629,000 hits, whereas Google Scholar

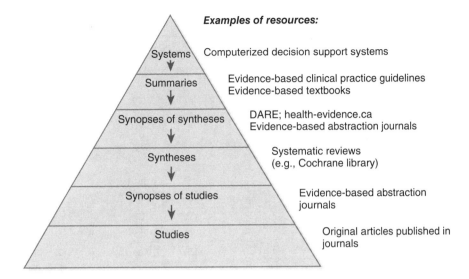

Figure 11-1 The 6S hierarchy of pre-appraised evidence

Reproduced from DiCenso, A., Bayley, L., & Haynes, R. B. (2009). Accessing pre-appraised evidence: Fine-tuning the 5S model into a 6S model. *Evidence Based Nursing, 12*(4), 99–101. https://doi.org/10.1136/ebn.12.4.99-b

returned 11,500. For focused searches that retrieve high-quality and relevant articles, citation databases such as PubMed, CINAHL, and Scopus are a better option due to their more sophisticated search and limitation capabilities. However, Google Scholar can be a good option to complement searches in citation databases, especially when comprehensiveness of the search is important. There is also the issue of access to the full text of journal articles to consider, although Google Scholar does have the capability to link out to the full text content of institutions via "Library links" in the Scholar Settings section.

EBP Core Competency: From Multiple Sources, Locate Evidence Summary Reports for Practice Implications in Context of EBP

Evidence summary reports are useful in that they can identify relevant research on a particular topic and usually include some sort of critical appraisal of the studies reviewed. In the 6S hierarchy of resources (DiCenso et al., 2009), evidence summaries are the second level of the pyramid, right under the systems level. Summaries draw from the lower level information sources such as systematic reviews and single research studies that are indexed in databases such as PubMed, CINAHL, and Scopus, but they then synthesize that information to provide a full range of evidence concerning the management of diseases or conditions. In this category, you find databases such as DynaMed, UpToDate, BMJ Best Practice, and clinical practice guidelines. Databases at this level are ideal for use at the point of care, as they are designed to locate the best available evidence quickly to inform patient care decisions. See **Table 11-1** for specific resources by category.

Table 11-1 6S Hierarchy of Information Resources

Haynes's Pyramid Levels	Free Resources	Subscription Resources
Systems	None	Institutional electronic health records with decision support link out to evidence-based resources

Summaries	ECRI Guidelines Trust
	guidelines.ecri.org
	Trip Database
	tripdatabase.com
		ACP PIER
		  aconline.org/clinical-information
		BMJ Best Practice
		  us.bestpractice.bmj.com/
		Clinical Evidence
		  bestpractice.bmj.com/info/evidence-information/
		Clinical Key
		  clinicalkey.com
		Clinical Key for Nursing
		  clinicalkey.com/nursing
		DynaMed
		  dynamed.com/home
		Joanna Briggs Institute EBPDatabase
		  know.lww.com/JBI-resources.html
		UpToDate
		  uptodate.com/home

Synopses of syntheses	Epistemonikos
	epistemonikos.org
		ACP Journal Club
		  acpjc.acponline.org
		Evidence-Based Nursing
		  ebn.bmj.com
		Evidence-Based Mental Health
		  ebmh.bmj.com
		Evidence-Based Medicine
		  ebm.bmj.com

Syntheses	AHRQ EPC Evidence-Based Reports ahrq.gov/research/findings/evidence-based-reports/index.html Epistemonikos epistemonikos.org Nursing + plus.mcmaster.ca/NP/ PubMed Clinical Queries for Systematic Reviews ncbi.nlm.nih.gov/pubmed/clinical TRIP Database tripdatabase.com/	Clinical Evidence clinicalevide nce.bmj.com Cochrane Database of Systematic Reviews cochranelibrary.com Joanna Briggs Institute EBP Database know.lww.com/JBI-resources.html
Synopses of single studies	Evidence Updates plus.mcmaster.ca/evidenceupdates/ PubMed Clinical Queries ncbi.nlm.nih.gov/pubmed/clinical TRIP Database tripdatabase.com	ACP Journal Club acpjc.acponline.org Evidence-based Nursing ebn.bmj.com Evidence-based Mental Health ebmh.bmj.com Evidence-based Medicine ebm.bmj.com
Studies	PubMed pubmed.ncbi.nlm.nih.gov TRIP Database tripdatabase.com Google Scholar scholar.google.com	CINAHL Plus Full Text ebscohost.com/nursing/products/cinahl-databases PsycINFO apa.org/pubs/databases/psycinfo Scopus scopus.com

EBP Core Competency: Using Existing Standards, Critically Appraise Evidence Summaries for Practice Implications in the Context

There are multiple resources available to aid in critically appraising the health science literature. The American Medical Association (AMA) has a comprehensive guide designed to help a scholar learn how to distinguish solid evidence, devise strong search strategies for clinical questions, critically appraise the medical literature, and then optimally apply that evidence-based information for patient care, which is called *The User's Guide to Medical Literature: A Manual for Evidence-Based Clinical Practice* (Guyatt et al., 2008). Originally published in the *Journal of the American Medical Association (JAMA)* as separate articles, they are now updated and compiled in a single edition. There is also "The How to Read a Paper" series, authored by Trisha Greenhalgh and published by the *British Medical Journal (BMJ)*, which explains how to read and interpret different kinds of research papers; the series includes helpful articles on topics such as statistics for the nonstatistician (Greenhalgh, n.d.).

There are also specific instruments and methods that have been developed to aid in critically appraising clinical practice guidelines, which are systematically developed statements that assist practitioners and patients in making decisions about appropriate healthcare for specific clinical circumstances (Grossman et al., 1990). The Appraisal of Guidelines Research and Evaluation II (AGREE II) instrument provides a framework to assess the quality of clinical practice guidelines, as well as providing a methodological strategy for developing guidelines and informing what information should be reported and how it should be reported. The AGREE II instrument replaces the original AGREE instrument, which was developed in 2003 by a group of international guideline developers and researchers (AGREE Collaboration, 2003). Composed of 23 items that cover six domains, AGREE II allows developers or reviewers a way to assign numeric values to a guideline's scope and purpose, stakeholder involvement, rigor of development, clarity of presentation, applicability, and editorial independence. Available in both print and electronic formats, AGREE II as well as training materials are available for use at www.agreetrust .org/agree-ii/.

The GuideLine Implementability Appraisal v.2.0 (GLIA) is another tool that can help those trying to implement guidelines to address identified barriers. The developers of GLIA define implementability as a set of characteristics that predict the relative ease of implementing guideline recommendations, and indicators of implementability focus on the ease and accuracy of translation of the guidelines into healthcare systems (Shiffman et al., 2005). The tool consists of 30 questions, and GLIA users should prepare to use the instrument by selecting those recommendations within a specific guideline for which implementation is planned. GLIA 2.0 is available in .pdf format at http://nutmeg.med.yale.edu/glia/login.htm, and a web-based version (eGLIA) is available by request.

The Grading of Recommendations Assessment, Development and Evaluation (GRADE) Working Group developed the GRADE approach to evaluate the quality of evidence and strength of recommendations for different types of evidence including evidence on intervention effects, test accuracy, prognosis, resources, and values and preference (Alonso-Coello et al., 2016). GRADE-CERQual can be used to assess the confidence in findings from qualitative data for systematic reviews of qualitative evidence. GRADE is currently used by over 100 organizations such as WHO and the Cochrane Collaboration, with many of these organizations having provided input into the development of the tool. Considered to be a standard in guideline development, GRADE provides an approach that assesses the certainty or quality of a body of evidence by outcome(s) while also providing an approach to moving evidence to a decision using Evidence to Decision (EtD) frameworks (Zhang et al., 2019). Reducing unnecessary confusion due to multiple systems for grading evidence and recommendations was another goal of the GRADE Working Group (www.gradeworkinggroup. org). Operational definitions used by the GRADE Working Group, consideration of domains that address certainty of evidence, the use of evidence summaries and decision criteria reinforce the strength of the evidence and add greater credibility to the evidence base supporting projects, and critical clinical decisions.

The Preferred Reporting Items for Systematic Reviews and Meta-Analyses (PRISMA) Statement, is an evidence-based minimum set of items for reporting in systematic reviews and meta-analyses (see **Table 11-2**). Although it was designed for developers, the 27-item checklist provides a comprehensive overview of items that are useful in evaluating systematic reviews and meta-analyses.

Going through the checklist to see if items are included or were reported correctly can help to determine the quality of the systematic review or meta-analysis if no other synopsis is available. More information and downloads are available at www.prisma-statement.org.

Table 11-2 Preferred Reporting Items for Systematic Reviews and Meta-Analyses (PRISMA)

Section/Topic	#	Checklist Item	Reported on Page #
TITLE			
Title	1	Identify the report as a systematic review, meta-analysis, or both.	
ABSTRACT			
Structured summary	2	Provide a structured summary including, as applicable: background; objectives; data sources; study eligibility criteria, participants, and interventions; study appraisal and synthesis methods; results; limitations; conclusions and implications of key findings; systematic review registration number.	
INTRODUCTION			
Rationale	3	Describe the rationale for the review in the context of what is already known.	

(continues)

Table 11-2 Preferred Reporting Items for Systematic Reviews
and Meta-Analyses (PRISMA)   *(continued)*

Section/Topic	#	Checklist Item	Reported on Page #
Objectives	4	Provide an explicit statement of questions being addressed with reference to participants, interventions, comparisons, outcomes, and study design (PICOS).	
METHODS			
Protocol and registration	5	Indicate if a review protocol exists, if and where it can be accessed (e.g., web address), and, if available, provide registration information including registration number.	
Eligibility criteria	6	Specify study characteristics (e.g., PICOS, length of follow-up) and report characteristics (e.g., years considered, language, publication status) used as criteria for eligibility, giving rationale.	
Information sources	7	Describe all information sources (e.g., databases with dates of coverage, contact with study authors to identify additional studies) in the search and date last searched.	
Search	8	Present full electronic search strategy for at least one database, including any limits used, such that it could be repeated.	
Study selection	9	State the process for selecting studies (e.g., screening, eligibility, included in systematic review, and, if applicable, included in the meta-analysis).	
Data collection process	10	Describe method of data extraction from reports (e.g., piloted forms, independently, in duplicate) and any processes for obtaining and confirming data from investigators.	
Data items	11	List and define all variables for which data were sought (e.g., PICOS, funding sources) and any assumptions and simplifications made.	
Risk of bias in individual studies	12	Describe methods used for assessing risk of bias of individual studies (including specification of whether this was done at the study or outcome level), and how this information is to be used in any data synthesis.	

Section/Topic	#	Checklist Item	Reported on Page #
Summary measures	13	State the principal summary measures (e.g., risk ratio, difference in means).	
Synthesis of results	14	Describe the methods of handling data and combining results of studies, if done, including measures of consistency (e.g., I2) for each meta-analysis.	
Risk of bias across studies	15	Specify any assessment of risk of bias that may affect the cumulative evidence (e.g., publication bias, selective reporting within studies).	
Additional analyses	16	Describe methods of additional analyses (e.g., sensitivity or subgroup analyses, meta-regression), if done, indicating which were prespecified.	
RESULTS			
Study selection	17	Give numbers of studies screened, assessed for eligibility, and included in the review, with reasons for exclusions at each stage, ideally with a flow diagram.	
Study characteristics	18	For each study, present characteristics for which data were extracted (e.g., study size, PICOS, follow-up period) and provide the citations.	
Risk of bias within studies	19	Present data on risk of bias of each study and, if available, any outcome level assessment (see Item 12).	
Results of individual studies	20	For all outcomes considered (benefits or harms), present, for each study: (a) simple summary data for each intervention group and (b) effect estimates and confidence intervals, ideally with a forest plot.	
Synthesis of results	21	Present results of each meta-analysis done, including confidence intervals and measures of consistency.	
Risk of bias across studies	22	Present results of any assessment of risk of bias across studies (see Item 15).	
Additional analysis	23	Give results of additional analyses, if done (e.g., sensitivity or subgroup analyses, meta-regression [see Item 16]).	

(continues)

Table 11-2 Preferred Reporting Items for Systematic Reviews and Meta-Analyses (PRISMA)   *(continued)*

Section/Topic	#	Checklist Item	Reported on Page #
DISCUSSION			
Summary of evidence	24	Summarize the main findings including the strength of evidence for each main outcome; consider their relevance to key groups (e.g., healthcare providers, users, and policy makers).	
Limitations	25	Discuss limitations at study and outcome level (e.g., risk of bias), and at review level (e.g., incomplete retrieval of identified research, reporting bias).	
Conclusions	26	Provide a general interpretation of the results in the context of other evidence and implications for future research.	
FUNDING			
Funding	27	Describe sources of funding for the systematic review and other support (e.g., supply of data); role of funders for the systematic review.	

Moher, D., Liberati, A., Tetzlaff, J., Altman, D. G., & The PRISMA Group. (2009). Preferred reporting items for systematic reviews and meta-analyses: The PRISMA statement. *PLoS Med, 6*(6), e1000097. https://doi.org/10.1371/journal.pmed1000097

For those in clinical practice who may want to carry out a more rapid appraisal of a systematic review, there is the 11-question Assessment of Multiple Systematic Reviews (AMSTAR; see **Table 11-3**). This validated tool was developed by building on empirical data collected from previously developed tools and expert opinion. It is designed to take about 15 minutes to administer and has good interrater reliability (Shea et al., 2009).

The tools mentioned thus far are for quantitative research, but what about tools that appraise qualitative research? When complex, multicomponent interventions are introduced into equally complex healthcare systems, both quantitative and qualitative research methods will be needed to effectively evaluate success (Berwick, 2008). Qualitative research is deeply rooted in descriptive modes of research and has the goal of uncovering truths that exist while developing an understanding of reality and how individuals perceive what is real (Williamson, 2009). Qualitative research serves as more of an umbrella term that covers different approaches arising out of the fields of anthropology, sociology, and psychology. Some of the commonly used study methods for health science research are ethnography, phenomenology, and grounded theory. Consequently, a consensus regarding quality criteria for qualitative research has yet to be determined. There are several published tools to help in critically appraising qualitative research (Duffy, 2005; Melnyk & Fineout-Overholt, 2011; Polit & Beck, 2011).

Table 11-3 The AMSTAR Measurement Tool

1. Was an "a priori" design provided? The research question and inclusion criteria should be established before the conduct of the review.	❏ Yes ❏ No ❏ Can't answer ❏ Not applicable
2. Was there duplicate study selection and data extraction? There should be at least two independent data extractors, and a consensus procedure for disagreements should be in place.	❏ Yes ❏ No ❏ Can't answer ❏ Not applicable
3. Was a comprehensive literature search performed? At least two electronic sources should be searched. The report must include years and databases used (e.g., Central, Embase, and MEDLINE). Key words and/or MESH terms must be stated, and where feasible, the search strategy should be provided. All searches should be supplemented by consulting current contents, reviews, textbooks, specialized registers, or experts in the field of study, and by reviewing the references in the studies found.	❏ Yes ❏ No ❏ Can't answer ❏ Not applicable
4. Was the status of publication (i.e., grey literature) used as an inclusion criterion? The authors should state that they searched for reports regardless of their publication type. The authors should state whether or not they excluded any reports (from the systematic review), based on their publication status, language, etc.	❏ Yes ❏ No ❏ Can't answer ❏ Not applicable
5. Was a list of studies (included and excluded) provided? A list of included and excluded studies should be provided.	❏ Yes ❏ No ❏ Can't answer ❏ Not applicable
6. Were the characteristics of the included studies provided? In an aggregated form, such as a table, data from the original studies should be provided on the participants, interventions, and outcomes. The ranges of characteristics in all the studies analyzed (e.g., age, race, sex, relevant socioeconomic data, disease status, duration, severity, or other diseases) should be reported.	❏ Yes ❏ No ❏ Can't answer ❏ Not applicable
7. Was the scientific quality of the included studies assessed and documented? "A priori" methods of assessment should be provided (e.g., for effectiveness studies if the author(s) chose to include only randomized, double-blind, placebo-controlled studies, or allocation concealment as inclusion criteria); for other types of studies alternative items will be relevant.	❏ Yes ❏ No ❏ Can't answer ❏ Not applicable
8. Was the scientific quality of the included studies used appropriately in formulating conclusions? The results of the methodological rigor and scientific quality should be considered in the analysis and the conclusions of the review and explicitly stated in formulating recommendations.	❏ Yes ❏ No ❏ Can't answer ❏ Not applicable

(continues)

Table 11-3 The AMSTAR Measurement Tool *(continued)*

9. Were the methods used to combine the findings of studies appropriate? For the pooled results, a test should be done to ensure the studies were combinable, to assess their homogeneity (i.e., Chi-squared test for homogeneity, I2). If heterogeneity exists, a random effects model should be used and/or the clinical appropriateness of combining should be taken into consideration (i.e., is it sensible to combine?).	❑ Yes ❑ No ❑ Can't answer ❑ Not applicable
10. Was the likelihood of publication bias assessed? An assessment of publication bias should include a combination of graphical aids (e.g., funnel plot, other available tests) and/or statistical tests (e.g., Egger's regression test).	❑ Yes ❑ No ❑ Can't answer ❑ Not applicable
11. Was the conflict of interest stated? Potential sources of support should be clearly acknowledged in both the systematic review and the included studies.	❑ Yes ❑ No ❑ Can't answer ❑ Not applicable

Reprinted from Shea, B. J., Hamel, C., Wells, G. A., Bouter, L. M., Kristjansson, E., Grimshaw, J., & Boers, M. (2009). AMSTAR is a reliable and valid measurement tool to assess the methodological quality of systematic reviews. *Journal of Clinical Epidemiology, 62*(10), 1013–1020. https://doi.org/10.1016/j.jclinepi.2008.10.009. Used with permission from Elsevier.

In addition, a recent literature review identified six questions to help guide the evaluation of qualitative research articles (Jeanfreau & Jack, 2010):

1. Did the qualitative research describe an important practice-related problem addressed in a clearly formulated research question?
2. Was the qualitative approach appropriate?
3. How were the participants selected?
4. What were the researchers' roles in conducting the study, and have they been taken into account?
5. What methods did the researcher use for collecting data, and are they described in appropriate detail?
6. What methods did the researcher use to analyze the data, and what measures were used to ensure that scientific rigor was maintained?

EBP Competency: Assemble Evidence Resources from Multiple Sources on Selected Topics into Reference Management Software

Early in the evidence-based movement, competencies regarding the management of information were being discussed and recommendations made. All professional decision-makers should have a system for storing the knowledge and evidence that is essential to their practice in a way that can be retrieved whatever the reason for the search; they should:

- Have, or have access to, a computerized reference management system
- Be able to input individual records to that system
- Be able to download the results of a search to their system
- Be able to perform searches on their system using more than one search item (Gray, 1997, p. 67)

When selecting a reference manager, the following functions should be supported (Gilmour & Cobus-Kuo, 2011, para. 2):

1. Import citations from bibliographic databases and websites
2. Gather metadata from PDF files
3. Allow organization of citations within the reference manager database
4. Allow annotation of citations
5. Allow sharing of the reference manager database or portions thereof with colleagues
6. Allow data interchange with other reference manager products through standard metadata formats (e.g., RIS, BibTeX)
7. Produce formatted citations in a variety of styles
8. Work with word processing software to facilitate in-text citation

While there are for-fee and free versions of reference management software, the choice of which one to use really depends on the needs of the user. RefWorks, Zotero, Mendeley, EndNote Basic, and EndNote Desktop are some common examples of reference managers, but there are others available. Some important considerations when choosing a package should include computer/device compatibility, ability to search external databases, citation styles supported, ability to collaborate with others, and compatibility with other software systems such as word processors or those that support systematic review development.

Regardless of which reference management option chosen, perhaps one of the more important things to emphasize is to use the software from the beginning of the information-gathering phase, because doing so will allow for organizing information into collections that can be easily accessed when the information needs to be used or formatted into some sort of finished product.

Summary

- Good information management skills are integral to implementing evidence in practice. The ability to locate relevant research to answer clinical questions and other information needs involves knowing what information resources will best answer your questions quickly and efficiently.
- Using higher level information resources that contain critically appraised summaries is ideal, but when the answers are not located in those resources, understanding what tools are available to help in the critical appraisal process of individual research studies, systematic reviews, meta-analyses, and clinical practice guidelines will be necessary.
- Organizing that information so that it is easily managed and accessible will also help to save time and allow for the sharing and dissemination of information among colleagues.
- Strengthening skills in these information management core competency areas will then ideally lead to stronger feelings of self-efficacy and capability beliefs, resulting in the better implementation of evidence from the research into practice.

Reflection Questions

1. What is the role of the CNL in information and outcomes management?
2. How does the CNL use information systems, technology, and skills to synthesize data, information, and knowledge in evaluating and improving patient outcomes?
3. What are the core competencies that have been identified for the master's-prepared nurse for evidence-based practice?

Learning Activities

1. With a group of peers (e.g., classmates, fellow nurses) select a systematic review and critically appraise the research evidence using one of the tools described in this chapter.
2. Select evidence-based guidelines (e.g., ECRI Guidelines Trust), and with your peers, critically appraise them.

References

AGREE Collaboration. (2003). Development and validation of an international appraisal instrument for assessing the quality of clinical practice guidelines: The AGREE project. *Quality & Safety in Health Care, 12*(1), 18–23.

Alonso-Coello, P., Oxman, A. D., Moberg, J., Brignardello-Petersen, R., Akl, E. A., Davoli, M., Treweek, S., Mustafa, R. A., Vandvik, P. O., Meerpohl, J., Guyatt, G. H., Schünemann, H. J., & GRADE Working Group. (2016). GRADE Evidence to Decision (EtD) frameworks: A systematic and transparent approach to making well informed healthcare choices. 2: Clinical practice guidelines. *BMJ, 353*. https://doi.org/10.1136/bmj.i2089

American Association of Colleges of Nursing. (2007). *White paper on the role of the clinical nurse leader*. http://www.aacn.nche.edu/publications/white-papers/cnl

Andermann, A., Ginsburg, L., Norton, P., Arora, N., Bates, D., Wu, A., & Larizgoitia, I. (2011). Core competencies for patient safety research: A cornerstone for global capacity strengthening. *BMJ Quality & Safety in Health Care, 20*(1), 96–101. https://doi.org/10.1136/bmjqs.2010.041814

Bandura, A. (1997). *Self-efficacy: The exercise of control*. Macmillan Publishers.

Bender, M. (2014). The Current Evidence Base for the Clinical Nurse Leader: A Narrative Review of the Literature. *Journal of Professional Nursing, 30*(2), 110–123. https://doi.org/10.1016/j.profnurs.2013.08.006

Berwick, D. M. (2008). The science of improvement. *Journal of the American Medical Association, 299*(10), 1182–1184. https://doi.org/10.1001/jama.299.10.1182

Cook, D. J., Mulrow, C. D., & Haynes, R. B. (1997). Systematic reviews: Synthesis of best evidence for clinical decisions. *Annals of Internal Medicine, 126*(5), 376–380. https://doi.org/10.7326/0003-4819-126-5-199703010-00006

Dang, D., & Dearholt, S. (2017). *Johns Hopkins nursing evidence-based practice: Models and guidelines*. Sigma Theta Tau International.

DiCenso, A., Bayley, L., & Haynes, R. B. (2009). Accessing pre-appraised evidence: Fine-tuning the 5S model into a 6S model. *Evidence Based Nursing, 12*(4), 99–101. https://doi.org/10.1136/ebn.12.4.99-b

Duffy, J. R. (2005). Critically appraising quantitative research. *Nursing & Health Sciences, 7*, 281–283. https://doi.org/10.1111/j.1442-2018.2005.00248.x

Gilmour, R., & Cobus-Kuo, L. (2011). Reference management software: A comparative analysis of four products. *Issues in Science and Technology Librarianship*. https://doi.org/10.5062/F4Z60KZF

GRADE. (2019). *What is GRADE?* https://www.gradeworkinggroup.org/

Gray, J. A. (1997). Evidence-based public health—what level of competence is required? *Journal of Public Health Medicine, 19*(1), 65–68.

Greenhalgh, T. (n.d.). *How to read a paper*. BMJ. http://www.bmj.com/about-bmj/resources-readers/publications/how-read-paper

Grossman, J. H., Field, M. J., & Lohr, K. N. (Eds.). (1990). Committee to advise the public health service on clinical practice guidelines, *Institute of Medicine. Clinical practice guidelines: Directions for a new program*. National Academies Press.

Guyatt, G., Rennie, D., Meade, M., & Cook, D. (2008). *Users' guides to the medical literature: Essentials of evidence-based clinical practice* (2nd ed.). McGraw-Hill Professional.

Iowa Model Collaborative. (2017). Iowa model of evidence-based practice: Revisions and validation. *Worldviews on Evidence-Based Nursing, 175–182.* https://doi.org/10.1111/wvn.12223

Jeanfreau, S. G., & Jack, L., Jr. (2010). Appraising qualitative research in health education: Guidelines for public health educators. *Health Promotion Practice, 11*(5), 612–617. https://doi.org/10.1177/1524839910363537

Klich-Heartt, E. (2010). *Entry-level clinical nurse leader: Evaluation of practice. Doctor of nursing practice (DNP) projects*. http://repository.usfca.edu/dnp/5

Liberati, A., Altman, D. G., Tetzlaff, J., Mulrow, C., Gøtzsche, P. C., Ioannidis, J. P. A., Clark, M., Devereaux, P. J., Kleijnen, J., & Moher, D. (2009). The PRISMA statement for reporting systematic reviews and meta-analyses of studies that evaluate health care interventions: Explanation and elaboration. *Annals of Internal Medicine, 151*(4), W–65. https://doi.org/10.7326/0003-4819-151-4-200908180-00136

Marshall, A. P., West, S. H., & Aitken, L. M. (2011). Preferred information sources for clinical decision making: Critical care nurses' perceptions of information accessibility and usefulness. *Worldviews on Evidence-Based Nursing, 8*(4), 224–235. https://doi.org/10.1111/j.1741-6787.2011.00221.x

Melnyk, B. M., & Fineout-Overholt, E. (2011). *Evidence-based practice in nursing and healthcare* (2nd ed.). Wolters Kluwer Lippincott Williams, Wilkins.

Melnyk, B. M., Gallagher-Ford, L., Zellefrow, C., Tucker, S., Thomas, B., Sinnott, L. T., & Tan, A. (2018). The first U.S. Study on nurses' evidence-based practice competencies indicates major deficits that threaten healthcare quality, safety, and patient outcomes. *Worldviews on Evidence-Based Nursing, 15*(1), 16–25. https://doi.org/10.1111/wvn.12269

Moher, D., Liberati, A., Tetzlaff, J., Altman. D. G., & The PRISMA Group. (2009). Preferred reporting items for systematic reviews and meta-analyses: The PRISMA statement. *PLoS Med, 6*(6), e1000097. https://doi.org/10.1371/journal.pmed1000097

Polit, D. F., & Beck, C. T. (2011). *Nursing research: Generating and assessing evidence for nursing practice*. Wolters Kluwer; Lippincott Williams, Wilkins.

Profetto-McGrath, J., Negrin, K. A., Hugo, K., & Smith, K. B. (2010). Clinical nurse specialists' approaches in selecting and using evidence to improve practice. *Worldviews on Evidence-Based Nursing, 7*(1), 36–50. https://doi.org/10.1111/j.1741-6787.2009.00164.x

Sackett, D. L. (1997). *Evidence-based medicine: How to practice and teach EBM*. Churchill Livingstone.

Sackett, D. L., Rosenberg, W. M., Gray, J. A., Haynes, R. B., & Richardson, W. S. (1996). Evidence based medicine: What it is and what it isn't. *British Medical Journal, 312*(7023), 71–72.

Sadoughi, F., Azadi, T., & Azadi, T. (2017). Barriers to using electronic evidence-based literature in nursing practice: A systematized review. *Health Information & Libraries Journal, 34*(3), 187–199. https://doi.org/10.1111/hir.12186

Shea, B. J., Hamel, C., Wells, G. A., Bouter, L. M., Kristjansson, E., Grimshaw, J., Henry, D. A., & Boers, M. (2009). AMSTAR is a reliable and valid measurement tool to assess the methodological quality of systematic reviews. *Journal of Clinical Epidemiology, 62*(10), 1013–1020. https://doi.org/10.1016/j.jclinepi.2008.10.009

Shiffman, R. N., Dixon, J., Brandt, C., Essaihi, A., Hsiao, A., Michel, G., & O'Connell, R. (2005). The GuideLine Implementability Appraisal (GLIA): Development of an instrument to identify obstacles to guideline implementation. *BMC Medical Informatics & Decision Making, 5*(1), 23–28.

Shorten, A., & Wallace, M. (1997). Evidence-based practice. When quality counts. *Australian Nursing Journal, 4*(11), 26–27.

Stevens, K. R. (2015). *Stevens Star Model of EBP: Knowledge Transformation*. San Antonio Academic Center for Evidence-based Practice (ACE), University of Texas Health Science Center, San Antonio. https://www.uthscsa.edu/academics/nursing/star-model.

Titler, M. (2007). Translating research into practice. *American Journal of Nursing, 107*(Suppl), 26–33. https://doi.org/10.1097/01.NAJ.0000277823.51806.10

Wallin, L., Boström, A. M., & Gustavsson, J. P. (2012). Capability beliefs regarding evidence-based practice are associated with application of EBP and research use: Validation of a new measure. *Worldviews on Evidence-Based Nursing, 9*(3), 139–148. https://doi.org/10.1111/j.1741-6787.2012.00248.x

Williamson, K. M. (2009). Evidence-based practice: Critical appraisal of qualitative evidence. *Journal of the American Psychiatric Nurses Association, 15*(3), 202–207. https://doi.org/10.1177/1078390309338733

Zhang, Y., Akl, E. A., & Schünemann, H. J. (2019). Using systematic reviews in guideline development: The GRADE approach. *Research Synthesis Methods, 10*(3), 312–329. https://doi.org/10.1002/jrsm.1313

EXEMPLAR

Using Evidence to Implement a Cost-Savings Initiative

David Wolf

The director of nursing (and liaison for the CNL team) at Texas Health Plano encouraged the CNL team to share cost-savings ideas with our unit managers that we could implement at our facility. Nurses were observed removing the thigh-high portion of the sleeves because patients were often uncomfortable in the thigh-high sequential compression devices (SCDs) sleeves. A proposal was submitted, by the CNL, to eliminate thigh-high SCDs in favor of knee-high SCDs at the facility.

This proposal was based on a best practice from another in our system that had already switched over from thigh-high to knee-high SCDs. A cost savings was associated with the switch (D. Banks, personal communication, July 2014). Research showed that knee-high SCDs were as effective as thigh-high SCDs, and patients were more compliant in wearing knee-high SCDs than thigh-high SCDs, thus further enhancing their effectiveness in preventing blood clots (Brady et al., 2007). Another study by Williams et al. (1996) showed that "compression of the thigh as well as the calf does not give extra benefit" (p. 1553). The unit manager agreed that this was a good practice change, and he submitted the idea to the hospital system. Texas Health Resources adopted the practice change at their 14 hospitals, and the associated cost savings was $1 million per year (B. Berdan, personal communication, December 17, 2015).

This is a value-added contribution by CNLs where scholarship is translated and integrated into practice. Additionally, multiple examples of organizational and systems leadership are evident directed at cost-effective care across the healthcare continuum.

References

Brady, D., Raingruber, B., Peterson, J., Varnau, W., Denman, J., Resuello, R., & De Contreaus, R., & Mahnke, J. (2007). The use of knee-length versus thigh-length compression stockings and sequential compression devices. *Critical Care Nursing Quarterly, 30*(3), 255–262.

Williams, A. M., Davies, P. R., Sweetnam, D. I., Harper, G., Pusey, R., & Lightowler, C. D. (1996). Knee-length versus thigh-length graduated compression stockings in the prevention of deep vein thrombosis. *British Journal of Surgery, 83*(11), 1553.

Changing Practice in Monitoring Arterial Sheaths in Patients Undergoing Percutaneous Coronary Interventions: Evidence-Based Practice

Gabriela Whitener

The CNL student introduced an evidence-based protocol for percutaneous cardiac intervention (PCI) to improve safe patient monitoring after a cardiac intervention. The new protocol aim was to improve the patient's recovery experience, to increase nursing satisfaction, and to reduce cost. The CNL initially completed a literature review that revealed a new procedure for arterial sheath monitoring post-procedure. Initially, the patient's arterial sheaths were left in place for extended periods of time and were connected using a transducer to monitor blood pressure and line patency. Medical practice has advanced and the use of platelet-inhibiting medication like bivalirudin (Angiomax), allows for timely sheaths removal within two to four hours. A further literature review revealed evidence-based data and new current standards of practice from AACN. The patients are recovered post-procedure and have their sheaths removed either in the Cardiac Catheterization Lab or Cardiac Step-Down Unit.

The CNL, in collaboration with the cath lab nurses, developed a protocol that evaluated whether capping the arterial sheaths after PCI in stable patients, without complications, increases the occurrence of complications such as bleeding, hematoma, and clot formation. The scope in practice change was to improve the patient's post-catheter recovery and to improve nursing satisfaction by reducing the training and energy required to set up and monitor an arterial line. The project included financial savings consisting of materials and nursing time. The intervention cardiology group agreed to participate. The project was presented at Unit Based Council and the staff meeting. The hospital nurse scientist reviewed the project protocol and the literature review to meet the EBP standards. The staff on both units received detailed information about the procedure and was educated about the project to ensure a high probability of success. The physicians evaluated each case and gave selective orders for monitoring arterial sheaths. The method consisted in monitoring post-PCI patient's vital signs using conventional noninvasive procedures and assessing the patients following patient assessment standards. This applied to stable patients, without complications, who would have their femoral arterial sheath removed in less than two hours. As a result, the uncomplicated patients had their arterial sheaths capped and pulled within two hours or less of the procedure time. After implementation, data was collected to determine the number of patients who had their sheaths capped and if any complications occurred.

During the project pilot time, the patients transferred from the Cardiac Cath Lab to the CSU unit for monitoring had their arterial sheaths capped (a 10-cc syringe with normal saline). This was a physician-accepted procedure. Within two hours of the intervention, the RN removed the sheath. No complications were encountered. The results were presented to the Cardiovascular Performance

Improvement Committee and the cardiology physician groups, who approved the change in practice. The information was disseminated to the Cath lab and CSU. Subsequently, the IT department met with representatives from nursing and cardiac administrative groups who agreed to make changes to the order sets that would reflect the new protocol. The patients who were unstable and/or had multiple comorbidities continued to be monitored post-intervention using the monitoring transducer setup. A cost-benefit analysis reveals financial savings for materials $34.88 and $112 for nursing time. The project was piloted for a month, and the cost-benefit analysis revealed $4,406.40 savings. Patient satisfaction was monitored using a patient's survey. The HCAPS score increased because of the change in practice. The nursing time saved for setting up the transducer was estimated by live monitoring the procedure. The transducer setup requires 9 minutes for an experienced RN, versus a novice RN (six months or less nursing experience) who requires 18 minutes.

The project is an example of the CNL's role as a system analyst, outcomes manager, information manager, and educator who reviewed the literature and improved the quality of nursing care delivered using EBP best practice concepts in clinical practice. Improving the patient experience and reducing the recovery time post-PCI intervention is consistent with the CNL patient advocate role.

EXEMPLAR

Utilizing Research to Improve Patient Outcomes and Decrease Length of Stay

Melanie Hanes

The facility recently received a Level II trauma certification. Shortly thereafter we received a female patient into the ICU who had jumped from a moving vehicle, suffering a traumatic brain injury (TBI). The patient was medically stabilized within three days, but her behavior continued to be erratic, aggressive, and impulsive. It was determined that she likely had an underlying psychiatric issue and a definitive substance abuse problem.

Her behavior continued to deteriorate, necessitating four-point restraints, as well as IV and oral antipsychotic agents. She was assigned 1:1 nursing care, yet continued to chew her way out of restraints, climb from the bed, and physically assault staff. This case frustrated the care team on many levels. Staff and management were weary of the physical abuse, and physicians were frustrated over the barrage of phone calls seeking assistance for behavior control. It quickly became apparent that as a new trauma service, the complex behavior issues that a complicated TBI patient presented were beyond our scope of experience. Eventually, the patient became so weak and confused that she could no longer make it to the toilet, eat in a chair at the bedside, or remember the names of her two small children.

The patient did not qualify for a higher level of care, a neurological rehab, and could not qualify for a psychiatric facility due to her TBI. Three referrals to the staff psychiatrist yielded three changes in the medication regimen and no change in behavior. Staff continued to be assaulted, and the patient remained in four-point restraints for over two weeks. Over the coming weekend, the CNL student began researching TBI, focusing on the care of young TBI patients, with substance abuse issues. This research yielded a surprising result—utilizing muscle relaxants in the place of antipsychotics had proven to be effective in TBI patients with substance abuse histories, in particular very young patients had exaggeratedly positive outcomes.

The following Monday, admission day 15, a new intensivist began overseeing the patient. He was approached with the "plan" and quickly jumped on board with a "what do we have to lose" attitude. All benzodiazepines and antipsychotics were discontinued in favor of scheduled muscle relaxants, the patient was moved to the end of a hallway, tape was placed on the floor to create boundaries, and free access was given to a shower and refrigerator. The goal was to remove the restraints, not approach the patient in any physically aggressive way, offer hugs routinely for a physical connection, encourage mobilization ad lib to regain lost strength, independently perform personal hygiene, and allow the brain to calibrate to its new normal. Admission day 16, the restraints were removed. Admission day 17, the patient was sitting at the nurse's station attempting to type on the computer and answer phone calls. Admission day 18, she asked for her children by name and was eager for a visit. Admission day 19, she knew her name, birth date, and where she was for the first time since the accident. On admission day 24, she left the ICU alert, smiling, and excited to go to neuro rehab.

Detailed TBI and substance abuse–specific research into multiple facets yielded remarkable results. Positive behavioral changes began within 24 hours after stopping antipsychotics, and removing physical boundaries allowed the patient to recalibrate at her own pace, likely cutting the length of stay by half.

This case example clearly illustrates the value of translating and integrating scholarship into practice. More specifically, two CNL competencies are evident, including: (1) facilitate practice change based on best available evidence that results in quality, safety, and fiscally responsible outcomes and (2) design care based on outcome analysis and evidence to promote safe, timely, effective, efficient, equitable, and patient-centered care.

EXEMPLAR

Improving Patient Medication Education Using EBP

Gabriela Whitener

On a 23-bed Cardiac Step-Down Unit, the CNL completed a microsystem assessment and diagnosed a nursing communication gap. EBP suggests that nurses should use every opportunity to educate the patients about their medications, who in return will be able to adhere to the treatment plan and remain in the community, thus reducing hospital readmission rates. The CNL developed a project to improve patient medication education that allows the nurses to address medication indications, doses, side effects, and compliance. The project consisted of dissemination of education materials for each patient, who received an individualized orange folder containing approved medication education information handouts. The CNL identified the caretaker, who would benefit from medication education, helping the patient after the hospital discharge. The nurses provided medication teaching during the med pass using the "teach-back" method, which has a dual benefit of allowing for the patient's health literacy-level evaluation and his or her knowledge about the medication prescribed (Tamura-Lis, 2013). Med passes, direct observations, and chart reviews helped demonstrate consistent and sustained teaching behaviors.

The CNL project success was evaluated using monthly patient satisfaction scores reflected by HCAHPS that were communicated to the staff. HCAHPS scores above 75 percentiles are directly correlated with project sustainability. Two months after the project implementation, the unit scores were in the 91 percentiles.

Reference

Tamura-Lis, W. (2013). Teach-back for quality education and patient safety. *Urology Series*, *33*(6), 267–271. https://doi.org/10.7257/1053-816X.2013.33.6.267

EXEMPLAR

Using Evidence to Guide Practice and Sustain Outcomes: Translating and Integrating Scholarship into Practice

Elizabeth Triezenberg

The orthopedic quality outcome team had a discussion on time of Foley catheter discontinuation following total joint replacement surgery. Earlier removal of the catheter reduces the risk of developing a CAUTI, increases ambulation, and allows for earlier assessment and intervention of postoperative urinary retention. The CNL suggested the electronic medical record (EMR) power plans be modified to direct Foley removal the evening of surgery rather than the current practice of removal the morning after surgery. The CNL further explained that the orthopedic literature and discussions at the National Association of Orthopedic Nurses (NAON) suggest avoiding the use of catheters all together for patients having total joint replacement. Several programs around the country had started trialing catheter-free total joint replacement and were having success. A short discussion followed and the power plan was changed for earlier catheter removal and approved for implementation. The CNL continued the monthly audit for time of catheter removal.

Within a month the audit showed a startling trend. One specific surgeon's patient was no longer having a catheter placed for surgery. When I approached the surgeon, he commented, "Well, you told me it was reasonable not to place the catheter, so I stopped." Randomized pre- and post-intervention data showed an almost 80% decrease in catheter days. A patient without a catheter does not develop a CAUTI!

Using Evidence to Improve Acute Delirium Interventions

Libby Skaggs

Acute delirium is an enormous problem in hospitals. Length of stay is prolonged due to agitation, stress chemicals, use of restraints, and impaired mobility. Nurses are not well educated on the safest interventions of acute delirium and may resort to interventions that can cause more harm, like restraints, for example. In the high acuity progressive care cardiac unit, the nurse manager, the shift supervisors, and the CNL student have been promoting implementation of EBPs in acute delirium for the last year.

An elderly male patient was transferred during the night to progressive care from an orthopedic floor. Originally, he had been admitted after a fall at work and had been to surgery for an open reduction internal fixation (ORIF) two days prior. He had become increasingly agitated, was confused and combative, and had decompensated clinically. His heart rate was high and exhibited tachypnea. Confusion Assessment Method—Non-ICU was positive the day before. The patient moved to progressive care during the middle of the night. The CNL student prepared for multidisciplinary briefings by reviewing patient charts at 6 a.m. The patient had been given sedatives multiple times for agitation and narcotics for pain control. He was in bilateral wrist restraints and still had his urinary catheter from surgery. He was clearly suffering from acute delirium. The CNL student wrote a clinician sticky note in the EHR that was viewable by all staff. The note said, "Acute delirium interventions: keep shades open for sunlight, avoid narcotics, and sedatives (including Benadryl), avoid restraints, seek removal of urinary catheter as soon as possible, keep out of bed." When the CNL student arrived to the unit later that morning, the day shift charge nurse and primary RN had the patient up in the chair at the door of the room for close monitoring. His restraints were off, and he had a weight-sensitive alarm under his bottom for extra falls protection. The primary RN removed the urinary catheter a bit later that morning. He was still very confused and impulsive. An order was obtained from the physician for a sitter to be assigned to sit with him. The nursing supervisor implemented the sitter, but no one was available for a few hours. Several staff members, including the patient care technician, the primary RN, the charge nurse, and the CNL student, took turns sitting next to him to keep close watch. During multidisciplinary briefings at 10 a.m., his needs were discussed, and staff was alerted to be aware of his high risk for falls. Gradually his mentation cleared. When he had poor urine output that afternoon, the nurses prompted him to drink water. They used a bladder scanner to check for retention. Another urinary catheter was never needed. The staff kept him awake and out of bed all day and the shades open. The next day, he was oriented and near baseline. Two days later, he was transferred to the orthopedic floor calm and oriented. He went to rehab upon discharge. This example demonstrates how powerful a multidisciplinary approach is for patient progression through the healthcare continuum.

CHAPTER 12

Using Project Management Basics for Sustained Improvement

Patricia L. Thomas

LEARNING OBJECTIVES

1. Identify project management tools for design, implementation, and evaluation.
2. Explore the role of the CNL in project management.
3. Describe elements of a microsystem assessment and SWOT analysis and how they fit with project management.
4. Illustrate alignment between problem identification, design, data collection, and evaluation.

KEY TERMS

Assessment	Quality improvement
Design	Rapid cycle change
Evaluation	Stakeholders
Evidence-based practice	Sustainability Value
Project management	

CNL ROLES

Horizontal leader	Risk anticipator
Information manager	Systems analyst
Outcomes manager	Team manager

CNL PROFESSIONAL VALUES

Accountability	Stewardship
Integrity	

CNL COMPETENCIES

Clinical and horizontal leadership	Outcomes manager
Designer and coordinator of care	Quality improvement and safety
Evidence-based practice	Systems thinking
Interprofessional team collaboration	Technology and informatics

Introduction

Batalden and Davidoff (2016) define quality improvement as: "the combined and unceasing efforts of everyone—healthcare professionals, patients and their families, researchers, payers, planners and educators—to make the changes that will lead to better patient outcomes (health), better system performance (care) and better professional development (learning)" (p. 2). Clinical microsystem research began in 2000 that emerged from studies of high-performing systems (Donaldson & Mohr, 2000). The significance for microsystem thinking and performance in the US healthcare system was highlighted by Berwick (2001), when sequential and interactive elements that needed to link together for high-quality care to be delivered was suggested. The patient and community as the primary unit interfaces with the microsystem of care delivery, which interacts with the macrosystem and functions in an environmental context. The microsystem is the essential block at the point that care delivery must work to improve the quality of the process outcomes (work of the professionals). The process can be complex, *but the purpose is the project that will change as the need to improve performance changes* (Gill & Mountford, 2012). Continuous quality improvement is the vehicle that helps organizations improve quality and safety, as discussed in Chapter 4.

Project management, defined by the Project Management Institute, is the "application of knowledge, skills, tools, and techniques to project activities to meet project requirements. Project management is accomplished through the application and integration of the process management process of initiating, planning, executing, monitoring and controlling, and closing" (Project Management Institute, 2013, p. 6). In addition to a detailed plan and schedule, project management combines tools, people, and systems to achieve defined goals (Harris, 2016).

Central to any practice, process, or project change is a team charter. This document establishes:

- Aim of the project
- Scope of the project
- Goals and objectives
- Team members and stakeholders
- Executive sponsors
- Specific clinical, financial, or organizational problem being addressed
- Ground rules and agreements about team behaviors, accountability, and conflict resolution
- Data collection, monitoring, and evaluation
- Quality improvement strategies (PDSA, QI tools)
- Expected outcomes (Digital Project Manager, n.d.; Harris, 2016).

CNLs are positioned in microsystems and act as leaders of teams who often identify process or system concerns. Through work with interdisciplinary colleagues, evidence-based interventions are endorsed to achieve practice improvements. Given the CNLs' knowledge of quality improvement strategies and tools and unique horizontal leadership capabilities, CNLs often lead projects to address clinical, financial, and satisfaction initiatives. As outcome managers, CNLs monitor quality and satisfaction data specific to unit goals or expected benchmark practices defined by accreditation, regulatory, payor, and professional organizations and identify when process or outcome indicators warrant attention. This monitoring and detection functions as a catalyst to engage project management, leadership, and quality improvement strategies achieved with evidence-based interventions that are positively linked to metrics viewed as stagnant, resistant to change, or shifting outside defined performance thresholds.

Continuous quality improvement principles, strategies, and interventions are the cornerstone vehicle for project work within organizations. An awareness of and embracing of an organization's quality philosophy and framework is essential. In US health systems, the IHI Model for Improvement and Lean Six Sigma frameworks are most commonly utilized. The Model for Improvement highlights the use of cyclical PDSA tests of change as teams work toward improvement as detailed in Chapter 4 (IHI, 2020a). Lean management focuses on defining value and eliminating waste, which is also discussed in Chapter 4.

Interprofessional and Organizational Team Leaders in Project Management

Identification of a need to correct a current process, or examine an existing problem in a complex system, requires an assessment. A foundation for project planning is a detailed needs, gap analysis, or microsystem assessment. Microsystem thinking examines the anatomy of a system where the problem or need arises and is a disciplined inquiry that supports change for sustained improvement. A comprehensive assessment prior to initiating a project leads to team success (Harris et al., 2016). All project team members require information for a unified and consistent approach to shape the project as it is defined. This supports efforts toward successful completion that includes measurable indicators of success (**Figure 12-1**).

There is a language in microsystem learning that provides a unifying framework to explore ideas regarding the process of a project being reviewed, and then improved. Problem identification and rapid cycle improvements through PDSA are the small cycles of change whereby team members engage in distinct evidence-based interventions in planned specific ways to achieve improvement (Harris et al., 2016; IHI, 2020b).

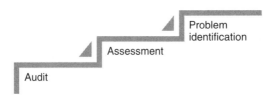

Figure 12-1 Process improvement ramp (Poyss)

Conducting Microsystem Assessments

Clinical microsystems require interdependent individuals to collectively share innovative ideas, techniques, and skills as care is provided for specific patient groups (IHI, 2020c). IHI identifies that microsystems are often embedded in larger organizations and offer examples of a neonatal intensive care unit or a spine center. While these examples help people recognize a microsystem, a traditional and limited view is provided. As unique care delivery systems and settings have emerged, a new appreciation for varied microsystems has materialized. Microsystems are no longer formed by physical space and distinct service areas within organizations. They are recognized as the environment that interdisciplinary healthcare team members and stakeholders accomplish the work of improving health outcomes.

There are promising configurations of microsystems that include clinicians, community leaders, policy makers, and constituents outside health services who have generated new microsystems to address social determinants of health and community-defined health needs. These configurations are gaining recognition and expand opportunities for CNLs. The skills and abilities that CNLs have in team leadership, outcomes management, appreciation for process and quality improvement, and managing complexity demonstrate impact, quantifiable outcomes, and sustainability (AACN, 2016; Williams et al., 2021). Beyond the scope of this chapter, but essential to future success, it is an imperative to embrace the promising frameworks of microsystem assessment that are responsive for transforming care delivery systems and improved patient/consumer health.

Another technique to perform a microsystem assessment includes the following. A project team member may have identified a problem or process change that requires action. Maybe an audit reveals the need for a change, or a true failure of a program has been identified in the service line. The mechanisms to identify what needs to done and actions to take that involve stakeholders of the microsystem or system require a formalized assessment.

Each microsystem has a mission, or core purpose. A microsystem is defined as a unit, clinic, or service area. Traditionally, a microsystem was defined by physical space or boundaries such as a unit or office. Recently, significant attention has occurred resulting in an expanded view and, as such, the microsystem is defined as the environment where providers provide service for patients or consumers. The microsystem has a patient or consumer and part of a population where professionals interact and perform distinct roles necessary to meet patient/consumer needs by engaging in direct care processes. The constant interactions yield patterns of critical results, referred to as "outcomes" (Godfrey et al., 2003). The patterns of results (outcomes) become part of the practice culture. The microsystem thus has a relationship with the larger system, and the relationship assists the microsystem in becoming a complex adaptive system (Nelson et al., 2007). Microsystems are evident in any setting where people engage with interprofessional team members to improve health and well-being.

Healthcare organizations are dynamic systems necessary to capture new payment models and develop innovative mechanisms that create efficient and improved quality and financial outcomes. The sustainability of process changes in projects is as important as the change itself. Improving a working system evolves from knowing the anatomy of the system and working parts of any system. The interconnectedness to the mesosystem is an important lens for project leaders to maintain at the core of project planning and management because a change in one part of a system impacts other parts of the system.

Utilizing a sequential dynamic analysis to frame the project and problem to solve allows a spiral process that yields new discoveries for the project leader and guides the project team to new discoveries that build the spirit of inquiry and evidence-based practices (Melnyk, 2016; Schön, 1983).

The one factor that is a top priority in project management for organizations is building and sustaining EBP into organizational culture. This is often referred to as a healthcare system's context. Shifting culture is a "character-building process." In building EBP culture, a spirit of inquiry must permeate the organization. CNLs are positioned to support this as clinicians are assisted to search and critically appraise evidence-based literature. This mentorship and skill generation for team members are worthwhile investments and provide the foundational skill necessary for use in future projects.

The CNL, as an advanced clinician with a systems lens, promotes the efforts toward improvement. Understanding the system in which a CNL works, leads to skillful, effective, and efficient care as change is implemented and aimed toward improved processes and outcomes. National mandates emphasize the need for advanced nurses, at the point of care, in order to provide clinical leadership that addresses critical problems in safety and quality. The CNL role focus fills the gaps in complex health organizations as the systems analyst/risk anticipator. Quality improvement elements possessed by a CNL emphasize competencies in gathering, analyzing, and evaluating data that promote safety and improvement for the patient, financial and clinical outcomes (AACN, 2011).

The IOM's 2001 report, *Crossing the Quality Chasm*, called for the creation of a 21st-century healthcare system built on the expectation of quality and safety. Expanding on the IOM's report, six specific aims are required for delivery of quality healthcare: safe, effective, efficient, timely, patient-centered, and equitable. A comprehensive microsystem assessment adds to the six aims, recognizing the importance of leadership of individuals and teams to create the conditions to continually improve the performance of frontline professionals and planning patient-centered outcomes. The challenge rests in creation of processes for safe and consistent interventions that lead to measurable improved outcomes requiring critical analysis in microsystems (Nelson et al., 2007).

The 5 P Assessment

An analysis within the smallest unit of the microsystem can be framed with the 5 Ps (Godfrey et al., 2003, p. 125). The 5 P framework helps organize and categorize fundamental elements in a microsystem assessment. When coupled with a SWOT analysis or gap analysis, areas of focus, where strengths can be leveraged, and gaps or weaknesses can be addressed or mitigated in the practice, or process change may be addressed. The 5P framework is as follows: the *purpose* of the microsystem, the *patient* subpopulation contained or served in the clinical microsystem, the *professionals* working in the microsystem, the *processes* delivering the service, and the *patterns* that characterize the function of the microsystem (Nelson et al., 2007, p. 126).

To begin a project, a comprehensive assessment of the system starts with a SWOT analysis.

- Strengths—special expertise, reputation, advantages; internal to the organization
- Weaknesses—limited service lines, staff problems, limited marketing; internal to the organization
- Opportunities—new technologies, new markets, new services; external to the organization

- Threats—new competition, insurance changes, economics; external to the organization (Harris et al., 2016).

Identifying the opportunities for change and threats to a change (or change process), allows the leader to analyze potential positive and negative processes that will influence the projected change. This assessment is vital for successful planning and implementation of a project. In a microsystem SWOT, the unit or service line examines known internal strengths, weaknesses, opportunities, and threats by internal and external forces (Harris et al., 2016) (**Figure 12-2**).

If one creates a 2 × 2 table and lists the strengths, weaknesses, opportunities and threats in separate categories, a visual depiction of relationships assist in identification of processes or personnel that might positively or negatively the microsystem (and organization). Questions in **Figure 12-3** must be answered by a team developing an assessment and listed on a board in a conference room so the team can address the questions for a complete and thorough microsystem assessment.

After the SWOT and microsystem assessment, aims of a change project are often clear because themes emerge. Different ways to organize the findings include storyboards or flowcharts so stakeholders can review the synthesized information and help narrow the focus or prioritize projects. The tools can be used during and after a change project to assist stakeholders in appreciating how inputs, ideas, and actions influenced work.

	Strengths	Weaknesses
Internal	Strengths are elements of the health system that work well, contributing to the achievement of system objectives and thereby to good system performance. Examples are the existence of training programs to improve human resource capacity or strong facility-level data collection and reporting capacity. Recommendations should build on the strengths of the system.	Weaknesses are attributes of the health system that prevent achievement of system objectives and hinder good system performance. Examples are lack of public health sector partnerships with the private sector, health worker dissatisfaction with salaries, or extensive staff turnover. Recommendations should suggest how to resolve system weaknesses.
	Opportunities	**Threats**
External	Opportunities are conditions external to the health system that can facilitate the achievement of system objectives. Examples are planned increases in donor funding or the existence of a vibrant private health sector with which to form partnerships. These factors can be leveraged when planning interventions.	Threats are external conditions that can hinder achievement of health system objectives. Examples are inadequate budget allocations to health or a currency devaluation that will depress health worker income. Recommendations should suggest how to overcome these threats.

Figure 12-2 Bergman's SWOT

Modified from Bergman, E. (2014, May/June). Big data: A brief SWOT analysis. *Information Outlook, 18*(3), 241–247.

I. What is the philosophy/organizing framework of the institution? Mission and vision statements? Look at the profile of the institution. What does the marketing department hail, or highlight? Is there an annual report? Describe the organization or institution (mesosystem). A general description of how the microsystem or unit demonstrates alignment with these statements is imperative. Who are the customers? Describe the microsystem you are assessing. How many employees? What is the breakdown (licensed staff, support services, housekeeping, unit clerk, tech, manager, educator)? Connect this microsystem to the organization (mesosystem).

II. Who is the leader? Roles and responsibilities should be described. The scope of responsibility focuses on the work of the unit. Does the appointed leader lead? Are there unappointed or informal leaders? Is there an annual report for the unit or department? What does this report highlight? Goals? Is the leader connected to the mesosystem?

III. Identify the team members. Not by name, but role and function. You can identify the skills of team members (i.e., RN, full or part time, unit clerk, housekeeping, receptionist, biller, etc.). Identify their skill expertise. Who is the "go-to" person, or the key informant, or the technical expert? Not every unit has these people, but a few conversations with key stakeholders, and you learn who has formal leadership and informal leadership. Identify the key decision maker if the identified leader is not the decision maker.

IV. Microsystem or unit morale/tone. Do people enjoy their work? What is the retention/turnover rate? What do people identify as the "thing that keeps them coming to work"? What is the employee satisfaction? What are they proud of? Do staff members demonstrate a sense of empowerment?

V. Budget. What is the budget for this unit? Is this unit on target? Always over budget and looking to figure out what to do? List the key personnel in the budget and salary information. What are the biggest costs? Does the manager have input into purchasing?

VI. Meetings. Are there scheduled meetings? Are councils or committees responsible for decision-making? Do meetings include interprofessional team members? Are there educational opportunities? Who goes to school? Who is not attending mandatory meetings/sessions?

VII. What are this year's goals for this unit or microsystem? Who determines what the goals are? Are the goals stated, highlighted, and communicated?

VIII. Summary and analysis. What are the strengths and opportunities for this microsystem? What needs attention? What experience has this microsystem had in making and sustaining change? What levers are available to support change?

Figure 12-3 Microsystem assessment steps

Many areas for improvement are identified in a microsystem assessment or SWOT analysis so it is beneficial to document all of these and engage stakeholders in the creation of a priority list. This enables stakeholders to participate in establishing priorities and generates support and buy-in for the project work.

Timelines need to be developed to engender a sense of urgency and enthusiasm around the priority project. The project leader should draft a written plan that frames the problem, project scope, goals and objectives, and a synthesis of best evidence for interventions from the literature. Once the project team is developed, the team members should review the project team charter and scope of work to endorse it for buy-in (referenced earlier in this chapter).

Examples of a SWOT After the Microsystem Assessment Is Completed

Figures 12-4 and **12-5** illustrate examples of SWOT after the microsystem assessment is completed.

Strengths:

- York Hospital is a non-profit facility and thus cares for all individuals regardless of financial stability or insurance coverage.

- York Hospital has a large behavioral health unit that serves the community.

- Constant improvement of care environments and willingness to improve services. I.E. - Current ED contruction to increase ED capacity and create a behavior health ED.

- Staff is encouraged to participate in shared decision-making, as well as patients and families.

Weaknesses:

- Due to York Hospital's non-profit status, profits go down because of self-pay and uninsured patients. Without a profit, the hospital would not be able to sustain.

- Since behavioral health is largely a community service, it has a low profit margin.

- Due to non-profit status the hospital is typically operating at an increased capacity due to patient volumes.

- The ongoing contruction creates detours and limits access to the helipad for trauma cases.

- Due to the high volume of committees and councils, units are paying increased non-productive education hours and nurses are at risk for spending more time in a meeting than at the bedside.

Opportunities:

- York Hospital can partner with outside medical companies to meet needs and limit loss of income and patients.

- York Hospital can partner with outside behavioral health contracts to increase income and decrease the chance of service loss.

- York Hospital is constantly improving it's appearance and care environments to stay up to date and appealing to consumers.

- With the proper balance of work and councils/committees, the hospital can encourage staff to become stakeholders and present valuable ideas.

Threats:

- Outside niche providers may draw insured patients away from York Hospital.

- Other large healthcare systems such as Pinnacle and Holy Spirit could align with nearby healthcare facilities and draw patients away from York Hospital.

- If the hospital continues to operate at maximum capacity, it may cause patients to want to go elsewhere due to lack of rooms and increased wait times.

Figure 12-4 Completed SWOT for microsystem assessment steps

Reproduced from Watson, L. (2015). *No pass zone: A process improvement* [Capstone project]. Drexel University.

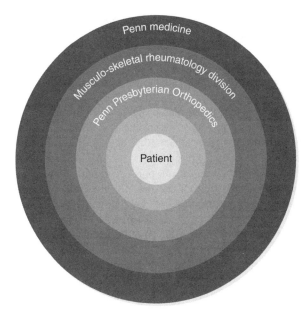

Figure 12-5 Microsystem assessment in a large urban trauma center

Reproduced from Robles, V. (2016). *Preventing readmission of hip replacement patients due to surgical site infections.* [Capstone project]. Drexel University.

Tool Selection for Quality Improvement and Project Management

Selecting tools in quality improvement projects demands process standardization and the gathering of data for visual depictions to help team members and stakeholders understand process and large volumes of data. The data collection tools should be easy to use and understand. Additionally, the tools need to transform data into a metric and visualization. The alignment between the project focus or problem identified and the selection of tools cannot be overstated. Chapter 4 provided details on several of the most-often-used improvement tools.

The presentation of the metrics requires a thoughtful process, engaging the team members into how the data can be translated into visual depictions and graphics. Tools useful to assist the project team begin with the aim of this project. What are you trying to do? Go back to the project objectives and allow the defined objective to guide the measures. How will the team know a change is effective? Identify the change—what creates the improvement? This becomes the engine for the PDSA cycle. You are mapping the process of change.

A process map is the visual diagram of the anatomy of the processes of care in a project. You develop symbols to visually document the flow of the change. Some suggested symbols include a box, as an activity step; an oval, as a process either beginning or end; and a cloud denoting "I don't know" (Nelson et al., 2007, pp. 298–300). Whatever visual symbols the project team uses, the visual steps or actions plotted on paper offer the steps in point of care processes that visually demonstrate where gaps, lapses, or redundances in activities exist in a care process.

At every step up the improvement process, deliberate PDSA cycles generate focused measures of success that lead the project team to the global aim of the improvement. Being cognizant of the end result (or global aim) coupled with a commitment to strategic goals ensures progress and momentum toward the outcome of the project. This provides the organization with deliverables that impact the function of the microsystem and moves the team toward continuous quality improvement.

A cause-and-effect diagram can support the specific aim of the outcome you want to achieve. This analysis tool can describe the possible causes for a single process outcome. Fishbone diagrams are most popular, especially in documenting failure of a change or process outcome (**Figure 12-6**). These diagrams can also be used in a gap analysis, visually diagramming what was dropped, or not communicated, impacting the outcome of a continuous quality improvement (CQI), or process improvement. The fishbone diagram can highlight a cause and effect, or offer information regarding a loss of people, equipment, materials, etc. It is a constant why question. Keep answering until all questions are answered (Nelson et al., 2007).

Recognizing the admission process as a problem, an in-patient admission cycle was tracked during this assessment, as described in **Figure 12-7**, and spanned a total of three hours.

Figure 12-8 illustrates an example of a run chart documenting Foley catheters.

Another example of a tool to use in quality improvement projects is a run chart (Figure 12-8). This chart documents a variable over time, as in falls. This metric is frequently documented, but the presentation may have little effect in documenting change over time. Microsystems use this tool for mandatory reporting, monthly reports, and to offer the stakeholders "how the unit" measures against the standard or benchmark of the system. If the microsystem is attempting to capture an event, or change in process of care, and the outcome can be documented with a run chart, then this measure is useful. A run chart can be

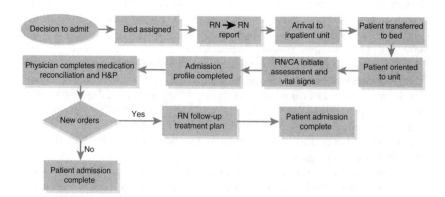

Figure 12-6 Fishbone diagram to document need for change in rounding procedures

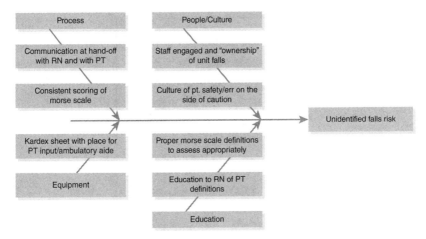

Figure 12-7 Microsystem assessment of a single clinical process (admission process)

Reproduced from Watson, L. (2015). *No pass zone: A process improvement.* [Capstone project]. Drexel University.

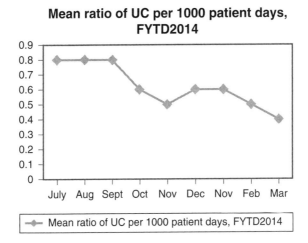

Figure 12-8 Example of a run chart of documenting Foley catheters

Reproduced from Cervini, C. (2014). *Decreasing indwelling urinary catheter use in the ICU: A model for improvement.* [Capstone project]. Drexel University.

superimposed with other control charts if several variables are required to be documented.

Gantt charts and Pareto charts (**Figure 12-9**) are bar graphs that can be plotted for the entire change in process or when improvement activities are documented for the desired outcome. Microsoft Excel is the program that is helpful to learn to make data useful in a presentation.

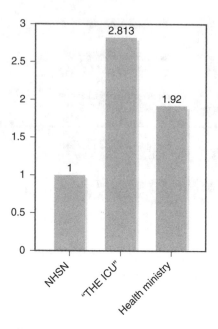

Figure 12-9 Example of a Pareto chart—benchmarking the microsystem (the ICU), against national standards

Reproduced from Cervini, C. (2014). *Decreasing indwelling urinary catheter use in the ICU: A model for improvement.* [Capstone project]. Drexel University.

Evaluation of the Improvement Plan

Completion of a project that includes process and quality improvement is derived in two ways. Evaluation is cyclic and continuous in PDSA and occurs when the goals or targets of the project are achieved based on the project plan established at the onset of the work.

The project team leader is responsible for communicating the results of the project to team members and stakeholders, typically done at regular intervals during the project and at a closing presentation to executive leaders, sponsors, and interdepartmental or organizational team members in committee or council presentations. Using the data and problem focus generated at the onset of the work, evaluation presentations need to use the data to guide the discussion. Starting with the problem and the data and microsystem assessment and SWOT analysis, the team leader uses the data, graphics, and measure to highlight how the team moved to success. Finally, the team leader offers a sustainability plan with trigger metrics to highlight the point at which the team will come back together to address backslide.

Conclusion

Leading continuous improvement is a complex process. The project leader and interdisciplinary team work toward common goals with the intent to improve quality, efficiency, satisfaction, costs, and results. The 5 P and microsystems assessment and improvement frameworks are often implemented in project management because they are flexible and comprehensive, recognize the interprofessional dependencies, and rely on current state analysis as the foundation for microsystem improvement team success.

Summary

- Project management requires deliberate and purposeful planning and documentation.
- Project scope, purpose, and intended outcomes must be defined prior to initiating improvement strategies using quantifiable data and findings from the microsystem assessment.
- Value is derived from sustainability centered on the six aims for quality in healthcare.
- Evaluation is ongoing in cyclical PDSA cycles and aligned with the defined problem and project aim.

Reflection Questions

1. How does assessing the clinical microsystem support the team leader in producing a clear vision for the process or project improvement?
2. What tools can a project leader use to keep the stakeholders engaged as the process toward improvement moves forward?
3. How can a team leader demonstrate sensitivity to the stakeholders and maintain project focus toward continued improvement?
4. Once the process/project improvement is implemented, what tools can help support sustained improvement?

References

American Association of Colleges of Nursing. (2007). *White paper on the education and role of the Clinical Nurse Leader.* http://www.aacn.nche.edu/Publications/WhitePapers/ClinicalNurseLeader07.pdf

American Association of Colleges of Nursing. (2011). *CNL job analysis study.* http://www.aacn.nche.edu/cnc/job-analysis-study

American Association of Colleges of Nursing. (2016). *Advancing healthcare transformation: A new era for academic nursing.* http://www.aacn.nche.edu/AACN-Manatt-Report.pdf

Batalden, P., & Davidoff, F. (2016). What is "quality improvement" and how can it transform healthcare? *Quality and Safety in Healthcare, 16*(1), 2–3.

Bergman, E. (2014, May/June). Big data: A brief SWOT analysis. *Information Outlook, 18*(3), 241–247.

Berwick, D. (2001). *Which hat is on?* General Address at the Institute for Healthcare Improvement's 12th Annual National forum, Orlando, FL.

Bortz, K. (2014). *Early mobility for geriatric head trauma patients.* [Capstone project]. Drexel University.

Cervini, C. (2014). *Decreasing indwelling urinary catheter use in the ICU: A model for improvement.* [Capstone project]. Drexel University.

Davis, D., & Dearman, C. (2010). Curriculum issue for academic CNL programs. In J. Harris, & L. Roussel (Eds.), *Initiating and sustaining the CNL: A practical guide* (2nd ed.). Jones & Bartlett Learning.

Digital Project Manager. (n.d.). *Write a project charter: How-to-guide and template.* https://thedigital projectmanager.com/project-charter/

Donaldson, M., & Mohr, J. (2000). *Exploring innovation and quality improvement in health care microsystems: A cross-case analysis.* Technical report for the Institute of Medicine Committee on Quality of Health Care in America. Institute of Medicine.

Gill, D., & Mountford, J. (2012). What is a quality improvement project? *British Journal of Hospital Medicine, 73*(5), 252–256.

Godfrey, M. (Ed.). (2010). *Microsystems at a glance.* The Dartmouth Institute for Health Policy and clinical practice. http://www.clinicalmicrosystem.org

Godfrey, M., Nelson, E., Wasson, J., Mohr, J., & Batalden, P. (2003). Microsystems in healthcare: Part 3. Planning patient-centered services. *Journal of Quality and Safety, 29*(4), 159–170.

Harris, J. (2016). Key foundations of successful project planning and management. In J. Harris, L. Roussel, C. Dearman, & P. Thomas (Eds.), *Project planning and management. A guide for nurses and interprofessional teams* (2nd ed.). Jones & Bartlett Learning.

Harris, J., Roussel, L., Dearman, C., & Thomas, P. (2016). *Project planning and management. A guide for nurses and interprofessional teams* (2nd ed.). Jones & Bartlett Learning.

Institute for Healthcare Improvement. (2020a). *How to improve.* http://www.ihi.org/resources/Pages /HowtoImprove/default.aspx

Institute for Healthcare Improvement. (2020b). *Clinical microsystem assessment.* http://www.ihi.org /resources/Pages/Tools/ClinicalMicrosystemAssessmentTool.aspx

Institute for Healthcare Improvement (2020c). *Plan-do-study-act (PDSA) worksheet.* http://www.ihi .org/resources/pages/tools/PlanDoStudyActworksheet.aspx

Melnyk, B. (2016). Culture eats strategy every time: What works in building and sustaining an evidence-based practice culture in healthcare systems. *Worldviews on Evidence-Based Nursing, 13*(2), 99–101. https://doi.org//10.1111/wvn.12161

Meyer, D. (2016). *Improving the admission process.* [Capstone project]. Drexel University.

Mountford, D. (2010). Toward an outcomes-based healthcare system: A view from the United Kingdom. *Journal of American Medical Association, 304,* 2407–2408.

Nelson, E., Batalden, P., & Godfrey, M. (Eds.). (2007). *Quality by design. A clinical microsystems approach.* Jossey-Bass.

Project Management Institute. (2013). *A guide to project management body of knowledge (PMBOK guide,* 5th ed.). Author.

Robles, V. (2016). *Preventing readmission of hip replacement patients due to surgical site infections.* [Capstone project]. Drexel University.

Schön, D. (1983). *The reflective practitioner: How professionals think in action.* Basic Books.

Stausmire, J. (2014). Quality improvement or research-deciding which road to take. *Critical Care Nurse, 34*(6), 58–63.

Watson, L. (2015). *No pass zone: A process improvement.* [Capstone project]. Drexel University.

Williams, M., Hardin, L., Radhakrishnan, N., & Thomas, P. (2021). How consumer demands and data are driving change. In P. Thomas, J. Harris, & B. Collins (Eds.), *How data frames quality, safety, innovation, and sustainability in interprofessional practice.* Springer.

EXEMPLAR

Post-Discharge Calls in the ED: Improving Quality and Efficiency

Megan Pashnik

According to Huber (2006), a microsystem can be defined as "a small group of people who work together on a regular basis to provide care to discrete subpopulations of patients" (p. 5). Microsystems produce performance outcomes and are often embedded in larger organizations (Huber, 2006). The role of the CNL is to maximize the potential of the microsystem so that the larger healthcare organization can provide the best care possible.

Much like a CNL, the priority for a CNL student is microsystem assessment. This requires a variety of techniques, including interview, direct observation, and data collection. The student must determine the overall aim of the microsystem and identify key processes within the microsystem. Data on the microsystem's quality improvement indicators and quality and safety metrics must also be considered. To achieve this goal, every aspect of the microsystem must be observed, evaluated, analyzed, and reviewed with a focus on value and patient outcomes. Identifying and improving even one area of waste, one aspect of patient care that is not adding value, or one process that is inefficient can lead to safer, more effective, and more affordable care for patients.

In the context of this student's assessment, the microsystem is a 44-bed Level II trauma center ED embedded within a larger 378-bed acute care organization in the Midwest. Based on the observation processes within the ED microsystem and interviews with nursing staff, post-discharge follow-up calls were identified as an area for quality improvement and a dissatisfier for nursing staff. Improving, developing, and revising the process for follow-up calls will serve as a scholarly project for this CNL student.

Nursing staff in the ED have been placing follow-up phone calls to its patients for seven years. When the calls were first initiated, the nursing staff received some initial education regarding the calls; however, the process has received very little attention since. As a consequence, there is great disparity between the standard of work and how the process is actually implemented day to day. Additionally, these calls are time-consuming and inefficient.

Nurses placing follow-up calls while caring for patients in the busy ED setting cannot perform the task of follow-up calls efficiently. Because nurses are engaged with caring for the patients who are physically present in the ED, they experience frequent interruptions while placing follow-up calls. Data from call tracking logs indicate that nurses spend as much as three times the number of minutes addressing issues identified in the follow-up calls compared to the actual time spent speaking with patients on the phone. While follow-up calls may take a nurse 15 minutes, it is not uncommon for it to take the remainder of the hour to address the concerns brought forward. As such, the time spent making the calls is far less than the actual time spent addressing concerns that are brought forward. This "lost" time may lead to increased costs for the ED as nurses are not able to perform the task efficiently.

Modifying the process for follow-up calls may improve the quality of the calls and decrease the amount of time necessary for placing the calls. These changes may also increase nurses' satisfaction with the follow-up call process, which could lead to increased nurse retention and, ultimately, better outcomes for patients (Andrews & Dziegielewski, 2005; Newman & Maylor, 2002; Newman et al., 2002). The purpose of this student's evidence-based practice protocol (scholarly project) is to revise the current standard of work in an effort to optimally and efficiently utilize nursing time, improve the quality of post-discharge calls, and improve job satisfaction for ED RN staff.

References

Andrews, D. R., & Dziegielewski, S. F. (2005). The nurse manager: Job satisfaction, the nursing shortage and retention. *Journal of Nursing Management, 13*(4), 286–295. https://doi.org/10.1111/j.1365-2934.2005.00567.x

Huber, T. P. (2006). *Micro-systems in health care: Essential building blocks for the successful delivery of health care in the 21st century* [PowerPoint slides]. https://www.google.com/url?sa=t&rct=j&q=&esrc=s&source=web&cd=5&ved=0ahUKEwj7gqCwi83JAhUE54MKHY0fBTIQFggzMAQ&url=http%3A%2F%2Fwww.dhcs.ca.gov%2Fprovgovpart%2Finitiatives%2Fnqi%2FDocuments%2FMicroSysHC.ppt&usg=AFQjCNEQlm4t4F3Wy3xtwB6ZSY_w7GX3Tw&sig2=GcXwskPCEq7iiGEWqvYeyg&bvm=bv.109332125,d.amc&cad=rja

Mercy Health. (2015). *Mercy Health St. Mary's campus, downtown Grand Rapids.* http://www.mercyhealthsaintmarys.com/saint-marys

Newman, K., & Maylor, U. (2002). The NHS plan: Nurse satisfaction, commitment and retention strategies. *Health Services Management Research, 15*(2), 93–105. https://doi.org/10.1258/0951484021912860

Newman, K., Maylor, U., & Chansarkar, B. (2002). The nurse satisfaction, service quality and nurse retention chain: Implications for management of recruitment and retention. *Journal of Management in Medicine, 16*(4/5), 271.

EXEMPLAR

CNL and Microsystem Assessment on a Trauma Unit

Tiffany Tscherne

Critical Thinking

The trauma program manager (TPM) is responsible for assessing the microsystem of the trauma patient to find out why poor outcomes have been obtained, and/or why evidence-based guidelines are not being adhered to. Through application of the chosen quality improvement model (PDCA), how it can be corrected is created by the TPM as the CNL student in consultation with the trauma medical director or multidisciplinary trauma operations committee.

The microsystem assessment can be as simple as interviews or as complex as workflow diagrams and retrospective analysis of charts and data from the trauma registry. Upon completion of the assessment through the CNL's clinical immersion experience, the CNL completed a new design for the corrections process and selected the outcome metrics, based on regulatory guidelines such as the American College of Surgeons or the state of Michigan, in concert with evidence-based practice.

Communication

In addition to e-mail, the CNL student must master both business and clinical venues of communication. The CNL student in the TPM role is responsible for developing high-level reports to senior leadership utilizing the A3 and other standard formats. Identifying the route of communication with the direct-care level provider is necessary for program operations. So, familiarity with marketing tools throughout the hospital as well as the staff communication venues allows the TPM (CNL student) to share everything from "kudos" to classes to educational tools.

Assessment

The CNL student's assessment focused on identification of the primary trauma population for the area served by the hospital. In my case, falls in those over the age of 55, with orthopedic injury are my primary population of interest. The information on falls was obtained through chart reviews, usage trends, the Michigan Hospital Association MIDAS database, and the hospital's central data warehouse.

Why is this knowledge so important? It allows us to focus on our injury prevention activities to the community that we serve. While handing out bicycle helmets to children is a noble cause, it doesn't help the seniors who are falling due to poor knowledge of fall risks. Anticipating the risk allows us to decrease the high mortality rates that often follow falls in those considered to be in their golden years.

Assessment of the microsystem, especially when poor outcomes or regulatory standards are not being met, is a primary job role of the TPM. Whether through the 5 Ps (purpose, patients, professionals, processes, and patterns), or a fishbone chart, the TPM utilizes tools to answer why this issue or outcome is occurring. This microsystem assessment, when done correctly, will yield valuable information and data to improve fall reduction outcomes for the elder population.

Health Promotion, Risk Reduction, and Disease Prevention

Injury prevention activities are a mandate for a trauma center according to the American College of Surgeons. As discussed, after an assessment of the primary trauma risks to the community, the CNL student evaluates EBP to develop a plan that best addresses the risk. The CNL student develops the outcome matrix tool, gathers the relevant data from the trauma registry, and then reports the findings to the trauma operations committee. No change in outcomes? Back into the PDCA it goes!

So who is responsible for delivering the programming? The CNL serves as the primary creator and the educator as well by going out into the community to give lectures, provide health fairs, and to also serve on committees throughout the community. This level of community involvement lends the CNL expertise to shape policy for health promotion, risk reduction, and disease prevention.

Illness and Disease Management

The CNL student served as the case manager for the trauma patient throughout the care spectrum. Yes, the CNL student served as one of the primary authors of the process, but she will also be the de facto case manager for the trauma patient through daily rounding, participating in multidisciplinary care planning, and applying both EBP and regulatory guidelines in order to shape a positive patient outcome.

Information and Healthcare Technologies

In addition to being a clinical care force, the TPM is responsible for the trauma registry. The trauma registry serves as a clinical repository for trauma patient care data on a myriad of data points ranging from demographics to procedures and even comorbidities. The CNL student is responsible for the operations of the data collection, creating the data collection process, data integrity, and the management of the trauma registry.

Healthcare Systems and Policy

Writing policy, managing all aspects of trauma center operations including staff and budget, are part of the CNL student's role expectations. A CNL student managed a team of two or more and assumed responsibility for office operations. The CNL student is responsible for the trauma services budget, which can include not only paper clips but on-call fees for physicians, as well as staff trauma training for an entire hospital.

The CNL student writes policy that affects not only trauma service, but the operations of the entire multidisciplinary team in regard to the trauma patient. Trauma policy must remain valid and applicable as the patient moves from the ED to diagnostic testing, to the inpatient realm, and upon discharge and transfer. Policies on trauma activations, transfer criteria, and even trauma education are crafted under the guidance of the CNL student.

Designer/Manager/Coordinator of Care

The CNL student bears the responsibility for the cornerstone of the trauma program for any hospital, of any size or designation: the process improvement/patient safety (PIPS) program. The PIPS program consists of daily activities, through trauma rounding and chart review, up to committee action by a physician peer review or the multidisciplinary operations committee. Whether a patient care failure or process failure, the issue moves through one of three levels of review, guided by the CNL student. The CNL student serves as the chief researcher, facilitator, and even outcomes manager for the issue in order to ensure loop closure.

EXEMPLAR

Health Promotion in an Acute Care Setting: A Quality and Process Improvement Initiative

Laurie Sayer and Kristin Mast

Influenza and pneumonia are major causes of hospitalization and death in the United States. As a clinician, the CNL promotes better health for populations by creating awareness, knowledge, and system changes to increase the adult inpatient immunization rate. This ensures improved compliance with the CMS quality-of-care measures and accountable care and will have a financial impact related to pay-for-performance standards. A higher immunization rate also aligns with the *Healthy People 2020* goal of increasing immunization levels and reducing preventable infectious diseases.

Our organization was not consistently meeting established benchmarks for pneumonia's quality core measures. In addition, a unit baseline audit indicated only 51% of patients actually received their ordered Pneumovax 23 (pneumococcal polysaccharides [PPSV]) vaccine and only 42% received the ordered influenza vaccine prior to discharge.

A CNL-led interdisciplinary task force was formed to look at current practice, analyze data, identify barriers, and develop a process improvement plan utilizing Lean principles. At a system-wide and microsystem level, CNLs support immunization processes through both formal and informal education, mentoring, system changes, data awareness, and accountability.

A root-cause analysis was performed with essential input from staff nurses to identify issues affecting immunization compliance. The team recognized several problems related to the immunization process and sought input from staff nurses to identify barriers to vaccine administration. Based on feedback from staff on all inpatient units, the team identified three main focus areas: education, accountability, and continual awareness of vaccine compliance.

CNLs were champions of the quality initiative. As outcome managers, unit CNLs received daily and monthly reports to monitor compliance and trends, and to evaluate gaps for unit-specific improvement opportunities. Inpatient CNLs have been instrumental in obtaining accurate patient immunization history. This has created an increased awareness of up-to-date immunizations. The CNLs provided education at unit staff meetings and mentoring on the units and obtained feedback from the nurses about barriers and gaps in the process, which was then taken back to the team to address. CNLs were also instrumental in eliminating duplicate vaccinations by researching patients' vaccine histories and updating immunization histories. The CNLs also received daily reports for active vaccine orders to ensure just-in-time education and compliance. Each unit's PPSV and influenza vaccine monthly data reports are posted on their quality boards for awareness and transparency.

With the CNL initiative, PPSV and influenza vaccines ordered and given increased from a baseline of less than 52% to 89.3%. Several initiatives at our organization have failed to improve and sustain pneumococcal and influenza rates for the adult inpatient populations, thus affecting the quality of care and safety of our patients. A CNL-led interdisciplinary initiative using process improvement methods and supported by an accountability model has played an instrumental role in improving and sustaining the overall vaccination rate for the organization. Ongoing efforts are directed toward accurately assessing and providing immunizations to every patient every time (100% of the time).

EXEMPLAR

Improving Glycemic Control

Ann Eubanks

Problem Statement

Surgical site infections, and particularly sternal and mediastinal infections, have implications for significantly increasing both morbidity and mortality, as well as their associated costs in both man hours and dollars spent. Postoperative hyperglycemia is associated with the development of surgical site infections among cardiac surgery patients. Adequate glycemic control has been shown to decrease the incidence of deep sternal wound infection. According to Furnary and colleagues (2003), continuous insulin infusion protocols should be the standard care for glycometabolic control in all patients undergoing cardiac surgical procedures. Furthermore, the CMS publicly reports on postoperative glycemic control as part of the SCIP. The goal of this project is to increase the percentage of cardiac surgery patients to at least 90% meeting SCIP criteria for adequate glycemic control, with serum glucose levels less than 200 mg/dL on the first and second postoperative days.

Multidisciplinary Team

A multidisciplinary team was formed to address the design and implementation of updated glycemic control strategies to conform to current evidence-based practices. The team consisted of the nurse manager, staff nurses, diabetic educators, a clinical pharmacist, information systems analysts, and a cardiovascular surgeon. These individuals were chosen based on expertise in their respective disciplines. A retroactive chart review was performed to obtain baseline data; it revealed that glucose targets were only met in 40% of heart surgery patients.

Project Processes and Evaluation Methods

A microsystem assessment was performed in the cardiac recovery unit to determine knowledge levels regarding glycemic control and current methods of glucose management. Brainstorming and cause-and-effect analysis methods were used to determine possible causes of poor glycemic control. A literature review of best practices for postoperative glycemic control was undertaken by the team, and numerous evidence-based protocols were evaluated. A mutually agreed on CII protocol was identified. Information systems analysts converted the protocol into an electronic form, which enabled bedside nurses to accurately titrate insulin infusion rates. The CII protocol was presented to the medical executive committee for approval as standing orders. The PDSA cycle was used to conduct tests of change using the agreed on protocol. Bedside nurses received comprehensive education on glycemic control and utilization of the new protocol prior to implementation.

Outcomes

Upon implementation of the new CII protocol, close supervision and clinical support was provided for all shifts. Data was monitored daily to ensure safety and to quickly identify problems. After the first quarter using the CII protocol, adequate glycemic control was achieved in 93% of patients.

Reference

Furnary, A. P., Gao, G., Grunkemeier, G. L., Ying Xing, W., Zerr, K. J., Bookin, S. O., & Starr, A. (2003). Continuous insulin infusion reduces mortality in patients with diabetes undergoing coronary artery bypass grafting. *Journal of Thoracic Cardiovascular Surgery, 125*, 1007–1021.

CHAPTER 13

Collecting, Analyzing, and Managing Projects and Improvement Data

James L. Harris, Patricia L. Thomas, and James M. Smith

LEARNING OBJECTIVES

1. Determine the range of improvement opportunities inherent in data and new technology within the fourth industrial revolution.
2. Define a problem in terms of objective, measurability, and quality data to achieve microsystem project-desired targets or goals.
3. Determine the information that needs to be collected to explore solutions.
4. Consider possible problem solutions, select an intervention, and design an improvement project.
5. Identify and describe tools for displaying data and converting them into meaningful information as CNLs manage microsystem projects.

KEY TERMS

Big data

Data analysis

Data collection

Data display and dissemination

Problem identification

CNL ROLES

Advocate

Catalyst

Integrator broker

Risk averter

CNL PROFESSIONAL VALUES

Accountability

Financial stewardship

Integrity

Interprofessional teams

Outcome management

Quality improvement

Social justice

CNL CORE COMPETENCIES

Assessment	Ethical decision-making
Communication	Information and healthcare
Critical thinking	technologies
Data analysis	Resource management
Design/Management/Coordination of care	

Introduction

One of the CNL's roles is to pursue clinical scholarship in the application of evidence to the clinical setting and the resolution of clinical problems. In this role, the CNL has accountability for the evaluation and improvement of outcomes, which includes not only using evidence-based practices but also striving to solve problems at the point-of-care setting. The keys to solving problems are knowing how to (1) identify and document problems from a needs assessment or gap analysis, (2) analyze processes to derive possible solutions, (3) design intervention strategies, and (4) collect and analyze outcome data. These tasks require a comfort level with data, quality improvement methodology, managing projects, and statistical concepts, as identified in the Clinical Nurse Leader Curriculum Framework Addendum to the AACN's *White Paper on the Role of the Clinical Nurse Leader* (AACN, 2007). The AACN *Competencies and Curricular Expectations for Clinical Nurse Leader Education and Practice* (2013), Essential 3, "Quality Improvement and Safety," implements quality improvement strategies based on current evidence, analytics, and risk anticipation; Essential 4, "Translating and Integrating Scholarship into Practice," applies improvement science theory and methods in performance measurement and quality improvement processes that underscore the need for clinical analysis and data management. CNLs are at the forefront in engaging teams and key stakeholders in improvement work.

However, the task does not stop there; dissemination of findings in an informative and user-friendly format is essential. Among the CNL's tasks are the education of healthcare team members and "practical experience in the dissemination of clinical knowledge such as grand rounds, case presentations, and journal clubs" (AACN, 2007, p. 8). The successful presentation and dissemination of information to other team members and to the organization at large (in charts, reports, posters, and formal and informal presentations) can be the determining factor in whether or not these results impact practices at the microsystem and organizational level.

Three aspects of data are critical to the improvement process. The three aspects include: (1) data to document the existence of a problem, (2) data on the processes that result in the problematic outcome, and (3) data to demonstrate that an improvement initiative resulted in actual improvement that is sustainable.

A new frontier to guide improvement projects has evolved as the importance of big data are constantly generated across multiple disciplines. Both big data and a range of new technologies link the physical, biological, and digital worlds together as the fourth industrial revolution evolves. The link is producing value across healthcare settings and is a catalyst for comprehensive administrative and clinical decisions. Big data and technology will inspire staff versus replacing them as innovative thought and meaningful project outcomes occur (Schwab, 2017).

Improvement and Timely Implementation

It is understood that the CNL and other staff in a healthcare setting want to improve care. Not only do staff want to improve care, they also want to improve it as soon as possible. Although this intention is laudable, it often leads to problems that can impede the process of improvement, if not derail it altogether.

How often have you heard someone define a problem in phrases such as: "Housekeeping needs to do a better job!" This may sound like a satisfactory problem statement—after all, lack of cleanliness in healthcare settings is not only aesthetically displeasing but also represents a serious risk of patient harm. Other versions of this type of problem statement are common in other areas as well: "The administration needs to build more parking!" or "The patients need to learn that they cannot miss their clinic appointments!"

Problem formulation arises from staff's laudable desire to fix problems, but, if one thinks about the problem statement, "Housekeeping needs to do a better job," it becomes apparent that it is actually a proposed solution to a perceived problem, not a problem statement. Often when staff perceive a problem, they immediately think of a way to solve it and then state the problem as not having implemented the perceived solution, which may or may not be the most effective and efficient solution. Perhaps housekeeping needs to do a better job, or perhaps staff and visitors need clearer cleanliness reminders/guidelines, or perhaps there should be more obvious and plentiful places to put trash.

In addition, these "solution-type" problem statements usually impute blame to someone for the problem. In the given examples, it is housekeeping's fault that the facility is not clean, or the administration's fault that there is not enough parking, or the patients' fault for missing their appointments. Acknowledging that fault exists is not exactly the best way to solve a problem. Blame should be absent and not essential in problem solving.

Two steps are common in problem identification. First, collect objective and measureable data on the problem. What observations led to the conclusion that the facility is not as clean as it should be? Does the completion of periodic observational checklists reveal that ward floors are not clean, that bathrooms have paper towels on the floor, or that the cafeteria has used dishes remaining on the tables? Obtaining observable and measurable data on a possible problem often requires the collaborative skills of the CNL, working together with staff from many different areas of the healthcare setting (e.g., unit, clinic, quality improvement, administrative, business office).

Once objective and measurable data on the problem have been obtained, the CNL must ask, "Compared to what?" In addition to objective and measurable data, all problem statements should have a clearly stated desired solution level, namely a target or goal. This target can be based on national standards, accreditation requirements, customer surveys, organizational performance goals, or the desires of the program leader or chief executive officer. The target needs to be stated clearly and explicitly. If the current state does not meet the target, a problem exists. The decision about whether to address this relates to how great the deviation is from the desired target and how great the impact is on patient care or facility operations. Chapter 12 provided more detail about project management in relation to how CNLs develop and manage improvement projects.

Causation

In a classic article published in *The New England Journal of Medicine*, Donald Berwick (1989) discussed the imprudence of trying to improve an organization by eliminating incompetent or unmotivated workers from the workforce. Poor employees do not cause the majority of problem outcomes. Directing improvement efforts at eliminating the organization of such employees will not create significant improvement, and will create coping behaviors that actually reduce performance. The vast majority of problematic outcomes are caused by deficiencies that occur in the sequence of processes that lead to the problematic outcome. This is as true of healthcare settings as it is of automobile manufacturers or insurance companies, or the local supermarket. Berwick notes that the most important investments in quality improvement are to study the complex production processes used in healthcare, noting, "We must understand them before we can improve them" (Berwick, 1989, p. 55).

To find a possible solution, a detailed assessment is needed to determine which process(es) contribute most to a problem outcome. In many instances, the solution will be readily apparent after reviewing the facts and meaningful data. It is reported that Willie Sutton, the famous bank robber, once said that he robbed banks "because that's where the money is!" Following Willie's example, the best strategy is to determine where the cost efficacy in the chain of processes that led to a problematic outcome. Stated another way, what are the specific point(s) in this process chain that, when changed, will produce the most dramatic improvement in outcome? Collect data on the processes, and the data will actually lead to a solution.

Process and Solution

There are various ways for the CNL to study processes (e.g., flow charts, fishbone diagrams, etc.), and multiple resources exist such as books on processes and tools of improvement, some specifically tailored to healthcare settings (Brassard & Ritter, 2008; Graban, 2011, 2019). An example of a problem resolution that illustrates the importance of focusing on the most critical elements of a process is provided. The authors of a study were interested in reducing delays in coronary thrombolysis for acute myocardial infarction patients in a 10-bed ICU (Bonetti et al., 2000). In a sample of 16 consecutively measured patients (patients 1–16), these delays averaged 57 minutes, as compared to an accepted standard of 30 minutes. To determine how to improve this process, staff carefully monitored the next five admissions requiring thrombolysis (patients 17–21) and also met as an interprofessional team to discuss the specific causes of delays that each had personally experienced. The monitoring and discussion revealed a total of 22 different causes of delays that were listed on a fishbone diagram. The most noteworthy of these causes were a lack of communication and cumbersome/inadequate guidelines in caring for this type of patient.

After implementing new communication and practice guidelines, door-to-needle time was tracked for the next 16 patients who required thrombolysis (patients

22–37); the results were a dramatic reduction in door-to-needle time. From a baseline intervention average time of 57 minutes (+/– 25.4), the post-intervention time fell to an average of 32 minutes (+/– 9.0). This change was statistically significant ($p < 0.002$). In the baseline, 0 of 16 patients met the 30-minute standard, whereas in the post-intervention phase, 10 of 16 patients met the standard.

The improvement example mentioned previously is the goal of any quality improvement initiative—an overall better level of performance and less variability. This dramatic improvement was achieved by addressing 22 critical causes of delay identified by the team in its process analysis.

A very simple test of whether or not an intervention introduced a statistically significant improvement over time is the run chart. The IHI has a brief but online resource on run charts, which includes an Excel template as well as instructions for interpretation (IHI, 2011). Control charts can also be used to test the significance of interventions over time (Carey & Lloyd, 2001; Kelley, 1999).

CNLs should remain mindful that when collecting data on process(es) is to collect the most detailed (granular) data that time and resources allow. For example, one facility had a problem with the system of escorts who took long-term care patients to clinics in the "main" hospital. There were complaints that escorts were late or sometimes did not arrive at all, and there was a feeling that a possible cause was that there were too many appointments in the afternoon. Had tallies of morning and afternoon appointments been kept, an increase in demand in the afternoon, but not a very dramatic one, would have been evident (see **Figure 13-1**).

Fortunately, much more detailed (granular) information was collected on the exact times that escorts were requested, so a much more precise analysis of the process could occur. **Figure 13-2**, drawn from exactly the same data but plotted for every half-hour interval of the day, displays a more detailed and informative picture of the fluctuation in demand for escorts.

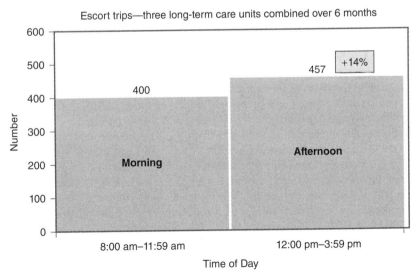

Figure 13-1 Number of escorts in the morning and afternoon

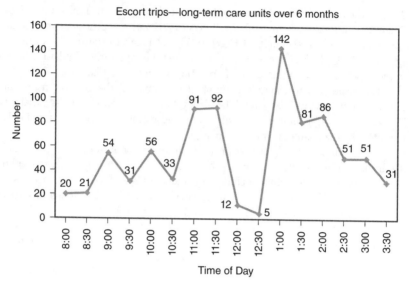

Time of day = 30-minute period starting with the time listed.

Figure 13-2 Number of escorts for every half hour during the day

By collecting data at this granular level, the healthcare setting was able to understand the process in more detail. These data, combined with additional analyses by day of week and the names of the specific clinics requiring escorts, allowed the setting to intervene strategically in the process by leveling peak demands, increasing supply during peak periods, or a combination of both. Thus, the value of granular data is evidence of positive and efficient results.

Additional Consideration

The need for data on the current status of the problem and data on the process steps that are involved in producing a problematic outcome was previously discussed. The following is a discussion of a third use of data—data collected to determine whether an intervention produced a real change in the outcome. However, before collecting outcome data, one of the most important questions the CNL should ask is, "If I find after analyzing the results that a real change occurred (i.e., one most likely not due to chance), can I be sure that the results are due to my intervention, or could they be due to something else?"

For example, based on patient feedback, a CNL is planning a small improvement project to assess the effectiveness of telephone reminders in reducing the percentage of missed appointments. Parenthetically, many companies, both large and small, evaluate "small bets" such as this before implementing an initiative on a larger scale (Sims, 2011). The project involved (1) collecting baseline data for a month, (2) introducing telephone reminders, and (3) collecting follow-up data after the introduction of the telephone reminders. This was a one-group pretest-posttest design. Although this type of design is classified as "preexperimental" or "nonexperimental," the problems associated with it (Campbell & Stanley, 1963; Heffner, 2004;

Lennon-Dearing & Neeley-Barnes, 2012) are frequently used in applied settings (as opposed to research settings) often due to forces requiring rapid responses.

The results of the study indicated that the percentage of missed appointments was reduced after the introduction of the reminders and that the results were unlikely due to chance (i.e., they were statistically significant). Could the CNL conclude that telephone reminders were the cause of the reduction in missed appointments? Poster presentations using a one-group pretest-posttest design would provide that conclusion.

More details about the missed appointment project are provided. The facility in question was located in the northeastern United States, the month without reminders was February, and the month with reminders was March. Is it possible a reduction in the number of missed appointments in March was caused by something other than the telephone reminders? How about the weather? Perhaps February was a particularly cold and snowy month. The director of these clinics was replaced on March 1. The former director was a very good physician, but was very businesslike and not particularly patient friendly. The new physician is very casual and patient friendly. Is it possible that the new and more patient-friendly director was the cause of the reduced number of missed appointments in March? The possible effects of the weather and the new director are considered threats to internal validity, namely, threats to the validity of conclusions a researcher may draw about an intervention. Other threats to the design relate to its external validity, namely, threats to the generalizability of its findings to other settings. The key message of this example is to show that even if statistically significant results exist, a poor design choice can leave the conclusion in doubt. Improvement outcomes may have statistical significance, but lack clinical significance and vice versa. Being a consumer of research and understanding basic statistical approaches are pivotal to a CNL's success when collecting, analyzing, mapping projects, and disseminating improvement data (Miller, 2019).

One may ask, Could the design of the project above have been improved? Yes. The most dramatic improvement would have been to randomly assign patients either to a "no reminder group" or a "reminder group" and then collect data for both groups over the entire two months. Both groups would be influenced by the weather factor and the new director factor (as well as all other factors, some of which may be unknown). Randomization, given a sufficient number of cases, is the great equalizer. If one has limited knowledge about this method and must employ the one-group pretest-posttest design, could it be improved? Yes—by doing all that can be done to avoid confounding factors. For example, scheduling an evaluation during a period when the weather would not be expected to have such a dramatic effect on missed appointments and by scheduling it during a period in which the clinics would not be undergoing any dramatic changes (in leadership, clinic location, etc.). This approach would not rule out any other factors (e.g., an unexpected reduction in copay starting in March), but it would at least reduce the possible effect of known or anticipated confounding factors (e.g., the weather and the appointment of a new director).

How to choose the best design for an evaluation can be problematic or difficult. Succinct descriptions of a number of basic design options (pre-experimental, quasi-experimental, and true experimental designs) may be found in several sources (Bordens & Abbott, 2018; Campbell & Stanley, 1963; Heffner, 2004; Lennon-Dearing & Neeley-Barnes, 2012; McGregor, 2017).

Analyzing Data: Tests of Statistical Significance

Quality data is a prerequisite prior to analysis. To enhance data quality, consider what meaningful uses of data would result in patient care outcomes. Quality data is a strong indicator of value and supports the ongoing processes and analysis of projects (Cai & Zhu, 2015). Big data or small microsystem information requires one to be aware of the data challenges that include volume, velocity, variety, and value, referred to as the 4 Vs. Volume is the vast amount of data present. Velocity is the speed at which data are generated. Variety is indicative of the diversity of data, whether structured or unstructured. And, value is the density of data. The greater the data, relative value is diminished (Katal et al., 2013).

As CNLs analyze improvement data, the 4 Vs are significant to data quality, integrity, and statistical significance. The following discusses data analysis and differences that exist among statistical tests and their significance.

In statistics, a basic distinction is made between "descriptive statistics" (mean, mode, median, correlation, etc.) and "inferential statistics" (those that lead to $p < 0.05$ type conclusions). Consider this scene that illustrates the latter—a father and his young daughter meet a friend whom they have not seen in a few years, and the following brief interaction ensues:

Father: "You remember my daughter, Maggie?"

Friend: "My, she's gotten big. What grade is she in? Third?"

Why would the friend guess the third grade? Probably because of the child's size (primarily her height). The friend probably has a small database in his head of children he knows who are third graders (his own children, relatives, neighbors, etc.), and he compared this child to that database to make an educated guess (an inference) that she is in the third grade based on his recollection of the average height of third graders (mean) and the fact that all third graders are not exactly the same height (deviations from the mean). Could he be wrong? Yes. Despite the fact that an educated guess based on height might place her in the third grade, she could actually be a tall second grader or a short fourth grader.

Inferences like this are common. Consider this statement, "I think I can leave work on time, stop for pizza, and still get Bobby to his soccer game on time to play." This inference is based on data that have been accumulated over the course of time, data on how likely it is that a person will be able to leave work on time, how long it takes to drive to the pizza parlor, how long it takes to cook the pizza, how long it takes to drive home and eat, how long it takes to drive to the soccer game, and whether the coach will allow Bobby to play even if he arrives a few minutes late. This line of thinking requires making a series of educated guesses, actually quite a complicated series, with the distinct possibility that these guesses could be wrong; that is exactly what inferences are—making decisions under conditions of uncertainty.

Take the previous example of the daughter, father, and friend, and suppose that the friend did not know any third graders; instead, someone gave him data on the heights of third graders. But instead of being given the heights of just a few third graders, he was given the heights of hundreds of third graders. Could an educated guess be made in this case? Yes, but there would be too much data to calculate in his head.

Consider the example of telephone reminders. An intervention (telephone reminders) was introduced, and then the evaluation was designed to preclude the results due to factors other than the reminders (e.g., weather or organizational or personnel changes). The evaluation was completed and the percentage of missed appointments for the period before reminders and the period after reminders was calculated. There was a reduction in the percent of missed appointments for the period after reminders. Can it be concluded that the reminders did in fact reduce missed appointments? No.

If data had been collected on missed appointments for each of the two months without introducing any change, and the average for each month was found, would these averages be exactly the same? This is highly unlikely, so the question remains, "Is the difference observed due to an intervention or is it due to the natural variability in the process?" Inferential statistics help answer the question, "How likely is it that chance (the natural variability of the process) caused the difference we observed?"

The majority of inferential statistics are built on a model of the normal curve, illustrated in **Figure 13-3** with hypothetical data on the height of third-grade girls with a mean of 50.0 inches and a standard deviation (SD) of 3.0 inches. As indicated, given these parameters, 68% of third graders would fall within +/–1 SD of the mean (i.e., from 47 to 53 inches), whereas 95% of third graders would fall within +/–2 SD of the mean (i.e., from 44 inches to 56 inches).

A conjecture of whether a girl of a certain height is likely to be in the third grade can be made based on the normal distribution of heights shown in Figure 13-3. If the height is more than 2 SDs above or below the mean, the probability of not being a third grader is high. Similarly, another conjecture about whether the difference between two means is indicative of a real difference is possible by comparing this difference to a normal distribution of mean differences with a mean of 0.0 and the standard error of the difference between two means ($SE_{mean difference}$, comparable to the SD in the third-grade example). If the obtained difference between means is more than 2 $SE_{mean differences}$ from the mean of 0.0, it is possible to conclude that the difference between the two means is a real difference, not one due to the natural variability of the process.

One of the tests commonly used to assess the likelihood that chance accounts for results is known as the student's t-test, which is an example of statistical inference. There are two types of t-tests—one that tests between groups composed of

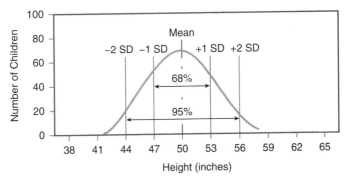

Figure 13-3 Hypothetical normal curve distribution for the height of third-grade girls

the same subjects tested before and after an intervention (known as a dependent t-test) and another that tests between two separate groups, one of which receives the intervention and one of which does not receive the intervention or that has the standard intervention (known as an independent t-test). Computing a t-test in Excel is easy; there are a number of resources that illustrate the process (Goldwater, 2007; Schmuller, 2009).

The Excel t-test results include the computed t-value and the exact probability of the result (i.e., the difference found between means) being due to chance. The values labeled as "two-tailed" should be used. Usually the chance (null) hypothesis is rejected if the exact probably of the result being a chance occurrence is less than 5 in 100 times (usually denoted as $p < 0.05$). In this instance, an inference that the result is not due to chance, but rather due to something else, presumably, the intervention if it is designed well, is possible.

There are many other tests of statistical significance based on the normal curve that are used in varying situations (e.g., when comparing means of more than two groups). In addition, some inferential tests are not based on the normal curve (e.g., when the data consist of counts or rankings). These "nonparametric" tests are simpler to compute than those based on the normal curve, are nearly as powerful in detecting differences, and in many instances can be done merely with a calculator and a set of reference tables. The classic and very practical text on nonparametric statistics, *Nonparametric Statistics for the Behavioral Sciences*, is still available (Siegel, 1956).

There are two areas of caution in inferential statistics. First, the conclusions are always probability statements. If it is more likely that the result was due to an intervention than to the natural chance variation of the process (the probability of the latter being 0.05 or less), there is still the remote possibility that the result was due to chance. For statisticians, conclusions become more firmly established by confirming results from multiple studies (i.e., from replications). Second, inferential statistics allow one to draw conclusions about whether the intervention produced a real effect, but cannot indicate whether this effect is important. Statistical significance is not the same as real-world importance.

Consider, for example, that statistical analysis indicated that telephone reminders did reduce missed appointments, from 14.7% in the "no reminder group" to 13.5% in the "reminder group"—this is an actual reduction of 1.2% and is statistically significant ($p < 0.05$). Also consider that the reminder system costs $10,000 per month to operate. Even though there is a reduction in missed appointments as a result of the reminder system, a manager must decide whether the reduction of 1.2% is worth the expenditure of $10,000 per month. Suppose that a new medication is more effective in reducing hypertension than other medications ($p < 0.05$) but is much more expensive or has a more problematic side-effect profile. The physician, in collaboration with the patient, must decide whether the more effective reduction in hypertension outweighs the cost and side effects. Inferential statistics does not make decisions. Decisions are made based on a variety of factors.

Analyzing Data: Correlations

Evaluation studies completed in applied settings involve correlations between two sets of data For example, ratings by two different raters on the same scale for the same patients, blood values on split samples analyzed by older and newer blood analyzers, or the amount of fish oil supplements consumed and cardiovascular risk score. For each of these examples, the scores in the two sets of data are "paired"—by patient, by blood sample, or by consumer.

Correlation, most commonly the Pearson product moment (linear) correlation, is a measure of the association between two sets of numbers (arrays). Correlations may range from +1.00 (high positive) to −1.00 (high negative). What does a correlation really mean? If a new piece of laboratory equipment correlates 0.98 with the old piece of equipment, is it safe to replace the old equipment with the new equipment? If the ratings of two raters are highly correlated, is it okay to use them interchangeably?

The principal size of a correlation is the relative positions of values in the two arrays. The highest positive correlations result when the highest values in one array are closely aligned (i.e., paired) with the highest values in the other array, and lowest with lowest. If these values are plotted in a scatter plot that has values for one array on the x-axis and values for the other array on the y-axis, the resulting scatter plot will be close to a straight line, sloping up from the lower left to the upper right (see **Figure 13-4**, scatter plot A). Conversely, the highest negative correlations result when the highest values in one array are closely aligned with the lowest values in the other array and, conversely, the lowest with the highest. If these values are plotted in a scatter plot that has values for one array on the x-axis and values for the other array on the y-axis, the resulting scatter plot will be close to a straight line, sloping down from the upper left to the lower right (Figure 13-4, scatter plot B).

In interpreting correlations, the size of the correlation is important (see **Table 13-1**). A note of caution—large sample sizes may produce statistically significant correlations that are so low as to be practically meaningless.

Computing a correlation in Excel is easy. Follow these steps:

1. Open an Excel spreadsheet and enter 10 values in two adjacent columns.
2. Select any empty cell on a sheet (somewhere below the two arrays is fine) and type in "=correl(."
3. Click and drag down the first column of numbers (dotted lines will now enclose the first array) and type in a comma.
4. Click and drag down the second column of numbers (dotted lines will now enclose the second array).
5. Complete by typing a closed parenthesis sign and press Enter.

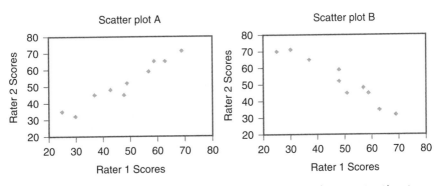

Figure 13-4 Scatter plots illustrating a high positive correlation (scatter plot A) and a high negative correlation (scatter plot B)

Table 13-1 Interpretative Guidelines for Size of Correlations

Size of Correlation	Interpretation
0.9–1.0	Very highly correlated
0.7–0.9	Highly correlated
0.5–0.7	Moderately correlated
0.3–0.5	Low correlation
< 0.3	Little if any correlation

The correlation will appear. Maintain the spreadsheet open for another use.

Another feature of computing correlations in Excel is if there are data sets with missing data (one data value or the other or both have data values missing), the correlation as computed in the listed steps automatically eliminate any data pair where one or the other or both data values are missing. There is no need to sort the data to get complete data set pairs.

There are two major cautions that should be kept in mind when interpreting correlations. First, a correlation, even a high correlation, explains nothing about the comparability of the means of the two groups. The reason is because by adding a constant no change was made in the relative positions of values in the two arrays in reference to each other—if the original correlation was relatively high, high scores on one are still associated with high scores on the other, and low scores on one are still associated with low scores on the other. A high correlation between readings on two pieces of laboratory equipment does not signify that they produce comparable values. The values on split blood samples for the two machines may be highly correlated, the new machine may indicate triglyceride levels that are two or three (or who knows how many) times higher than the old equipment. A second caution about correlations is that a high correlation does not mean that one variable (*A*) causes the other variable (*B*). Correlation does not mean causation. *A* may cause *B*, or *B* may cause *A*, or both may be caused by some other factor.

An example of drawing erroneous conclusions occurred in correlation studies of hormone replacement therapy and the risk of developing coronary heart disease (CHD). This 1991 meta-analysis of multiple epidemiological studies of women taking postmenopausal estrogens concluded that there was a reduced risk of CHD, which was "unlikely to be explained by confounding factors." Based on this finding, the Food and Drug Administration approved a label change, which included the prevention of heart disease as an indication for hormone replacement therapy (Lawlor et al., 2004). Subsequent to these correlational studies, two large randomized trials found either no effect on CHD or a slightly increased risk (Hulley et al., 1998; Rossouw et al., 2002), and many have speculated on the possible confounding factors in the earlier epidemiological studies (Barrett-Connor, 2004; Kuller, 2004; Lawlor et al., 2004; Petitti, 2004; Vandenbroucke, 2004). Despite problems associated with epidemiological (correlational) studies, they remain a valuable tool in identifying possible areas for more controlled trials.

Presenting Data

Although narratives and tables can be very useful in conveying results, charts are one of the most effective means of communication when selected and designed correctly. As Roam noted in a broader context, "The mechanism for making good verbal communication great is to add the visual" (2011, p. 51). It is not uncommon to view posters of improvement projects that were well designed and well executed with truly meaningful results that were hindered in the exposition by the use of poorly developed charts.

Microsoft Office offers an array of chart choices; there are 11 types of charts and numerous variations of each. The challenge is to pick the correct chart for the data from among this vast array of 73 chart types/variations. Naomi Robbins suggests a simple rule for selecting the most effective chart: "One graph is more effective than another if its quantitative information can be decoded more quickly or more easily by most observers" (2005, p. 6). When the rule is applied to data that are typically presented in a healthcare setting, a minimum number of the 73 chart types/variations meet the criterion of being able to convey information quickly and easily to most observers.

The first step in choosing a chart type is to select and format a chart that conveys the information that (the subject-matter expert deems) is most important. It is a poor decision to provide raw data to an expert in chart design and delegate this decision to the expert. Consider the example of a CNL in a hypothetical South Beach clinic who was concerned about declining patient satisfaction. The CNL desired to know whether this was affecting the number of patients enrolling and dropping out of the clinic (enrollees and attrition). The CNL requested that the data expert construct a chart of monthly data on enrollees and attrition over the past year. The data are presented in **Figure 13-5**. What conclusion can be drawn from this chart? How convincing is the conclusion?

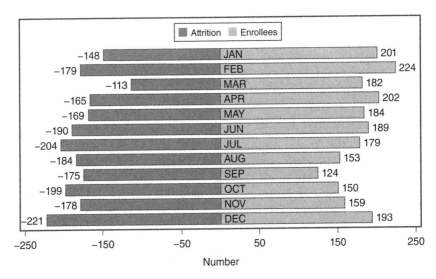

Figure 13-5 South Beach clinic: Enrollees and attrition by month

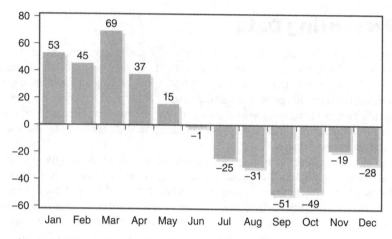

Figure 13-6 South Beach clinic: Net change by month

Consider if instead of asking for a chart of enrollees and attrition, the data expert was told that the information of most interest was whether the clinic was gaining or losing patients each month (i.e., enrollees minus attrition). The data are presented in **Figure 13-6**. What conclusion could be drawn? How convincing is the conclusion? Both charts were drawn from exactly the same data; Figure 13-5 presents data, and Figure 13-6 presents information of value to management.

Other pitfalls in chart design to avoid are poor title(s) for charts or axes (vague or incomplete), chart junk (e.g., distracting or space-wasting pictures or templates, shading/color for no purpose), and the use of the third dimension (e.g., depth of field effects in columns, bars, line, or pie charts), which conveys no information and makes the chart much more difficult to read and interpret (Smith, 2012).

Types of Charts

Here are some guidelines for different types of charts:

1. *Column (vertical) and bar (horizontal) charts:* These are ideal for displaying values for independent categories on the x-axis, for example, different hospitals, and different departments. Column charts (but not bar charts) can also be used to show a trend over time (e.g., years, months) but should not be used to convey a trend over long time intervals (more than approximately eight time intervals). Never truncate the y-axis (the value axis) in a column or bar chart. Bar charts are particularly useful when the x-axis labels (categories) are lengthy.
2. *Line charts:* Line charts are ideally suited to displaying trends over time for either short- or long-term intervals. The value axis (y-axis) of line charts may be truncated. Stacked lines are difficult to interpret by most observers and should be avoided.
3. *Pie charts:* Despite the widespread use of these charts, most experts in chart design agree that they should not be used. Observers cannot easily compare angular quantities in a pie chart much less compare angles in a group of pie charts. Tufte (1983) wrote, "A table is nearly always better than a dumb pie chart; the only worse design than a pie chart is several of them, for then the viewer is asked to compare quantities located in spatial disarray both within

and between pies" (p. 178). Few (2007) wrote that, "Of all the graphs that play major roles in the lexicon of quantitative communication...the pie chart is by far the least effective. Its colorful voice is often heard, but rarely understood. It mumbles when it talks" (p. 1). If the goal is to display the distribution of data from numerous categories adding up to a total number or percentage (the typical use of a pie chart), use a column or bar chart, preferably arranged in a Pareto format (highest value first progressing to the lowest value). If one uses a pie chart, the possibility to improve it is by arranging the segments in increasing or decreasing order of magnitude.

4. *Scatter charts:* These are used when both the x-axis and the y-axis are composed of continuous values (e.g., scores 0 through 100 or 5.0 through 45.0). These are typically used to display a relationship between two sets of continuous variables. Use the "scatter with only markers" chart; do not use scatter charts with lines.

In general, area, stock, surface, donut, or bubble charts are of limited utility in most applications in a healthcare setting. Radar charts may be effective in certain instances, for example, in displaying performance on a number of variables in relation to targets that are different for each of the variables. There are a number of resources on chart design; basic texts include those by Zelazny (2001) and Robbins (2005).

Summary

- The vast majority of problems result from issues in work processes that result in a problematic outcome. Poor employee performance accounts for only a small percentage of these problems.
- Before attempting to find and implement a solution, objective and measurable data should be obtained on current performance. This data should be compared to a clear and an explicit desired target or goal.
- Data on the processes that produce problematic outcomes are the key to solutions. If one analyzes these processes closely, coupled with data, the solution will be readily apparent.
- Designing an evaluation strategy to assess a proposed solution requires care to ensure that the results of the evaluation are as unambiguous as possible.
- Dissemination of findings in an informative and user-friendly format is essential and may be the determining factor in whether these results impact practices at the program and organizational level. Charts are one of the most useful formats for presenting data. It is essential that the correct chart be selected to ensure that the most critical information is clearly displayed.

Reflection Questions

- How open is your organization to identifying problems? How willing is it to commit time and energy to solving them?
- If you observed a problematic outcome, how would you approach getting a team involved in finding a solution? How would you respond to a staff member who said that this was always the way it had been and that things could not be improved?

Learning Activities

1. Consider a problem outcome that occurs frequently in a work setting. List the processes involved in an outcome and consider how to collect data on these process steps.
2. Review a published evaluation study. What design was used? What are the risks of this design? Did the authors adequately address them?
3. Select five published evaluation/research articles that used charts to display findings. Were the findings presented clearly so that they could be understood immediately? Was the correct chart selected for the data presented? Did these charts avoid the basic pitfalls of chart design?

References

American Association of Colleges of Nursing. (2007). *White paper on the role of the Clinical Nurse Leader.* Author. https://nursing.uiowa.edu/sites/default/files/documents/academic-programs/graduate/msn-cnl/CNL_White_Paper.pdf

American Association of Colleges of Nursing. (2013). *Competencies and curricular expectations for clinical nurse leader education and practice.* http://www.aacn.nche.edu/cnl/CNL-Competencies-October-2013.pdf

Barrett-Connor, E. (2004). Commentary: Observation versus intervention—what's different? *International Journal of Epidemiology, 33*(3), 457–459.

Berwick, D. M. (1989). Continuous improvement as an ideal in healthcare. *New England Journal of Medicine, 320*(1), 53–56. https://doi.org/10.1056/nejm198901053200110

Bonetti, P. O., Waeckerlin, A., Schuepfer, G., & Frutiger, A. (2000). Improving time-sensitive processes in the intensive care unit: The example of "door to needle time" in acute myocardial infarction. *International Journal for Quality in Healthcare, 12*(4), 311–317.

Bordens, K., & Abbott, B.B. (2018). *Research design and methods: A process approach* (10th ed.). McGraw-Hill.

Brassard, M., & Ritter, D. (2008). *The memory jogger II: Healthcare edition.* Goal/QPC.

Cai, L., & Zhu, Y. (2015). The challenges of data quality and data assessment in the big data era. *Data Science Journal, 14,* 2. https://doi.org/10.5334/dsj-2015-002

Campbell, D. T., & Stanley, J. C. (1963). *Experimental and quasi-experimental designs for research.* Rand McNally.

Carey, R. G., & Lloyd, R. C. (2001). *Measuring quality improvement in healthcare: A guide to statistical process control applications.* ASQ Quality Press.

Few, S. (2007, August). Save the pies for dessert. *Visual Business Intelligence Newsletter,* 1–14. http://www.perceptualedge.com/articles/08-21-07.pdf

Few, S. (2009). *Now you see it: Simple visualization techniques for quantitative analysis.* Analytics Press.

Goldwater, E. (2007). *Using Excel for statistical data analysis—caveats.* http://people.umass.edu/eva-gold/excel.html

Graban, M. (2011). *Lean hospitals: Improving quality, patient safety, and employee engagement* (2nd ed.). CRC Press.

Graban, M. (2019). *Measures of success: React less, lead better, improve more.* Constancy, Inc.

Heffner, C. L. (2004). Experimental design. *Research Methods.* http://allpsych.com/researchmethods/experimentaldesign.html

Hulley, S., Grady, D., Bush, T., Furberg, C., Herrington, D., Riggs, B., & Vittinghoff, E. (1998). Randomized trial of estrogen plus progestin for secondary prevention of coronary heart disease in postmenopausal women. Heart and Estrogen/progestin Replacement Study (HERS) Research Group. *Journal of the American Medical Association, 280*(7), 605–613.

Institute for Healthcare Improvement. (2011). *Run chart tool.* http://www.ihi.org/knowledge/pages/tools/runchart.aspx

Katal, A., Wazid, M., & Goudar, R. (2013). Big data: Issues, challenges, tools and good practices. *Procedures of the 2013 Sixth International Conference on Contemporary Computing, Noida, IEEE,* 404–409.

Kelley, D. L. (1999). *How to use control charts for healthcare.* ASQ Quality Press.

Kuller, L. H. (2004). Commentary: Hazards of studying women: The oestrogen oestrogen/progesterone dilemma. *International Journal of Epidemiology, 33*(3), 459–460.

Lawlor, D. A., Smith, G. D., & Ebrahim, S. (2004). Commentary: The hormone replacement-coronary heart disease conundrum: Is this the death of observational epidemiology? *International Journal of Epidemiology, 33*(3), 464–467.

Lennon-Dearing, R., & Neeley-Barnes, S. L. (2012). Quantitative research. In H. R. Hall & L. A. Roussel (Eds.), *Evidence-based practice: An integrative approach to research, administration and practice* (pp. 3–21). Jones & Bartlett Learning.

McGregor, S. L. T. (2017). *Understanding and evaluating research. A critical guide.* Sage.

Miller, R. J. (2019). Evaluating statistical approaches in nursing. In C. R. King, S. O. Gerard, & C. G. Rapp (Eds.), *Essential knowledge for CNL and APRN nurse leaders* (pp. 283–295). Springer.

Petitti, D. (2004). Commentary: Hormone replacement therapy and coronary heart disease: Four lessons. *International Journal of Epidemiology, 33*(3), 461–463.

Roam, D. (2011). *Blah, blah, blah: What to do when words don't work.* Penguin Group.

Robbins, N. B. (2005). *Creating more effective graphs.* John Wiley & Sons.

Rossouw, J. E., Anderson, G. L., Prentice, R. L., LaCroix, A. Z., Kooperberg, C., Stefanik, M. L., Jackson, R. D., Bersford, S. A. A., Howard, B. V., Johnson, K. C., Kotchen, J. M., Ockgene, J., & Writing Group for the Women's Health Initiative Investigators. (2002). Risks and benefits of estrogen plus progestin in healthy postmenopausal women: Principal results from the Women's Health Initiative randomized controlled trial. *Journal of the American Medical Association, 288*(3), 321–333.

Schmuller, J. (2009). *Statistical analysis with Excel for dummies.* Wiley Publishing, Inc.

Schwab, K. (2017). *The fourth industrial revolution.* Penguin Random House.

Siegel, S. (1956). *Nonparametric statistics for the behavioral sciences.* McGraw-Hill.

Sims, P. (2011). *Little bets: How breakthrough ideas emerge from small discoveries.* Free Press.

Smith, J. M. (2012). *Problems with 3D charts.* http://blog.indezine.com/2012/08/problems-with -3d-charts-by-james-m-smith.html

Stampfer, M. J., & Colditz, G. A. (1991). Estrogen replacement therapy and coronary heart disease: A quantitative assessment of the epidemiologic evidence. *Preventive Medicine, 20*(1), 47–63.

Tufte, E. R. (1983). *The visual display of quantitative information.* Graphics Press.

Vandenbroucke, J. P. (2004). Commentary: The HRT story: Vindication of old epidemiological theory. *International Journal of Epidemiology, 33*(3), 456–457.

Zelazny, G. (2001). *Say it with charts: The executive's guide to visual communication.* McGraw-Hill.

Changing the System for Vulnerable Patients: A Population Approach

Lauran Hardin

High-cost, high-needs patients are the focus of national attention as healthcare systems shift strategy to population health. CNLs can have an important impact on successful outcomes in risk-based contracts and global payment. In 2012, Mercy Health Saint Mary's in Grand Rapids, Michigan, supported a change in focus from the CNL competencies applied in the microsystem of a unit to application in a population of complex, vulnerable patients.

A Complex Care Center, led by a CNL, was created to analyze and intervene with the population. Approximately 1,200 patients have participated in the program since its inception in 2012. Only 17% are uninsured, while 19% are dual eligible, and 35% have Medicaid insurance. The majority (91%) of the population is less than 65 years old with a high degree of psycho/social issues including addiction (59%), homelessness (19%), trauma (43%), and psychiatric diagnoses (70%). Several of the patients (28%) have a medical home outside of our network yet use Mercy Health Saint Mary's for their hospital services.

All patients have a root-cause analysis performed on a retrospective 10-year review of their medical record. A multidisciplinary conference is conducted that results in the creation of a complex care map and plan of care that is used to manage the patient at both ED visits and hospital admissions. The care map brings forward the patient's story and links providers to the cross-continuum team and evidence-based recommendations for care through an alert in the EMR.

In addition to clinical intervention, the Complex Care Center implements process improvements and community interventions to change the root cause for populations. Most programs for complex patients focus on changing the patient by adding additional care management resources. The focus of the Complex Care Center is to change the system by improving the delivery and coordination of existing resources.

Following intervention, patients in the program for two years ($n = 252$) have seen a 62% reduction in inpatient admissions, a 66% reduction in LOS, and a 43% reduction in emergency room and urgent care visits. An increase in operating margin of $373,000 and a 32% decrease in direct expenses/case was also observed in the population. Applying the CNL competencies of leadership for patient-care practices and delivery, synthesis of data/evidence to evaluate and achieve optimal outcomes, integration of care for cohorts of patients, and collaboration across disciplines and systems resulted in important improvements for population health.

The project was undertaken as a clinical QI initiative at Mercy Health and as such was not formally supervised by the Mercy Health Institutional Review Board per their policies.

CHAPTER 14

Using Informatics and Healthcare Technologies to Guide CNL Practice

Julia Stocker Schneider

LEARNING OBJECTIVES

1. Discuss the role and current state of informatics in healthcare.
2. Describe informatics competencies specific to CNL practice.
3. Examine how information technology (IT) can be used to support CNL practice.

KEY TERMS

Algorithm
Clinical decision support
CPOE
Data
EHR
EHR maturity
Health information exchange
Health IT
HITECH Act

Informatics
Interoperability
Meaningful use
mHealth
Patient safety
Privacy and security
Systems life cycle
Telehealth

CNL ROLES

Client advocate
Educator
Information manager
Member of a profession

Outcomes manager
System analyst and risk anticipator
Team member

CNL PROFESSIONAL VALUES

Accountability

Altruism

Human dignity   Social justice
Integrity

CNL CORE COMPETENCIES

Communication assessment   Information and healthcare
Critical thinking   technologies
Designer/Manager/Coordinator of care   Resource management
Ethical decision-making

Introduction

Healthcare organizations have invested heavily in health information technology (IT) in recent years. The resulting widespread adoption of health IT has transformed how nurses and healthcare providers do their work. Through the support of these powerful tools at the point of care, nurses and other healthcare providers now have easy access to necessary information, as well as decision support and communication tools. CNLs should be knowledgeable and proficient with the use of health IT as they lead microsystem team members to achieve better care outcomes for the population they serve. Most aspects of the CNL role rely heavily on the use of data, information, and knowledge. CNLs with a solid mastery of informatics principles and practice will be better equipped to leverage health IT to support high-reliability care processes that lead to better care.

Nursing Informatics

Biomedical and health informatics is the science of making use of data, information, and knowledge to improve health and the delivery of healthcare services (AMIA, 2020). Nursing informatics is a subset of biomedical and healthcare informatics, and a nursing specialty that integrates nursing science with information and analytic sciences to "identify, define, manage, and communicate data, information, knowledge, and wisdom in nursing practice" (ANA, 2015).

Nursing informatics (NI) is concerned with data, information, knowledge, and wisdom. These major concepts of the NI specialty are characterized according to increasing levels of complexity, with each of the simpler concepts serving as building blocks to the most complex. Data serves as the fundamental concept from which information is derived, information serves as the basis of knowledge, and knowledge is requisite to the generation of wisdom. Data are defined as discrete entities that are objectively described without interpretation. Information refers to data that are interpreted, organized, or structured; knowledge is the synthesis of information that leads to the identification and formalization of relationships. Wisdom is the use of knowledge to manage and solve human problems. The goal of nursing informatics is to support nurses, patients, and other care providers in their decision-making in all roles and across various settings (ANA, 2015).

Role of IT in Healthcare

Health IT has been implemented to support the delivery of high-quality healthcare. The use of health IT benefits providers, patients, and healthcare organizations by providing the information infrastructure to support the flow of information needed for the delivery of care. Healthcare providers use health IT to access pertinent patient information when and where it is needed and to record and communicate patient health information that has been gathered and care that has been delivered. Patients and providers use health IT to communicate and share information with one another and, increasingly, as a tool through which care can be delivered. Providers rely on decision support features and alerts to assist them in providing safer care. Healthcare organizations use health IT to monitor care delivery and outcomes, and to build knowledge for process improvement (ONC, 2020a).

Electronic Health Record

The EHR serves as the centerpiece in leveraging health IT. It is known as an enterprise solution since it incorporates information management features that support direct care activities, and those that support indirect activities such as scheduling and billing functions. An EHR is a longitudinal patient health record that is created, stored, and accessed in an electronic format. It contains patient health information generated at the point of care in any care delivery setting and serves as the complete record for that clinical encounter (Douglas & Celli, 2015). Ideally, an EHR would provide access to the complete longitudinal health record for any given patient across all clinical encounters.

The EHR automates clinical information and streamlines the clinician's workflow. It enhances patient safety through alerts and decision support. EHR core functions include:

1. Documentation and retrieval of health information and data
2. Results management such as lab or X-ray results
3. Computerized provider order entry (CPOE) and order management
4. Clinical decision support (CDS)
5. Electronic communication and connectivity (to improve care coordination)
6. Patient education and support
7. Administrative processes such as scheduling and billing
8. Reporting and population health management (Barey et al., 2018; IOM, 2003)

Barriers to Health IT Adoption

The first use of a computer system to support patient care occurred more than 50 years ago (Shortliffe, 2005). Despite long-standing recognition of the benefits of informatics and technology use in healthcare, barriers to adoption have persisted over the years. Shortly after the IOM (now the National Academy of Medicine) released *To Err Is Human* (1999) and *Crossing the Quality Chasm* (2001), it published *Patient Safety: Achieving a New Standard for Care* (2004). The 2004 report recognized the need for the broad implementation of EHRs to support improved patient safety by providing immediate access to patient information and decision support tools. Further, it called for the creation of a national health information infrastructure to support safer patient care. During that year, the Office of the National Coordinator for Health Information Technology (ONC) was created with the primary goal to support widespread adoption of EHR throughout the United States (Bergman et al., 2016). Despite this initiative, numerous barriers to health IT adoption persisted including concerns related to cost, time, lack of computer skills, concerns about confidentiality, and knowledge and attitudinal barriers (AHRQ, n.d.).

HITECH Act

During the economic downturn of 2008–2009, funding to jump-start the significant investment needed for widespread adoption of health IT was included in the American Reinvestment and Recovery Act of 2009. The bill, known as the Health Information Technology for Economic and Clinical Health (HITECH) Act, contained several provisions designed to stimulate investment and expansion of health IT in the United States. Key initiatives of the program included an EHR incentive program designed to encourage hospitals and providers to adopt and meaningfully use EHRs, and an EHR certification program that set a national standard of functionalities, so that hospitals and providers could ensure that their EHR was capable of supporting meaningful use (Bergman et al., 2016; Blumenthal & Tavenner, 2010).

The unprecedented investment in health IT ushered in the quickest uptake of health IT that the United States has ever seen. In 2008, only 9.4% of non-federal acute care hospitals had adopted a basic EHR system (includes patient demographics problem lists, medication lists, discharge summaries, medication CPOE, and lab, radiology, and diagnostic test results). By 2016, hospital adoption of basic EHRs grew to 83.8%. Further, in the years immediately following the implementation of the EHR incentive and certification programs, the number of hospitals adopting EHR technology certified to meet federal requirements grew from 71.9% in 2011 to 96% in 2015. Additionally, office-based physicians achieved a 78% certified health IT adoption rate by 2015 (Charles et al., 2015; Henry et al., 2016; HHS & ONC, 2018).

Meaningful Use

The meaningful use program was designed to build on the EHR incentive program to be sure that the EHR hardware and software that was purchased by healthcare systems and providers were not only adopted but were also used in meaningful ways to support patient safety. The HITECH Act established three incremental goals for meaningful use as follows:

- Stage 1: Data capture and sharing
- Stage 2: Advanced clinical processes
- Stage 3: Improved outcomes (ONC, 2013)

In essence, these requirements were designed to ensure that healthcare organizations and providers were capable and performing basic tasks with their EHR including using a certified EHR, exchanging health information, and reporting quality measures (Bergman et al., 2016). The EHR certification process has elevated the capabilities of EHRs, since they were required to perform a number of standard functions from basic, such as recording vital signs, to more complex, like exchanging clinical information electronically. Each new iteration of the certification criteria has made EHRs more functional and interoperable for users (Barey et al., 2018). The EHR incentive meaningful use programs have demonstrated success in that EHR adoption has reached near universal levels, and that EHRs are increasingly more robust (Henry et al., 2016; Soriono & Hunter, 2019).

EHR Maturity

In 2005, the Healthcare Information and Management Systems Society (HIMSS) created an EMR adoption and maturity model to assist healthcare organizations in achieving adoption of high-level health IT. The eight-stage Electronic Medical Record Adoption Model (EMRAM) measures adoption and utilization of health IT functions within the EMR. The model was updated in 2016 to include more of a focus on e-health and less on technology, and with privacy and security added to combat increasing data breaches (Green, 2016).

In 2007, more than 70% of US hospitals were at stage 2 or below, with none achieving stage 7. By 2014, 90% were at a stage 3 or above, with 3.7% at stage 7 (Hersh et al., 2018). Using the updated model, more than 80% of 5,487 US hospitals achieved a stage 4 or greater, with 6.4% achieving a stage 7 (Cohen, 2018). It is clear from the achievement of hospitals on the EMRAM that EHRs adopted in practice are becoming more robust with more features and tools to better support safe patient care. Given the progress, and to better target health IT adoption in other areas, HIMSS has added additional adoption and maturity models including the Adoption Model for Analytics Maturity, Continuity of Care Maturity Model, Clinically Integrated Supply Outcomes Model, Digital Imaging Adoption Model, Infrastructure Adoption Model, and Outpatient EMR Adoption Model (HIMSS Analytics, 2017b).

Emerging Health IT Tools and Applications

As technology evolves, additional innovations are being introduced into the health IT space to support care delivery functions. Some of these innovations have become available as part of the EHR, while others are add-on tools that can be integrated into the EHR. Many of these emerging health IT tools target both patient and providers as end users.

Tablets

The capability and availability of tablets has supported their adoption as part of a broader health IT solution. Procedure consents have been slower to transition to electronic due to challenges with signature capture. While signature capture devices have been successfully integrated with desktop computers in health systems, there was still a need at the point of care. Tablet technology is beginning to fill that void to support the consent process and capture signatures at the bedside (Jayasinghe et al., 2019; MITRE, 2014). Tablets are also increasingly being implemented with patients for completion of questionnaires and patient histories and to update medication lists (Abernethy et al., 2008; Kripalani et al., 2019; Lee Ventola, 2014). During the COVID-19 pandemic, tablets took on several important uses including connecting patients to their loved ones while no-visitor policies were in place to minimize COVID-19 spread (Martineau, 2020).

Patient Education and Engagement

Many health systems have implemented digital health education solutions that are integrated with the EHR. These platforms allow nurses to assign patient education videos to the patient's in-room TV via the EHR in a manner that supports patient education. These add-in solutions support important nursing workflow processes while also engaging patients in learning and with digital health. Patient portals have been implemented widely across health systems and providers as a mechanism to connect patients with their health providers and with their EHR. Although patient portals were envisioned as a mechanism for patient engagement with health IT, which was a goal of meaningful use, portal use by patients and families has remained relatively low (Furukawa et al., 2014). Since these digital tools provide an important mechanism for patients and providers to communicate, it is hopeful that patient use will increase during the COVID-19 pandemic (Brock, 2020). With encouragement and education on how to use these tools, patients and families may begin to use them.

Telehealth

Capabilities for telehealth have long been available for distance delivery of healthcare, though widespread adoption has not occurred despite improvements in technology to support telehealth. Barriers have existed due to a lack of comfort with technology use, privacy and security concerns, licensing and regulation limitations, and lack of reimbursement. With the outbreak of COVID-19, licensing and regulation concerns have been relaxed and reimbursement for telehealth has increased. Trends indicate a significant initial uptake of telehealth utilization, particularly for non-COVID-19 patient visits. It is hopeful that the increased acceptance of telehealth will remain beyond the pandemic, and that the delivery of care via telehealth technology will be utilized for the visits it is most suited for (HHS, 2020; Hollander & Carr, 2020; Koonin et al., 2020; ONC, 2020b).

mHealth

Mobile health or mHealth refers to the use of mobile devices such as phones, tablets, wearable devices, and monitoring devices to support health objectives (Care Innovations, 2020; Park, 2016). Since more than 90% of US adults own cell phones, and there is a wide variety of health-related education, tracking, and other apps available, there is good potential for engaging patients in this manner (IMedicalApps, 2020; Pew Research Center, 2015). Many patients have initiated use of apps themselves as a tool to assist them in meeting health goals. Healthcare providers are increasingly incorporating them as part of a patient education and self-care strategy.

Algorithms/Machine-Learning Models

One of the benefits of EHRs is the ability to capture large volumes of complex data. Subtle patterns can then be detected within that "big data" using machine-learning algorithms, so that insights can be gleaned related to early warning signs, process variation, care efficacy, and patient outcomes (Dananjayan & Raj, 2020). Through this process, early warning systems can be created based on patterns detected using machine learning such as sepsis prediction in the ICU (Nemati et al., 2018). The IHI began support for the use of early warning systems to implement rapid response teams during its 100,000 lives campaign (IHI, 2020). EHRs are key to the creation and implementation of such algorithms through data capture necessary for machine learning. Further, the early warning systems can be implemented within the EHR, so that the nurse is alerted when a concerning score threshold is achieved. Examples of algorithms that have been implemented include Modified Early Warning Score (MEWS) and Pediatric Early Warning Score (Mathukia et al., 2015; PEWS: Gold et al., 2014).

Informatics Competencies

As health IT has become more integrated and standard to the delivery of healthcare, the need for nurses to be proficient in the use of this technology has been increasingly recognized. Staggers et al. (2001) identified three major categories of nursing informatics competencies including computer skills, informatics knowledge, and informatics skills. The TIGER Initiative (2007) built on that work to develop a Nursing Informatics Competencies Model structured around: (1) basic computer competencies, (2) information literacy, and (3) information management. The TIGER Initiative identified competencies for each portion of the model coupled with resources to support nurses in achieving them. Recent efforts have been focused on the creation of an interprofessional competency model. To that end, the TIGER Initiative has joined forces with HIMSS in an international competency synthesis project to develop recommendations for health informatics core competencies.

CNL Informatics Competencies

Informatics competencies specific to CNL practice build on identified nursing and healthcare competencies to support implementation of the CNL's role. Essential CNL competencies for informatics and healthcare technologies were identified by AACN (2013) to include the following:

1. Use IT, analytics, and evaluation methods to:
   a. collect or access appropriate and accurate data to generate evidence for nursing practice;
   b. provide input in the design of databases that generate meaningful evidence for practice;
   c. collaborate to analyze data from practice and system performance;

    d. design evidence-based interventions in collaboration with the health professional team;

    e. examine patterns of behavior and outcomes; and

    f. identify gaps in evidence for practice.

2. Implement the use of technologies to coordinate and laterally integrate patient care within, across care settings and among healthcare providers.
3. Analyze current and proposed use of patient-care technologies, including their cost-effectiveness and appropriateness in the design and delivery of care in diverse care settings.
4. Use technologies and information systems to facilitate the collection, analysis, and dissemination of data including clinical, financial, and operational outcomes.
5. Use information and communication technologies to document patient care, advance patient education, and enhance accessibility of care.
6. Participate in ongoing evaluation, implementation and integration of healthcare technologies, including the EHR.
7. Use a variety of technology modalities and media to disseminate healthcare information and communicate effectively with diverse audiences (AACN, 2013, pp. 15–16).

Core Healthcare Informatics Knowledge, Skills, and Abilities for CNL Practice

The importance of informatics knowledge, skills, and abilities (KSAs) by CNLs in practice were measured as part of the most recent CNL job analysis, which was conducted by the CNC (2016). The analysis was conducted by using subject matter experts to identify KSAs, then having them ranked by CNLs in practice. The resulting core set of 14 healthcare informatics KSAs for CNL practice are as follows:

1. Assess, critique, and analyze information sources
2. Design care utilizing informatics and patient care technology
3. Apply multiple sources of systems data in designing processes for care delivery
4. Evaluate clinical information systems to provide feedback related to efficient and accurate documentation
5. Apply ethical principles in the use of information systems
6. Evaluate the impact of new technologies on patients, families, and healthcare delivery
7. Identify and assess the relationships among information systems, accurate communication, error reduction, and healthcare system operation
8. Analyze and disseminate healthcare information among the interprofessional team and across the care continuum
9. Validate accuracy of consumer-provided information regarding culturally relevant health issues from multiple sources
10. Utilize technology for health promotion and disease prevention
11. Collaborate with quality improvement and IT teams to design and implement processes for improving patient outcomes

12. Utilize current technology to anticipate patient risk
13. Demonstrate to other healthcare providers the efficient and appropriate use of healthcare technologies to maximize healthcare outcomes
14. Access, critique, and analyze information from multiple sources (CNC, 2016, pp. 168–169).

CNL Informatics Competency Themes

CNL informatics competencies were analyzed along with core CNL practice knowledge, skills, and abilities. Major themes that were identified are described next.

Use of Technology to Support Patient Care

One of the key features of the EHR is to provide an electronic method of easily recording patient information and care provided in a manner that is immediately accessible by other care providers. To achieve maximal health IT support for patient care, it is best that the EHR solution selected is user-friendly, well organized, and easy to navigate. Hardware should be available at the point of care (e.g., computers-on-wheels, at the patient's bedside, tablets, etc.), and software should support recording of patient data as part of the clinician workflow. The user interface (the screens that the users interact with) and local implementation by the organization should make clear to users where within the EHR specific types of data should be documented and retrieved. As additional documentation requirements are imposed, there has been a tendency for users to be required to navigate through more and more screens. While drop-down menus are often used on these screens to speed data entry and standardize responses for better aggregation and retrieval of data, clinicians may have a harder time connecting these data points to clearly convey or receive the patient's story. While technology can support that picture, many vendor systems may not easily provide that function. CNLs should be involved in selection and implementation to maximize EHR system support for patient care.

Clinical Decision Support

CDS is the process of enhancing health-related decisions and actions through the use of relevant, organized clinical knowledge and patient information to improve health and healthcare quality and outcomes (Osheroff et al., 2012). EHRs often contain decision support features to provide clinicians or patients with pertinent clinical knowledge and patient-related information within the EHR in a timely manner to enhance patient care. Common forms of CDS found in EHRs include the use of charts to simplify complex information (e.g., growth charts), EHR templates, medication prescribing and administration alerts and reminders, medication formularies, clinical guidelines, and health literature databases (e.g., CINAHL; Dowding et al., 2009; Ross Kraft & Androwich, 2015).

The key purposes of CDSs are to:

1. assist in problem solving of semi-structured problems,
2. support (rather than replace) the judgment of a manager or clinician, and
3. improve the effectiveness of the decision-making process.

CDS features can deliver powerful support to providers by delivering knowledge at the point of care that enhances care delivery. CDS systems can deliver active alerts (push) or allow the user to query the desired information (pull). In addition to knowledge-based CDS, some EHRs may have predictive CDS, where the system recognizes patterns in the data to make predictions based on the trajectory of previous such occurrences in the database (Berner & LaLande, 2007). CNLs should advocate for and support CDS use that provides clinicians with the knowledge they need at the point of care to provide the safest and highest quality of care possible. CDS has become much more available in practice areas across the continuum as full EHR implementation is achieved, and as the systems implemented become more mature. Full CDS is part of stage 6 in the EMR Adoption Model, and as of 2017, over 40% of registered US hospitals had achieved stage 6 or better (Cohen, 2018).

Understanding and Evaluating Data

Data input by users into the EHR are collected and stored in a secure data warehouse, which is made up of a number of databases. A database is a collection of related objects, including tables, forms, queries, and reports. Once data are entered, they are organized into tables so that they can be stored and retrieved in an organized way. The tables are connected by identical key fields that relate the tables to one another. A query is the mechanism that is used to ask questions of the data from one or more related tables. Reports are used to display information generated from the query. Through the query process, desired data are aggregated and organized in a way that generates information. Interpretation of the information in the context of clinical practice by clinicians turns the information into knowledge. The application of the knowledge to the provision of care by the clinician or nurse creates and involves wisdom (Joos & Nelson, 2015).

In most EHRs, clinical managers and staff may have access to report functions that allow clinicians to run specified queries for the monitoring and evaluation of the information of interest. Custom queries may often be generated by the IT department according to the way the data are structured and stored. Analytics can offer insight beyond that of simple reporting; it involves the aggregation and retrieval of more complex data including data from multiple databases (such as those in a data warehouse) that yields a more detailed understanding of the problem (Kimmel, 2015).

Communicating and Disseminating Healthcare Information

The EHR includes basic tools to support care coordination in the inpatient setting, through electronic communication tools, and EHR documentation that supports care coordination. In addition to vendor-included coordination screens, organizations can customize EHR support for care coordination in conjunction with their vendor. Since the CNL leads care coordination at the point of care, it is important for the CNL to determine the extent to which the organization's EHR solution supports coordination, and advocate for the inclusion of tools in the EHR to support the activity. CNLs are tasked with lateral integration, which means patient care is coordinated among all independent and interdependent care providers across the healthcare continuum (Nelson, 2016); it is important that electronic coordination tools extend beyond the acute care setting.

Healthcare reform, and the establishment of the patient-centered medical home, has provided a model to better support patient care coordination across the continuum. Available and developing technology to support care coordination were identified by Demiris and Kneale (2015) to include CDS, use of registries, technology to support team care (often EHR), telehealth, personal health records, and patient-centered measurement. Other technology developments to support care coordination include the HIE, which will allow patient care data to be securely exchanged across health systems and providers in a way that retains the data meaning. Success with HIE is dependent on the adoption of standards that support interoperability. The establishment of interoperability is a key strategic goal of the ONC (HIMSS, 2020c; ONC, 2020a).

Patient Safety, Risk Management, and Care Improvement

Many EHR functions exist to support patient safety. The following integrations are key to the support of safe patient care.

CPOE

CPOE refers to an electronic order management system that consists of electronic order selection, transmittal, and decision support functions. Whether occurring in an inpatient or outpatient setting, CPOE is often contained and integrated within an EHR. In some cases, CPOE may have been adopted prior to EHR implementation due to the important safety features it provides including elimination of illegible orders and improved decision support (i.e., drug and dosing guidance, allergy and drug interaction warnings, order accuracy checking; Barey et al., 2018).

Technology to Support Medication Administration

Given the alarming frequency of adverse drug events in the United States (5% of all hospitalized patients and likely > 5% for ambulatory patients), several technology solutions are often used to support safe medication administration. In addition to CPOE, these include the electronic medication administration record (eMAR) automated dispensing cabinets (e.g., Pyxis), smart pumps, and barcode-assisted medication administration (BCMA). These point-of-care technologies have been implemented to provide additional protection against errors involving wrong patient, wrong drug, wrong route, wrong dose, and wrong time. BCMA utilizes radio frequency identifiers to verify the correct patient and drug and dose given and record the time and nurse administering the medication. More mature EHRs (stages 6 and 7) include a closed-loop medication system (CLMS) that integrates these functions seamlessly together to reduce the occurrence of adverse drug events (Burkoski et al., 2019; Grissinger & Mandrack, 2015; HIMSS Analytics, 2017a).

Systems Life Cycle

The process of planning, developing, implementing, and maintaining an information system is known as the systems life cycle. The main phases of the cycle include:

- planning,
- system design or selection,

- implementation, and
- maintenance.

The systems life cycle begins with a needs assessment to determine the gap between the current health IT state and the current and future needs of the organization. This assessment should include an evaluation of information needs for clinical care and administrative support processes (e.g., billing, bed management, etc.), and should consider the process workflow. To truly understand information needs and process workflow, stakeholders should be consulted including those doing the work in each of the affected job functions, as well as patients receiving care.

Once current needs and deficits are identified, the representative team charged with developing a solution should brainstorm solutions based on the organization's information needs requirements. The solution will include both hardware (physical machines, monitors, wiring, and infrastructure) and software (the instructions for what the computer will do, includes locally installed and web-based programs). A solution decision should be made based on the established selection criteria according to the solution that best addresses the information needs and according to the most desirable delivery features and costs. The solution may be homegrown (typically have high development and maintenance costs and aren't certified), or a vendor solution (may have high licensing fees, but no development fees, and may be certified).

Once an information system solution is identified, it is important that an implementation plan is developed and executed. Care should also be taken to thoughtfully integrate the new information system solution efficiently into the work process. Solutions with poor implementation strategies have higher rates of failure and means that the information need remains unaddressed despite the investment of time and monetary resources to solve the problem.

The maintenance phase involves periodic evaluation of how the informatics solution is being used and how well it is addressing the organization's information management needs, including those it was intended to address and any new needs that may have arisen. Further, it is helpful to examine the impact the information system use has had on patient outcomes like medication errors, prehospitalization rates, and length of stay, and other organizational outcomes such as time efficiency, staff satisfaction, and patient satisfaction. Gaps noted in the evaluation begin the system life cycle over again (Douglas & Celli, 2015; McBride & Newbold, 2016).

Privacy and Security

As technology has become more integrated in our society, threats to privacy and security have become increasingly prevalent. Health data are particularly attractive to hackers because they contains robust personal information that includes financial and health information. According to a recent cybersecurity survey, most healthcare organizations are experiencing significant security incidents. Phishing by cybercriminals to obtain financial information, employee information, and patient information were the most commonly reported incidents (HIMSS, 2020a). While health IT is a powerful tool, it carries with it significant privacy and security risk. CNLs must support processes that protect patient privacy and data security including adherence to HIPAA guidelines and best practices in healthcare cybersecurity (HIMSS, 2020b; ONC, 2019).

Summary

- Health IT supports safe, high-quality care by providing secure access to patient data and decision-making tools at the point of care.
- The current state of health IT includes near universal EHR adoption with systems that are increasingly more feature laden and mature
- Achievement of CNL health informatics competencies requires knowledge and skills related to:
  - Use of technology to support patient care
  - Clinical decision support
  - Understanding and evaluating data
  - Communicating and disseminating healthcare information
  - Patient safety, risk management, and care improvement
  - Systems life cycle
  - Privacy and security

Reflection Questions

1. Evaluate your own competence with informatics. What areas do you need to learn more about, and where can you gain the necessary knowledge?
2. How well do you manage information within your microsystem? Identify ways that you might more fully leverage informatics in your microsystem to support quality, safe, and efficient care.

Learning Activities

1. Evaluate where your organization is in the systems life cycle. Identify any information needs that you have that need a technological solution. Consider what health IT option would best address your need.
2. Speak with your organization's nurse informaticist, systems analyst, or IT department to find out what reports can be generated from your EHR. Discuss which queries you can run yourself, and the steps required to run them. Inquire about the availability of having additional reports run, and what your organization's process is to request these queries.
3. What patient outcomes or microsystem issues are you aware of that could benefit from the use of CDS? Formulate a question that can be asked of the data and determine the data elements you would likely need to answer the question.

Websites That Address Healthcare Informatics

- https://digital.ahrq.gov/ (Agency for Health Research and Quality [AHRQ] Digital Healthcare Research)
- https://www.amia.org/ (American Medical Informatics Association)

- https://www.ania.org/ (American Nursing Informatics Association)
- https://www.allianceni.org/ (Alliance for Nursing Informatics)
- https://geekgirls.com/ (Geek Girls Plain English Computing)
- https://www.himss.org/ (Healthcare Information Management and Systems Society)
- https://www.healthit.gov/ (The Office of the National Coordinator for Health Information Technology)
- https://www.himss.org/what-we-do-technology-informatics-guiding-education -reform-tiger (The TIGER Initiative)
- https://nnlm.gov/mcr/training/technology-program/electronic-health-records -ehrs (National Library of Medicine—Electronic Health Records
- https://www.nursing.umaryland.edu/academics/pe/events/sini/ (Summer Institute in Nursing Informatics)

References

Abernethy, A. P., Herndon, J. E., Wheeler, J. L., Patwardhan, M., Shaw, H., Lyerly, H. K., & Weinfurt, K. (2008). Improving health care efficiency and quality using tablet personal computers to collect research-quality, patient-reported data. *Health Services Research, 43*(6), 1975–1991. https://doi .org/10.1111/j.1475-6773.2008.00887.x

Agency for Health Research & Quality. (n.d.). *Barriers to HIT implementation.* https://digital .ahrq.gov/health-it-tools-and-resources/health-it-costs-and-benefits-database/barriers-hit -implementation

American Association of Colleges of Nursing. (2013). *Competencies and curricular expectations for Clinical Nurse Leader education and practice.* https://www.aacnnursing.org/Portals/42/AcademicNursing /CurriculumGuidelines/CNL-Competencies-October-2013.pdf

American Nurses Association. (2015). *Nursing informatics: Scope and standards of practice* (2nd ed.). Author.

AMIA. (2020). *What is informatics?* https://www.amia.org/fact-sheets/what-informatics

Barey, E. B., Matrian, K., & McGonigle, D. (2018). The electronic health record and clinical informatics. In D. McGonigle & K. Mastrian (Eds.), *Nursing informatics and the foundation of knowledge* (4th ed., pp. 566–618). Jones & Bartlett Learning.

Bergman, D. M., McBride, S., & Tietze, M. (2016). National health care transformation and information technology. In S. McBride & M. Tietze (Eds.), *Nursing informatics for the advanced practice nurse* (pp. 82–101). Springer.

Berner, E. S., & LaLande, T. J. (2007). Overview of clinical decision support systems. In E. S. Berner (Ed.), *Clinical decision support systems* (Vol. 6, pp. 463–477). Springer.

Blumenthal, D., & Tavenner, M. (2010). The "meaningful use" regulation for electronic health records. *New England Journal of Medicine, 363*(6), 501–504.

Brock, J. (2020). Using tech to improve patient engagement in the new normal. *Becker's Hospital Review.* https://www.beckershospitalreview.com/using-tech-to-improve-patient-engagement-in -the-new-normal.html

Burkoski, V., Yoon, J., Solomon, S., Hall, T. N. T., Karas, A. B., Jarrett, S. R., & Collins, B. E. (2019). Closed-loop medication system: Leveraging technology to elevate safety. *Nursing Leadership, 32*(SP), 16–28. https://doi.org/10.12927/cjnl.2019.25817

Care Innovations. (2020). *What is mHealth? How is it different from telehealth?* https://news.care innovations.com/blog/what-is-mhealth-how-is-it-different-from-telehealth

Charles, D., Gabriel, M., & Searcy, T. (2015). Adoption of electronic health record systems among U .S . non-federal acute care hospitals: 2008–2014. *ONC Data Brief,* 23. https://www.healthit .gov/sites/default/files/data-brief/2014HospitalAdoptionDataBrief.pdf

Cohen, J. K. (2018). How many hospitals are on each stage of HIMSS Analytics' EMR Adoption Model? *Becker's Health IT.* https://www.beckershospitalreview.com/ehrs/how-many-hospitals-are -on-each-stage-of-himss-analytics-emr-adoption-model.html

Commision on Nurse Certification. (2016). *Clinical Nurse Leader (CNL) 2016 job analysis summary and certification examination blueprint.* http://www.aacnnursing.org/Portals/42/CNL/CNL-Exam-Content-Outline-2017.pdf

Dananjayan, S., & Raj, G. M. (2020). Artificial intelligence during a pandemic: The COVID-19 example. *International Journal of Health Planning and Management, 35*(5), 1260–1262. https://doi.org/10.1002/hpm.2987

Demiris, G., & Kneale, L. (2015). Informatics systems and tools to facilitate patient-centered care coordination. *IMIA Yearbook, 10*(1), 15–21. https://doi.org/10.15265/IY-2015-003

Douglas, M., & Celli, M. (2015). System life cycle: A framework. In V. K. Saba & K. A. McCormick (Eds.), *Essentials of nursing informatics* (6th ed.). McGraw-Hill Education.

Dowding, D., Randell, R., Mitchell, N., Foster, R., Lattimer, V., & Thompson, C. (2009). Clinical decision support systems in nursing. In B. Staudinger, V. Höß, & H. Ostermann (Eds.), *Nursing and clinical informatics: Socio-technical approaches* (pp. 26–40). IGI Global.

Furukawa, M. F., King, J., Patel, V., Hsiao, C. J., Adler-Milstein, J., & Jha, A. K. (2014). Despite substantial progress in EHR adoption, health information exchange and patient engagement remain low in office settings. *Health Affairs, 33*(9), 1672–1679. https://doi.org/10.1377/hlthaff.2014.0445

Gold, D. L., Mihalov, L. K., & Cohen, D. M. (2014). Evaluating the pediatric early warning score (PEWS) system for admitted patients in the pediatric emergency department. *Academic Emergency Medicine, 21*(11), 1249–1256. https://doi.org/10.1111/acem.12514

Green, L. (2016). Refreshing HIMSS EMRAM requirements. *HIT Leaders and News.* https://us.hitleaders.news/refreshing-himss-emram-requirements/

Grissinger, M. C., & Mandrack, M. M. (2015). The role of technology in the medication-use process. In V. K. Saba & K. A. McCormick (Eds.), *Essentials of nursing informatics* (6th ed., pp. 419–428). McGraw-Hill Education.

Healthcare Information and Management Systems Society. (2020a). *Cybersecurity survey.* https://www.himss.org/resources/himss-healthcare-cybersecurity-survey

Healthcare Information and Management Systems Society. (2020b). *HIMSS healthcare cybersecurity survey.* https://www.himss.org/resources/himss-healthcare-cybersecurity-survey

Healthcare Information and Management Systems Society. (2020c). *Interoperability in healthcare.* https://www.himss.org/resources/interoperability-healthcare

Henry, J., Pylypchuk, Y., Searcy, T., & Patel, V. (2016). Adoption of electronic health record systems among U.S. non-federal acute care hospitals: 2008–2015. *ONC Data Brief, 35,* 1–11. https://dashboard.healthit.gov/evaluations/data-briefs/non-federal-acute-care-hospital-ehr-adoption-2008-2015.php

Hersh, W. R., Boone, K. W., & Totten, A. M. (2018). Characteristics of the healthcare information technology workforce in the HITECH era: Underestimated in size, still growing, and adapting to advanced uses. *JAMIA Open, 1*(2), 188–194. https://doi.org/10.1093/jamiaopen/ooy029

HIMSS Analytics. (2017a). *Electronic Medical Record Adoption Model.* https://www.himssanalytics.org/emram

HIMSS Analytics. (2017b). *Healthcare provider models.* https://www.himssanalytics.org/healthcare-provider-models/all

Hollander, J. E., & Carr, B. G. (2020). Virtually perfect? Telemedicine for COVID-19. *New England Journal of Medicine, 382*(18), 1679–1681. https://doi.org/10.1056/nejmp2003539

IMedicalApps. (2020). *Reviews of medical apps & healthcare technology.* https://www.imedicalapps.com/#

Institute for Healthcare Improvement. (2020). *Early warning systems: Scorecards that save lives.* http://www.ihi.org/resources/Pages/ImprovementStories/EarlyWarningSystemsScorecardsThatSaveLives.aspx

Institute of Medicine. (1999). *To err is human: Building a safer health system.* National Academies Press.

Institute of Medicine. (2001). *Crossing the quality chasm: A new health system for the 21st century.* National Academies Press.

Institute of Medicine. (2003). *Key capabilities of an electronic health record system.* National Academies Press. https://doi.org/10.17226/10781

Institute of Medicine. (2004). *Patient safety: Achieving a new standard for care.* National Academies Press.

Jayasinghe, N., Moallem, B. I., Kakoullis, M., Ojie, M. J., Sar-Graycar, L., Wyka, K., Reid, M. C., & Leonard, J. P. (2019). Establishing the feasibility of a tablet-based consent process with older adults: A mixed-methods study. *Gerontologist, 59*(1), 124–134. https://doi.org/10.1093/geront/gny045

Joos, I., & Nelson, R. (2015). Data and data processing. In V. K. Saba & K. A. McCormick (Eds.), *Essentials of nursing informatics* (6th ed., pp. 83–100). McGraw-Hill Education.

Kimmel, K. C. (2015). Healthcare analytics. In V. K. Saba & K. A. McCormick (Eds.), *Essentials of nursing informatics* (6th ed., pp. 513–524). McGraw-Hill Education.

Koonin, L. M., Hoots, B., Tsang, C. A., Leroy, Z., Farris, K., Jolly, B., Antall, P., McCabe, B., Zelis, C. B. R., Tong, I., & Harris, A. M. (2020). Trends in the use of telehealth during the emergence of the COVID-19 pandemic—United States, January–March 2020. *Morbidity and Mortality Weekly Report, 69*(43), 1595–1599. https://doi.org/10.15585/mmwr.mm6943a3

Kripalani, S., Hart, K., Schaninger, C., Bracken, S., Lindsell, C., & Boyington, D. R. (2019). Use of a tablet computer application to engage patients in updating their medication list. *American Journal of Health-System Pharmacy, 76*(5), 293–300. https://doi.org/10.1093/ajhp/zxy047

Lee Ventola, C. (2014). Mobile devices and apps for health care professionals: Uses and benefits. *Pharmacy and Therapeutics, 39*(5), 356–364. https://www.ncbi.nlm.nih.gov/pmc/articles/PMC4029126/

Martineau, P. (2020, April). iPads are crucial health care tools in combating COVID-19. *Wired.* https://www.wired.com/story/ipads-crucial-health-tools-combating-covid-19/

Mathukia, C., Fan, W., Vadyak, K., Biege, C., & Krishnamurthy, M. (2015). Modified early warning system improves patient safety and clinical outcomes in an academic community hospital. *Journal of Community Hospital Internal Medicine Perspectives, 5*(2), 26716. https://doi.org/10.3402/jchimp.v5.26716

McBride, S., & Newbold, S. (2016). Systems development life cycle for achieving meaningful use. In S. McBride & M. Tietze (Eds.), *Nursing informatics for the advanced practice nurse* (pp. 191–223). Springer.

MITRE. (2014). Electronic consent management: Landscape assessment, challenges, and technology. *ONCReport.* https://www.google.com/url?sa=t&rct=j&q=&esrc=s&source=web&cd=&ved=2ahUKEwiis4Xa-9DtAhWYKs0KHUC6Cd4QFjAHegQIDxAC&url=https%3A%2F%2Fwww.healthit.gov%2Fsites%2Fdefault%2Ffiles%2Fprivacy-security%2Fecm_finalreport_forrelease62415.pdf&usg=AOvVaw3QxfwL_5BbNPV3

Morawski, T. S. (2020). *Health informatics.* https://www.himss.org/resources/health-informatics

Nelson, S. T. (2016). Lateral integration. In C. R. King & S. O. Gerard (Eds.), *Clinical Nurse Leader certification review* (2nd ed., pp. 71–77). Springer.

Nemati, S., Holder, A., Razmi, F., Stanley, M. D., Clifford, G. D., & Buchman, T. G. (2018). An interpretable machine learning model for accurate prediction of sepsis in the ICU. *Critical Care Medicine, 46*(4), 547–553. https://doi.org/10.1097/CCM.0000000000002936

Office of the National Coordinator for Health Information Technology. (2013). *What is meaningful use?* https://www.healthit.gov/faq/what-meaningful-use

Office of the National Coordinator for Health Information Technology. (2019). *Privacy, security, and HIPAA |.* https://www.healthit.gov/topic/privacy-security-and-hipaa

Office of the National Coordinator for Health Information Technology. (2020a). *2020–2025 federal health IT strategic plan.* http://www.afpe.org.uk/physical-education/wp-content/uploads/afPE-Strategic-Plan-2016-2020.pdf

Office of the National Coordinator for Health Information Technology. (2020b). *Telemedicine and telehealth.* https://www.healthit.gov/topic/health-it-health-care-settings/telemedicine-and-telehealth

Osheroff, J. A., Teich, J. M., Levick, D., Saldana, L., Velasco, F. T., Sittig, D. F., Rogers, K. M., & Jenders, R. A. (2012). *Improving outcomes with clinical decision support: An implementer's guide* (2nd ed.). HIMSS.

Park, Y. T. (2016). Emerging new era of mobile health technologies. *Healthcare Informatics Research, 22*(4), 253–254. https://doi.org/10.4258/hir.2016.22.4.253

Pew Research Center. (2015). *American demographics of digital device ownership.* https://www.pewresearch.org/internet/2015/10/29/the-demographics-of-device-ownership/

Ross Kraft, M., & Androwich, I. M. (2015). Incorporating evidence: Use of computer-based decision support systems for health professionals. In V. K. Saba & K. A. McCormick (Eds.), *Essentials of nursing informatics* (6th ed., pp. 569–582). McGraw-Hill Education.

Shortliffe, E. H. (2005). Strategic action in health information technology: Why the obvious has taken so long. *Health Affairs, 24*(5), 1222–1233. https://doi.org/10.1377/hlthaff.24.5.1222

Soriono, R., & Hunter, K. (2019). Electronic health record systems. In T. L. Hebda, K. Hunter, & P. Czar (Eds.), *Handbook of informatics for nurses & healthcare professionals* (6th ed., pp. 112–134). Pearson.

Staggers, N., Gassert, C. A., & Curran, C. (2001). Informatics competencies for nurses at four levels of practice. *Journal of Nursing Education, 40*(7), 303–316.

TIGER. (2007). *Overview informatics competencies for every practicing nurse: Recommendations from the TIGER collaborative.* http://www.tigersummit.com

US Department of Health and Human Services. (2020). *Telehealth: Delivering care safely during COVID-19.* https://www.hhs.gov/coronavirus/telehealth/index.html

US Department of Health and Human Services & Office of the National Coordinator for Health Information Technology. (2018). *2018 Report to Congress—Annual update on the adoption of a nationwide system for the electronic use and exchange of health information.* https://www.healthit.gov/sites/default/files/page/2018-12/2018-HITECH-report-to-congress.pdf

---

EXEMPLAR

Simulation to Improve Knowledge and Skills Related to Meaningful Use and New Core Measure Data Sets

Cathy Coleman

The American Recovery and Reinvestment Act of 2009 led to federal funding for the Health Information and Technology for Economic and Clinical Health Act (King & Gerard, 2016, p. 228). This strategic initiative directed by the CMS includes financial incentives for adoption and "meaningful use" (MU) of certified electronic health information systems by hospitals and eligible professionals. Three stages of MU range from 2010–2021 and gradually accelerate the utilization and exchange of information to improve multiple outcomes. The processes related to program registration, data entry, and attestation can be tedious for busy professionals and hospital staff. This exemplar introduces the complexity and reality of using electronic data to document existing meaningful use measures and to anticipate new core measure sets recently introduced by CMS (2016).

The majority of CNLs will never earn incentive dollars associated with these federal programs. However, they are likely functioning across different microsystems as information managers with direct impact on teams that influence data collection, entry, and outcomes. The AACN has recognized the critical importance of nursing informatics and health technologies by defining a specific domain within the *Graduate-level QSEN Competencies* (AACN, 2012) and through dissemination of *Competencies and Curricular Expectations for CNL Education and Practice* (AACN, 2013).

In the simulation exercise, student pairs are allotted 45 minutes to review and discuss three CMS websites that provide: (1) an introduction to MU (https://www

.cms.gov/regulations-and-guidance/legislation/ehrincentiveprograms/basics.html),
(2) practice entering proxy MU data (https://www.cms.gov/apps/stage-2-meaningful
-use-attestation-calculator/), and (3) knowledge about new measures (https://www
.cms.gov/Medicare/Quality-Initiatives-Patient-Assessment-Instruments/Quality
Measures/Core-Measures.html) that will essentially transition the MU measures to
seven new core measure sets in 2017. CNLs gain an appreciation for measure spec-
ifications, entry of electronic data, and comparison of MU metrics with new core
measure sets.

References

American Association of Colleges of Nursing. (2012). *Graduate-level QSEN competencies: Knowledge,
    skills and attitudes*. http://www.aacn.nche.edu/faculty/qsen /competencies.pdf
American Association of Colleges of Nursing. (2013). *Competencies and curricular expectations
    for CNL education and practice*. http://www.aacn.nche.edu/cnl /CNL-Competencies-October
    -2013.pdf
Centers for Medicare and Medicaid Services. (2016, February 16). *Core measures*. https://www
    .cms.gov/Medicare/Quality-Initiatives-Patient-Assessment-Instruments/QualityMeasures
    /Core-Measures.html
King, C., & Gerard, S. (2016). *Clinical Nurse Leader Certification Review* (2nd ed.). New York, NY,
    Springer Publishing.

EXEMPLAR

Utilizing Informatics to Improve Patient Outcomes

Alex Nava

In May 2014, a southwestern healthcare organization redesigned its care management process to include the CNL's role to improve quality outcomes and to enhance
seamless care coordination. The care redesign process included the CNL/Patient
Care Facilitator (PCF) team completing a readmission assessment with all patients
within 24 hours of their arrival.

In 2014, CMS imposed financial penalties upon a southwestern suburban hospital concerning their 30-day readmission rate. Within this hospital, nine nurses
enrolled in their healthcare organization's academic partnership program with a
local college to attain their graduate degree specializing in the CNL role.

In May 2015, the hospital formed a readmission steering committee to decrease their number of 30-day readmissions. The hospital's chief medical officer
asked a CNL to preside over the Readmission Data Analysis subcommittee to identify issues and trends. The goal of the subcommittee was to decrease the number of
30-day readmissions by 10%.

The CNL modified an existing EHR database query to list all 30-day readmission patients admitted into any of the CNL units within the last seven days.
The list and corresponding data was saved in a spreadsheet. The CNL team and
retail pharmacist met weekly to review each readmission case to determine the
following:

- What was the category of the readmission case (e.g., new acute condition, acute on chronic heart failure, etc.)?
- Could the readmission have been prevented by either the patient, family, nursing facility, nursing staff, ancillary staff, or physician?
- Did the patient utilize the pharmacy concierge service during their initial admission? The retail pharmacist provided this information.

During the weekly meeting, the CNL team discussed relevant readmission assessment data that may have provoked the readmission and whether all appropriate staff implemented best practices related to communication, education, discharge, and care transitions.

Beginning in May 2015, the CNL/PCF team disseminated information regarding preventable readmissions with their respective units to avert similar incidents. The chairperson reported all trends concerning readmission categories, facilities/agencies, and successful interventions to the steering committee. For example, the CNL chairperson reported how the hospital's pilot of the pharmacy concierge service decreased the number of 30-day readmissions within two acute care units. The steering committee responded by authorizing the use of the discharge service in all acute care units for specific key performance indicator diagnoses and high risk for readmission patients. The PCF chairperson updated and archived the spreadsheet for future reference and analysis.

As evidenced previously, the value of using IT and evaluation methods is an essential function of CNL practice. CNLs are positioned to analyze current and proposed use of patient-centered technologies, including cost-effectiveness and appropriateness in the design and delivery of care in diverse care settings and use technologies and information systems to facilitate the collection, analysis, and dissemination of data including clinical, financial, and operational outcomes.

EXEMPLAR

Using Informatics and Healthcare Technologies to Guide CNL Practice Patient-Centeredness/Team Collaboration/Efficiency

Elizabeth Triezenberg

Patients who had total knee replacement surgery were sent home from the hospital with lengthy and confusing discharge instructions. Prior to the patient leaving the hospital, the surgeon would edit the template provided through the EMR to reflect surgeon-specific care preferences. The discharge information given to the patient varied by surgeon, was wordy, and often had significant grammatical errors resulting from quick edits. The discharging nurse was left to review pages of disorganized paragraphs and highlight the essential information for the patient. As a result, patients often verbalized uncertainty related to posthospital care.

The CNL worked with the physician team and using the interdisciplinary team created a new template utilizing the information in the existing EMR patient discharge education. The surgeon-specific additions were reviewed for common trends and variances. Information that was standard to all surgeon preferences was added to the new template. The template was divided into several sections emphasizing the care necessary for the 7 to 10 days between hospital discharge and office follow-up. Variances in care were presented to the orthopedic surgeons for discussion and consensus. The benefits of clarity of patient discharge information as well as simplifying the process of entering discharge instructions into the EMR was enough to drive consensus on finite details.

Utilizing adult learning principles, the template was designed to become a reference tool for the patient rather than a novel of information. The template saved as a two-sided front/back PDF and entered into the EMR as well as printed on cardstock in color and given to the patients on admission.

The modified template has streamlined discharge instruction and has helped to clarify postoperative care. A three-month random sample pre- and post-intervention showed an improvement from 60 to 97% of accuracy of discharge information sent home with patients. Nurses report less time is needed for review of discharge instructions, and patients are verbalizing understanding of instructions prior to final moments of hospitalization.

EXEMPLAR

Collaboration of a CNL and CNS

Mary Harnish

A hospital system seeking to improve the care of patients with diabetes facilitated the collaborative work of its CNL for diabetes and its CNS for medicine, diabetes, and renal service line. The CNL and CNS roles complemented and enhanced one another through the joint efforts to implement evidence-based practice to improve efficiency and patient safety. Both the CNL and CNS were integral members of a hospital-wide diabetes operations team.

The CNL and CNS joined forces to attain The Joint Commission accreditation for advanced in-patient diabetes care for the hospital. The CNS performed a gap analysis to determine the current state prior to beginning the process of accreditation. The CNL, also a certified diabetes educator, utilized her knowledge and expertise of diabetes while simultaneously applying her knowledge of systems to work toward meeting the needs identified in the analysis. The CNL developed a standardized tool to assess the comprehension and competencies of patients with regard to their diabetes to facilitate educating patients to meet these identified needs. The CNL and CNS collaborated on developing education material for patients and staff. They educated multiple disciplines on best practices. The hospital was the first in the state to receive The Joint Commission accreditation for advanced in-patient diabetes care.

The CNL and CNS collaborated on implementing the use of computer software to assist in dosing of intravenous insulin. The prior process involved a paper protocol and through the use of software a computerized system for documentation was an option. The result evidenced a decrease in hypoglycemic rates from 2.1% to less than 0.5%.

EXEMPLAR

Partnerships for Patient Quality and Safety

Kevin Hengeveld and Lauran Hardin

In 2010, over 50% of psychiatric medical unit admissions were dementia patients need-ing treatment for behavior control. Assessment completed by the CNL revealed staff injuries, staff fear and lack of knowledge, extended length of stay, and patient deaths.

With mentoring, the staff unit-based council developed an evidence-based guideline for care. Advanced dementia patients cannot self-report pain, fear, or bowel, bladder, and environmental concerns. The guideline taught staff how to treat and anticipate needs in this vulnerable population, increasing their confidence in care and decreasing injuries from patient agitation.

CNLs then collaborated to assess the root cause of outcomes involving psychiatry, medicine, and palliative care. Families of dementia patients are challenged with making complex end-of-life decisions regarding code status and feeding tubes. A process was developed to trigger the integration of palliative care for decision-making support from the day of admission, giving families time to develop relationships and struggle through complex issues. Complex issues were solved sooner, patients were transferred to the appropriate setting in less time, and average LOS decreased from 14 to 10 days.

Analysis of deaths found that some patients did not really need to be admitted to the unit in the first place. Hospice patients and near end-of-life patients were not best served in a locked psychiatric unit. The act of transferring the patient was often traumatic near the end of life. A collaborative process between CNLs was engaged to create risk assessment at entry points to the hospital (intake coordinators and

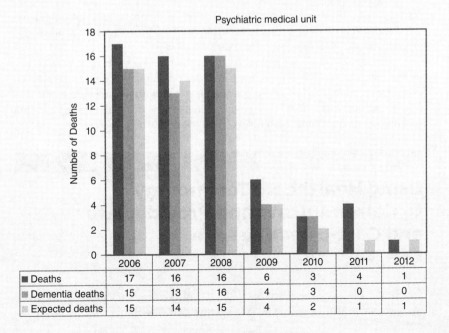

	2006	2007	2008	2009	2010	2011	2012
■ Deaths	17	16	16	6	3	4	1
■ Dementia deaths	15	13	16	4	3	0	0
■ Expected deaths	15	14	15	4	2	1	1

the ED). Clinical support was offered to get patients the services they needed in the setting they were already in. CNLs partnered with hospices from the community to improve outcomes for the population. These combined efforts decreased dementia deaths in the unit to zero. Data for the unit is shown in the figure.

Implementing Safe Insulin Infusion Dosing with a Computer Software Tool

Mary Harnish

Hyperglycemia in hospitalized patients increases infection rates, mortality, and LOS. In turn, better glycemic control in hospitalized patients causes a decrease in LOS, infections rates, and mortality. Patients often require intravenous (IV) insulin infusion to maintain optimal glycemic control. Standardization of how IV insulin is titrated decreases blood glucose variability and maintains blood glucose in acceptable and preferred target ranges.

As a CNL for diabetes, I am a member of our hospital's diabetes operations team that works to improve glycemic care in our institution. A need to standardize titration of IV insulin was identified by this team. Various software tools were researched, and the team's clinical members made a choice.

In collaboration with a CNS, I implemented this new insulin titration software tool in the critical care unit. The rollout of this software tool challenged us with educating physicians, especially the intensivists, on use of this tool. Nursing staff were given hands-on training, along with "at-the-elbow" guidance during the initial few weeks of "going live" with the software.

After implementation of this software tool, critical care data on patients receiving insulin drips indicated a drop in the rate of hypoglycemia (blood glucose < 70 mg/dL) in patients on insulin drips from 2.1 to 0.5%. The rate of severe hypoglycemia (blood glucose < 50 mg/dL) decreased from 0.6 to 0.08%.

After the software tool proved useful in the critical care area, it became apparent that there was also a need for insulin drip standardization in step-down units. I assisted the cardiac step-down unit to go live with the software six months after the critical care unit. One year after initiating the use of the insulin titration software, all acuity adaptable units were trained and using the software.

Using Healthcare Technology to Communicate and Provide Safe and Cost-Effective Care

Rebecca Valko

One of the CNL key competencies is the use of healthcare technologies to assure we have safe patient-centered and cost-effective care. The use of a secure messaging system has had mixed reviews with the interdisciplinary team. It is no surprise that communication between consulting and primary teams is sometimes difficult. A patient was ordered an MRI of his foot by the medicine team on a patient who was at high risk of limb loss. Unfortunately, he did not tolerate lying still and conscious sedation with anesthesia was scheduled the next morning. Knowing that this would create additional safety and team utilization and cost, the CNL (as team manager) began to investigate. The consulting orthopedic team who would perform the amputation did not mention awaiting MRI results in the EHR and was ready to perform surgery. The CNL constructed a secure message with the attending medicine service, the orthopedic surgeon, and primary RN—questioning the need for the MRI. The orthopedic surgeon responded they never needed the MRI. The medicine team quickly canceled the MRI, the patient was scheduled for a below-the-knee amputation, and a test that was never needed was averted. Placing all the members of the care team on the same message was a quick and effective strategy using technology, thus, highlighting the fact that clear communication is needed to keep our cost of care as low as possible.

CHAPTER 15

Transitions in Care

Linda A. Roussel

LEARNING OBJECTIVES

1. Describe distinctions between transitional care and transitions of care.
2. Define transitions of care and their impact on quality and safe patient outcomes.
3. Identify common elements of the transitional care models.
4. Identify root causes of ineffective transitions of care.
5. Outline transitions of care models describing the major component of the most used frameworks.
6. Integrate CNL competencies with effective care transition.
7. Describe how communication, documentation, evidence-based practices, and relationships enhance transitions of care.
8. Discuss how informatics and technology can increase efficiency and efficacy of transitional care.

KEY TERMS

Comprehensive planning
Cultural sensitivity
Illness prevention
Lateral integration
Multidisciplinary communication
Patient engagement
Population health

Readiness for change
Secondary prevention
Self-care
Self-management
Shared accountability
Wellness

CNL ROLES

Client advocate
Clinician
Educator

Lifelong learner
Outcomes manager
Team manager

CNL PROFESSIONAL VALUES

Accountability   Healthcare systems and policy
Altruism   Human dignity
Communication   Illness and disease management
Disease prevention   Integrity
Health promotion   Social justice

CNL COMPETENCIES

Assessment   Healthcare systems and policy
Communication   Human diversity
Design/Management/Coordination   Illness and disease management
   of care   Member of a profession
Disease prevention   Provide and manage care
Health promotion   Risk reduction

Introduction

What does it mean to provide transitional care for patients from setting to set-ting? From one patient's care experience to the next? Naylor and colleagues (2009) describe transitional care as a period of *limited* services and settings (situations) that *complement primary care* and are developed to ensure healthcare continuity and reduce avoidable poor outcomes among *at-risk* populations moving from one level of care to another, among multiple providers and across settings. The National Translations of Care Coalition (NTCC) defines care transition as being related but different from care coordination. One perspective of care coordination refers to the interaction of providers to ensure optimal care for a patient. Care transitions re-quire coordination of care, which includes the broader perspective of assessment of the patients' needs, developing and implementing a care plan, and evaluation of the care experience.

Transitions of care are core to the work of the CNL. Specifically, the CNL provides oversight for care coordination of a distinct group of patients and ac-tively delivers direct patient care in complex situations, transitioning as appropri-ate to care systems that uniquely meet the patient's needs. The CNL incorporates evidence-based practice into action to ensure that patients take advantage of the latest innovations in care delivery. As part of care coordination and lateral integra-tion, the CNL collects and evaluates patient outcomes, assesses cohort risk, and has the decision-making authority to change care plans when appropriate. As a lateral integrator, the CNL is part of an interdisciplinary team who communicates, plans, and implements care directly with other healthcare professionals, including physi-cians, pharmacists, social workers, clinical nurse specialists, and nurse practitioners (AACN, 2004).

The CNL's role in transitions of care are aligned with the Master's Essentials and the CNL competencies. Eight of the nine CNL competencies underpin the critical responsibilities of the CNL centered on care transitions. For example, Es-sential 2, Competency 2, "Organizational and Systems Leadership," note that the

CNL takes on a leadership role of an interprofessional healthcare team directed toward patient-centered care. The primary purpose focuses on assessing quality care and cost-effectiveness across the healthcare continuum. The CNL uses systems theory in the assessment, design, delivery, and evaluation of healthcare within complex, high-reliability organizations. Another example of the alignment of the Essentials and CNL competencies is found in Essential 5, "Informatics and Healthcare Technologies." This competency provides excellent direction for the CNL to use informatics and healthcare technologies essential to coordinating and laterally integrating patient care within and across care settings, and among healthcare providers. The CNL analyzes current and recommended evidence-based patient-care technologies to include cost-effectiveness and appropriateness in the design and delivery of care in diverse care settings. The CNL uses technologies and information systems to facilitate quality improvement and expedite clinical, financial, and operational outcomes management to include collection, analysis, and dissemination of outcomes (AACN, 2013).

Essential 8, "Clinical Prevention and Population Health for Improving Health," is also significant in transitions of care for the CNL. Essential 8 embraces the CNL's ability to engage the community and social service delivery systems that recognize new models of care and health services delivery. Being informed and conversant with various care transition models advances the CNL's knowledge of strategies and principles that are useful in supporting successful outcomes. Advancing population health, the CNL participates in the design, delivery, and evaluation of clinical prevention and health promotion services that are patient-centered and culturally appropriate. This is a critical component of the CNL's role in transitions of care. As the competency purports, the CNL monitors the outcomes of comprehensive plans of care that address the health promotion and disease prevention needs of patient populations. As a lateral integrator, and a key player in transitioning patients, the CNL takes into account social determinants of health and population health incorporating public health concepts to inform equitable and efficient preventive services and policies. As such, these policies facilitate population health as well as forge partnerships at multiple levels of the health system. This is critical to effective coordination, delivery, and evaluation of clinical prevention and health promotion interventions and services across the care continuum. The CNL uses epidemiological, social, ecological, and environmental data from local, state, regional, national, and international sources to reach conclusions regarding the health risks and status of populations, to promote and sustain healthy lifestyles. The CNL uses evidence in developing and implementing teaching and coaching strategies to preserve health in patient populations. In addition, the CNL provides leadership to the healthcare team to promote health, facilitate self-care management, optimize patient engagement, and prevent future decline including progression to higher levels of care and re-admissions (AACN, 2013).

Care transitions describe the movement (transition) patients make between healthcare practitioners and settings as healthcare conditions and care needs change during the episodes and course of a chronic or acute illness (Allen et al., 2014). To illustrate, in an episode of an acute exacerbation of an illness, a patient might receive care from a primary care provider (PCP) or specialist in an outpatient setting, then transition to a hospital physician and interprofessional team during an inpatient admission. This transition may occur before moving on to another interdisciplinary care team at a skilled nursing facility or a freestanding rehabilitation hospital. Last, the patient may be discharged home, to receive care from a visiting nurse through a home health agency. Each of these episodes or shifts from care providers and settings defines care transition (AHRQ, 2015; Coleman et al., 2006; Kurtz, & Pauly, 2009; Naylor, Ouchida, et al., 2009; Zander, 2001).

Care transition (or the lack of transitions of care) has received the attention of policy makers for some critical reasons:

1. Twenty-one percent of hospitalized patients 65 or older are discharged to a long-term care or other institution (Epstein, 2009).
2. It is estimated that by 2025, chronic diseases will affect 164 million Americans—nearly half (49%) of the population. Additionally, between 2000 and 2030 Americans with chronic conditions will demonstrate an increase by 37 percent, approximately 46 million people (Wu & Green, 2000).
3. The complexity of their illness may involve up to 16 different physicians providing care for them in one year (Garrido et al., 2005).
4. Re-admissions to a hospital continue to be problematic with approximately 25% coming from Medicare SNFs (Kripalani et al., 2007).
5. Medicare patients admitted to a hospital in 2003 (41.9–70%) received services from 10 or more physicians during their stay (Sebelius, 2010).

These are but a few examples that point to fragmented, duplicative services, waste, and poor coordination and transitions of care. Fragmentation leads to high costs and dissatisfaction of patients, family, and providers (Guterman et al, 2010; The Joint Commission Center for Transforming Healthcare, 2010).

The American Geriatrics Society (2003) defines transitional care as a set of actions created to ensure the continuity and coordination of healthcare delivery as patients move between different locations or different levels of care within the same location. This may include (but is not limited to) hospitals, subacute and post-acute nursing facilities, the patient's home, primary and specialty care offices, and long-term care facilities. The phenomenon of transitional care has at its underpinnings of comprehensive care planning and accessible and available healthcare providers well prepared in chronic care. These systems and providers also have current information about the patient's goals, preferences, and clinical status. This may include logistics of the living arrangements, environments of care, education of the patient and family, and collaboration and coordination among the health professionals involved in the transition. Coleman (2003) describes transitional care as integrating the sending and the receiving aspects of the transfer that are essential aspects to successful outcomes for persons with complex care needs. The CNL is particularly poised to lead patients through transitions of care. This is clearly articulated in the Essential 4, "Translating and Integrating Scholarship into Practice," and Essential 7, "Interprofessional Collaboration for Improving Patient and Population Health Outcomes." Using translational science, the CNL communicates current quality and safety guidelines and nurse sensitive indicators, including validation processes to the interprofessional healthcare team, patients, and caregivers. By applying improvement science theory and methods in performance measurement and quality improvement processes, the CNL leads change initiatives to reduce or eliminate discrepancies between actual practices and evidence-based practice standards of care. Through disseminating changes in practice and improvements in care outcomes to internal and external audiences, the CNL facilitates sustainable innovations. Additionally, the CNL designs care based on outcome analysis and evidence to promote the six aims of quality, specifically, care that is safe, timely, effective, efficient, equitable, and patient-centered (IOM, 2001). The CNL is educated to design and implement transitional care models that engage the patient and family and improve the overall patient experience (AACN, 2013).

Transitional care is described as a broad range of time-limited services created to ensure healthcare continuity, avoid preventable poor outcomes among at-risk populations, and facilitate the smooth safe and timely transfer of patients from one level of care to another or from one type of setting to another (Naylor & Sochalski, 2010). Transitional care aligns with, but is different from, other aspects of care delivery including primary care, care coordination, discharge planning, disease management, or case management. *Primary care* focuses on specific patient concerns addressing one-to-one healthcare needs for the patient. *Care coordination* is broader in scope and includes interaction of providers in addressing complex care needs of the patient. *Discharge planning* may be an end point of an episode of care, focused on the final requirements of the patients moving to the next level of care, which may be home or a skilled-nursing or assisted-living facility (Holland & Hemann, 2011). *Disease management* is based on the population health model, which involves identifying, treating, and slowing the progression of chronic diseases by developing and activating patients over time. Active symptom management, patient education, and care coordination using a variety of tools (screenings, assessments, and evidence-based protocol) are interventions employed in disease management. *Case management* is personalized care with an intensive emphasis on collaborative assessment, planning, facilitation, and advocacy for services to meet individual patient care needs (Naylor & Sochalski, 2010).

Major aspects of transitional care, which transcend any one model, include working with chronically ill, highly vulnerable patients throughout critical transitions in health and healthcare and the time-limited nature of services. There is an intense focus on educating patients and family caregivers attending to health literacy and readiness to make modifiable lifestyle changes. Transitional care addresses root causes of poor outcomes and ways to avoid preventable rehospitalizations (Naylor et al., 2011).

Developing care transition models can be challenging when organizational systems are steeped in hierarchical, traditional structures. Systems with positive impact on re-admission supported by transitions of care included the support of leadership, interprofessional collaboration, evidence-based methods of transitioning patients through thoughtful handoffs, person-centered care with active family involvement, and technology that enhances communication.

Examples such as those from MD Anderson, in which patients receiving treatments at its Houston facilities for a wide range of cancers, incorporate the previous and other activities into the development of its primary team nursing model that result in positive transitions. Specifically, four 12-bed cohorts (from a 48-bed unit) have been developed with each cohort assigned a team led by a CNL. This model has expanded to four demonstration units with the goal of increasing patient satisfaction scores. Activities implemented within the CNL-led patient care delivery model are interdisciplinary communication, aligning support and accommodations after discharge, and advanced education aimed at the patient's specific condition, taking into account health literacy and environments of care (AACN, 2013; The Joint Commission Center for Transforming Healthcare, 2010).

Distinction Between Transitional Care and Transitions of Care

There may be confusion around care coordination, transitional care, and transitions of care. Care coordination is the methodical organization of patient care activities among two or more participants (including the patient and/or the family) to support the essential delivery of healthcare services. The business of organizing care involves coordinating personnel and resources to follow through on all necessary and appropriate patient care activities. This can be managed by the interchange of information among participants responsible for different aspects of the care. Transitions of care can be defined as patient flow among healthcare locations, providers, or different levels of care within the same location as their conditions and care needs change. Transitions of care can occur in the following ways:

1. Within settings, for example, including primary care to specialty care, or ICU to medical surgical units.
2. Between settings, may include hospital to subacute care, or ambulatory clinic to senior centers of day program. An example of a between settings transition includes psychiatric day care services.
3. Across health states, would include curative care to palliative care or hospice, or personal home to assisted living.
4. Between providers, could be a generalist to a specialist practitioner, or acute care provider to a palliative care specialist (National Transitions of Care Coalition, 2010).

Transitions of care are a set of actions developed to facilitate coordination and continuity. These actions should be grounded in a comprehensive care plan and the availability of well-trained practitioners who have current information about the patient's treatment goals, preferences, and health or clinical status. Actions may include logistical arrangements, patient, and family education, as well as coordination among health professionals involved in the transition. In summary, transitions of care are a subpart of a broader concept of care coordination. Using innovative strategies and technology, the CNL can advance actions to promote timely care and follow-up. Specifically, the CNL implements the use of technologies to coordinate and laterally integrate patient care within and across care settings and among healthcare providers (AACN, 2013). By analyzing current and proposed use of patient-care technologies, including their cost-effectiveness and appropriateness in the design and delivery of care in diverse care settings, the CNL exposes providers and patients to a wide array of options to facilitate best care delivery practices (AACN, 2013).

Transitions in Care and Their Impact on Quality and Safe Patient Outcomes

Transitions in care significantly impact quality and safe patient outcomes. As noted, a key component of transitioning care is to determine patients who are at risk for complications and possible re-admissions (National Quality Forum, 2006). CNLs are engaged in working with patients, families, and professionals in assessments. A comprehensive assessment may include the following considerations:

- Older, frail elders with chronic conditions and comorbidities.
- Inadequate home environment or homeless.
- History of previous admissions and re-admissions for all preventable causes.
- Numerous medications leading to potential over- or underdosing.
- Multiple care providers, particularly specialists who may have limited knowledge of the patient's overall plan of care, family, and environmental challenges.
- Financial hardship (The Joint Commission Center for Transforming Healthcare, 2010).

Comprehensive assessments that point to the vulnerability of high-risk patients for fragmented care underscore the need to consider evidence-based transitional care models. CNLs are prepared to complete assessment and as importantly work with key providers in translating assessment data to determine best evidence-based strategies to address the many concerns that face the patient and family caregivers. Naylor and her University of Pennsylvania colleagues, through their research over time, have created the TCM (Naylor & Sochalski, 2010). Essential components of the TCM include the following:

- A TCN is a centerpiece for the model, which provides consistent provider care across the entire episode of care. The TCN is a master's prepared nurse with a skill set that includes understanding complex disease states, coordination of care, strong communication and relationship base care, being able to lead and work in teams. The CNL is exquisitely positioned to assume this role.
- Strong physician-nurse collaboration.
- Comprehensive in-hospital patient assessment.
- Multidisciplinary approach to care planning and coordination to include multiple providers, the patient, and caregivers.
- Using evidence-based practice protocols in preparing patient care delivery experiences.
- Regular home visits by the TCN, including ongoing telephonic support (seven days a week) through an average of two months' postdischarge.
- Continuity of medical care between hospital and primary care providers facilitated by the TCN. The TCN accompanies each patient to his or her first follow-up visit to assure a comprehensive holistic focus. This can be particularly challenging given the many providers and disease management protocols.
- Communication among the many stakeholders including the patient, family, informal caregivers, and the often many healthcare providers and professionals.
- Active engagement of patients and their family through education, support, and emphasis on early identification and responses to healthcare risks and symptoms to activate longer-term positive outcomes and avoid complications and untoward episodes that lead to re-admissions (Naylor, Feldman, et al., 2009).

The CNL is educated and socialized into the role to assume the TCN role, specifically focused on working with and through others to understand complex disease states, coordinate care, provide strong communication and relationship-based care, and leading and working in teams. The CNL can readily assume a leadership role of an interprofessional healthcare team with emphasis on the delivery of patient-centered care and the evaluation of quality and cost-effectiveness across the healthcare continuum. Additionally, the CNL integrates his or her understanding of systems theory in the assessment, design, delivery, and evaluation of healthcare within complex organizations in which patients and family caregivers find themselves in. By using business and economic principles and practices, including cost-benefit analysis, budgeting, strategic planning, human and other resource management, marketing, and value-based purchasing, the CNL addresses the aims for quality, which include effective, efficient, timely, and equitable care (AACN, 2013; IOM, 2001).

The AHRQ (2015) in a systematic review on transitional care interventions to prevent re-admission for people with heart failure, describe transitional care interventions and the efficacy of these strategies. Specifically, the following transitional care and heart failure interventions were identified:

- Home-visiting programs
- Structured telephone support
- Telemonitoring
- Outpatient clinic-based interventions
- Multidisciplinary HF clinics
- Nurse-led HF clinics
- Primarily educational interventions

The AHRQ's (2015) systematic review purported that home-visiting programs and multidisciplinary HF clinic–based interventions for patients with HF reduced all-cause re-admissions with a high level of research strength and mortality (moderate level of evidence) over three to six months. Also reported to be effective was structured telephone support, which reduced HF-specific re-admissions (high strength of evidence) and mortality (moderate strength of evidence) over three to six months. The authors noted that structured telephone support did not reduce all-cause re-admissions over three to six months similar (moderate strength of evidence). Furthermore, there was limited evidence regarding the efficacy of telemonitoring interventions, nurse-led HF clinic–based interventions, and primarily educational interventions. The researchers noted that direct evidence was insufficient to permit conclusions about whether one type of intervention was more efficacious than any other.

Root Causes of Ineffective Transitions of Care

Research evidence supports the positive effects of well-organized and coordinated transitions of care. Making a case for transitional care includes high rates of medical errors, serious unmet patients and family caregiver needs, the patients' dissatisfaction with care experiences, high rates of preventable re-admissions, and extensive human and cost burden are causes of ineffective care. These causes are foundational to making a case for transitional care. Adding to these challenges consist of providers, fragmentation of care, and a lack of a comprehensive approach to the patient and family caregivers. Outcomes that have been measured to determine effective care transitions involve increased patient engagement, activation of self-management strategies, and preventable re-admissions (The Joint Commission Center for Transforming Healthcare, 2010). One root cause of ineffective care transition is communication breakdowns. Specifically, risk factors related to communication breakdowns include differing expectations between senders and receivers of patients in transition and an organizational culture that does not promote successful handoffs due to lack of teamwork and respect. Other risk factors contributing to ineffective handoffs are inadequate amount of time provided for successful handoff and lack of standardized procedures in conducting successful handoff, such as the use of SBAR. Risk factors may include lack of timely communication, which may be incomplete at best (The Joint Commission Center for Transforming Healthcare, 2010). Other root causes include patient education breakdowns such as receiving conflicting recommendations, confusing medication regimens, and unclear instructions about follow-up care. There may be a lack of sufficient understanding of the medical condition or the plan or care, possibly the patient not being convinced of the significance of following the care plan, or inadequate knowledge or skills to do so. Another root cause of ineffective transition of care includes accountability breakdowns. For example, when multiple providers are involved, there may be no one provider that assumes responsibility for coordinating the patient's healthcare across various settings and among different providers. Often when multiple specialists are involved, there may be a lack of collaboration or limited communication, often creating confusion for the patient and those responsible for transitioning the care of the patient to the next setting or provider. There may be limited discharge planning and risk assessment especially when primary care providers are not identified by name or area of specialization. This may delay discharge planning and critical risk assessments. A comprehensive plan that does not identify steps to assure that sufficient knowledge and resources are available will likely delay discharge and transition of care. Primary care providers are sometimes not identified by name, therefore, limiting discharge planning and risk assessment due to lack of collaboration and cooperation (Naylor & Sochalski, 2010).

Transitions of Care Models: Major Components of the Most Commonly Used Frameworks

There are several transitional care models that have been tested and provide evidence-based strategies for managing transitions of care. Overall goals for evidence-based translation models are generally consistent and include improving care for patients and family caregivers, promoting patient engagement, reducing negative outcomes (readmission, length of stay, medication error, costs, ineffective care delivery), and increasing positive outcomes (care coordination, patient satisfaction, patient self-management). The Care Transition Model (CT; "Coleman Model"), and TCM ("Naylor Model") are likely the most written about regarding transitioning care. The CT model promotes care coordination and continuity of care, using health coaches who are a wide array of individuals with strong interpersonal skills. Health coaches facilitate skill transfer so that patients can do more for themselves. Developing a personal health record and teaching red flags for symptom management are part of the work of the health coach (Coleman, Parry, Chalmers, & Min, 2006). The TCM uses a TCN, an advanced practice nurse with a master's of science in nursing (MSN) with advanced knowledge and skills in providing care for older adults. Follow-up home visits over a specific time (two months) and attending the first follow-up visit with a provider are also included in the TCN's responsibilities (Naylor & Sochalski, 2010).

Other models in the literature include Better Outcomes for Older Adults through Safe Transitions (BOOST), which focused on elders and pre- and postdischarge strategies. Using "teach back" is an important educational strategy to engage patients and family caregivers using simple language, return demonstrations, and individualizing a patient care plan with 72-hour follow-up (Project BOOST, 2010). The Bridge Model is a hospital to home transition model specifically focused on patients over 60 years of age. The Bridge Model is primarily staffed by social workers emphasizing reducing caregiver stress, increasing consumer safety, reducing ED visits, and increasing older adult and caregiver satisfaction. Telephonic follow-up calls (at least 48 hours and additional if needed) are included in the Bridge Model (Bridge Model, n.d.).

Care transition models have been developed that focus on reducing hospital re-admissions. An example of this type of model is Project Re-Engineered Discharge (RED), which developed and tested strategies through a research group at Boston University Medical Center. This model proposed to improve the hospital discharge process that facilitates patient safety and decreases rehospitalization rates. The RED intervention was developed on 12 discrete, mutually reinforcing concepts and have demonstrated a reduction in rehospitalizations correlating with high rates of patient satisfaction. Virtual patient advocates were tested in conjunction with RED. Also noted with Project RED is that this model has been implemented at other hospitals serving diverse patient populations. Project RED has also moved into the transitional care space, particularly from inpatient to outpatient care of specific populations (i.e., those with depressive symptoms). Project RED has also started a patient-centered project to create a tool that hospitals can use to discover factors (i.e., medical legal, social, etc.) in patients' re-admissions. Also, Project RED was supported by grants from the AHRQ, NIH—National Heart, Lung and Blood Institute (NHBLI), the Blue Cross Blue Shield Foundation, and the Patient-Centered Outcomes Research Institute.

A model that outlines interventions to address acute care transfers is the Interventions to Reduce Acute Care Transfers (INTERACT) framework. INTERACT has been described as a quality improvement program that is publicly available whose centerpiece is the management of acute change in resident condition. It includes clinical and educational tools and strategies for use in everyday practice in long-term care facilities. According to Ouslander and colleagues (2014), INTERACT was updated from a tool kit concept to a quality improvement program that centers on improving the management of acute changes in residents' healthcare conditions. Using this systematic management approach, hospitalizations are avoided or minimized in situations that can be realistically and safely addressed in the nursing home. INTERACT implementation is based on five fundamental strategies (Ouslander et al., 2014):

1. *Principles of quality improvement:* Incorporates an interdisciplinary team facilitated by designated champions and strong leadership support. Additional quality improvement principles include measurement, tracking, and benchmarking of clearly defined outcomes with feedback to all staff. Root-cause analyses of hospitalizations with continuous learning and improvement based on them is also a quality improvement strategy included in the INTERACT model.
2. *Early identification and evaluation of changes in residents' healthcare conditions:* Includes strategies that evaluate risk in order to mitigate poor outcomes such as transfer to acute care.
3. *Management of common changes in residents' healthcare conditions:* With early identification and evaluation of residents' healthcare status, evidence-based practices to manage changes would follow the plan.

4. *Improved advance care planning:* Incorporates the use of palliative or hospice care when indicated and the choice of the resident (or their healthcare proxy) as an alternative to hospitalization.
5. *Improved communication and documentation:* Having evidence-based systems and principles in place for the nursing home staff and families and between the nursing home and the hospital provides a "road map" and language that promotes consistent approaches to reducing acute care transfers.

According to Ouslander and colleagues (2014), the INTERACT model is concerned with improving the identification, evaluation, and management of acute changes in condition of nursing home residents. The authors note that effective implementation has been linked with substantial reductions in hospitalization of nursing home residents. Along with assisting nursing homes to eliminate or minimize unnecessary hospitalizations and their related complications and costs, by the ongoing focus of becoming effective partners for hospitals, healthcare systems, managed care plans, and accountable care organizations (ACOs), effective INTERACT implementation will assist nursing homes in meeting the new requirement for a robust QAPI program, which is being rolled out by the federal government over the next year. Additionally, INTERACT has been adopted by many nursing homes throughout the United States, and is also being used in other countries including Canada, the United Kingdom, and Singapore. Ouslander and colleagues (2011) note that active implementation of the INTERACT program has been associated with up to a 24% reduction in all-cause hospitalizations of nursing home residents over a six-month period. Furthermore, the authors state that use of the model would result in over $100,000 in Medicare savings annually in each nursing home successfully implementing and sustaining the program. INTERACT necessitates the importance of interprofessional team leadership, including major players such as directors of nursing, administrators, and medical directors. Buy-in from primary care clinicians (including physicians, nurse practitioners, and physician assistants) is also essential to garnering support and ongoing effectiveness. This model's express intent is to eliminate or minimize acute care transfers that could best be handled from safety and quality perspectives within the residents' care setting.

CNLs consider evidence-based practices and models in transitioning care of patients within their microsystems. The principles of care coordination, collaboration, leadership, and managing complex care are the heart of the work. CNLs are exquisitely educated to do this critical work in managing patient populations and systems of care. Transitioning care is the cornerstone of CNLs' work and is evident in their ability to lead a team, manage change, laterally integrate, and use evidence-based practice strategies in working with and through interdisciplinary teams.

Summary

- CNLs require an understanding of transitions of care as an executive role as care coordinators and lateral integrators.
- The importance of transitions of care and their impact on quality and safe patient outcomes are the cornerstone to the CNLs' competencies in leading care coordination across the continuum.
- Knowing the CNLs' competencies and being able to align these skills facilitates the CNLs' influence and impact when using technologies and information

systems to facilitate quality improvement and expedite clinical, financial, and operational outcomes management including collection, analysis, and dissemination of outcomes.

- Identifying common elements of the transitional care models and how to translate these elements through communication, documentation, and use of informatics and technology advances the CNL as an effective lateral integrator.
- By determining root causes of ineffective transitions of care and being able to mitigate these risks increases the CNLs' efficacy in leading interprofessional team care transitions.
- The CNL's knowledge of transitions of care models and the major component of frequently used frameworks informs the CNL in the unique role as care coordinator and lateral integrator.
- CNLs integrate core competencies with effective care transition.

Reflection Questions

1. As a CNL student, how would you answer the question, "What is your role (CNL) in care transition?"
2. Describe the advantages and disadvantages of the various care transitions models. Would one model be preferred over another in acute versus chronically ill patients?
3. Identify readiness for implementing a transition of care model. How would you know that your microsystem was ready to integrate care transition as part of discharge planning within your system?

Learning Activities

1. Outline core features of transitional care cross-referencing specific CNL competencies to carrying out evidence-based transitions of care.
2. Consider a variety of settings in which your microsystem transitions patients in your daily work. For example, if you are hospital-based, do you transition patients to skilled-nursing facilities? Freestanding rehabilitation hospitals? Home? If you are in a long-term care facility, do you transition your residents to acute care? Home? Select at least two transitions and describe how you would carry out the core features of transitional care.
3. With a trusted CNL and staff nurse colleague, role-play communication and relational skills that enhance effective care transition. Use the examples in question 2 as the case study for "trying out" best communication and relationship-based practices.
4. A comprehensive assessment of an individual's health status, goals, and care preferences is critical to effective care transitions. Identify risk-assessment tools that are primarily used with your patient population. For example, if you are in an acute care setting, fall and pressure ulcer risks are likely part of your evidence-based standards for practice. Using a variety of tools, describe how knowing risk scores (levels) assist in risk mitigation and smooth care transition to the next setting.
5. Using the examples from question 2, outline a plan of care that is based on sound evidence supporting positive outcomes (patient and family satisfaction, reduced length of stay, and re-admission).

6. Using any one of the evidence-based transitional care models, walk through your current care transition practices comparing a tested model (Naylor, Coleman, Project RED, INTERACT). Describe what you learned as you completed this process. What recommendations would you make to your microsystem team?

References

Agency for Healthcare Research and Quality. (2015). *Transitional care interventions to prevent readmissions for people with heart failure.* https://effectivehealthcare.ahrq.gov/products/heart-failure-transition-care/clinician

Allen, J., Hutchinson, A. M., Brown, R., & Livingston, P. M. (2014). Quality care outcomes following transitional care interventions for older people from hospital to home: A systematic review. *BMC Health Services Research, 14*(346). http://www.bimedcentral.com/1472-6963/14/346\

American Association of Colleges of Nursing. (2004). Clinical Nurse Leader talking points. https://www.aacnnursing.org/CNL/About/Talking-Points

American Association of Colleges of Nursing. (2011). *The essentials of master's education in nursing.* http://www.aacn.nche.edu/educationresources/MastersEssentials11.pdf.

American Association of Colleges of Nursing. (2013). *Competencies and curricular expectations for clinical nurse leader education and practice.* http://www.aacn.nche.edu/cnl/CNL-Competencies-October-2013.pdf

American Association of Colleges of Nursing CNL Steering Committee. (2009). *Statement on post-master's CNL Certificate Program.* http://www.aacn.nche.edu/cnl/pdf/Post-Masters-Certificate-Programs-Statement.pdf

American Geriatrics Society. (2003). *Improving the quality of transitional care for persons with complex care needs.* AGS.

Bridge Model. (n.d.). Illinois Transitional Care Consortium. http://www.transitionalcare.org/the-bridge-model

Care Transitions Program. (n.d.). http://www.caretransitions.org/documents/CTM_FAQs.pdf

Coleman, E. A., Parry, C., Chalmers, S., & Min, S. J. (2006). The care transitions intervention: Results of a randomized controlled trial. *Archives of Internal Medicine, 166*(17), 1822–1828.

Coleman, E. A., & Williams, M. V. (2007). Executing high-quality care transitions: A call to do it right. *Journal of Hospital Medicine, 2*(5), 287–290.

Epstein, A. M. (2009). Revisiting readmissions—changing incentives for shared accountability. *New England Journal of Medicine, 360*(14), 1457–1459.

Garrido, T., Jamieson, L., Zhou, Y., Wiesenthal, A., Liang, L., & Kaiser Foundation Health Plan. (2005). Effects of electronic health records in ambulatory care: Retrospective, serial, cross sectional study, *British Medical Journal, 330*(7491), 581–584.

Guterman, S., Davis, K., Stremikis, K., & Drake, H. (2010). Innovations in Medicare and Medicaid will be central to health reform's success. *Health Affairs, 29*(6), 1188–1193.

Holland, D. E., & Hemann, M. A. (2011). Standardizing hospital discharge planning at the Mayo Clinic. *The Joint Commission Journal on Quality and Patient Safety, 37*(1), 29–36.

Institute of Medicine. (2001). *Crossing the quality chasm.* National Academies Press.

The Johns Hopkins Bloomberg School of Public Health: Guided Care. (n.d.). http://www.guidedcare.org.

The Joint Commission Center for Transforming Healthcare. (2010). *Improving transitions of care: Hand off communications.* http://www.centerfortransforminghealthcare.org/assets/4/6/CTH_Handoff_commun_set_ Final_2010.pdf.

Kripalani, S., LeFevre, F., Phillips, C. O., Williams, M. V., Basaviah, P., & Baker, D. W. (2007). Deficits in communication and information transfer between hospital and primary care physician: Implications for safety and continuity of care. *Journal of Medical Association, 297*(8), 831–841.

National Quality Forum. (2006). *NQF-endorsed definition and framework for measuring care coordination.* Author.

National Transitions of Care Coalitions. (2010). *Health professional resources.* http://www.ntocc.org/WhoWeServe/HealthCareProfessionals.aspx

Naylor, M. D., Aiken, L. H., Kurtzman, E. T., Olds, D. M., & Hirschman, K. B. (2011). The importance of transitional care in achieving health reform. *Health Affairs, 30*(4), 746–754.

Naylor, M. D., Feldman, P. H., Keating, S., Koren, M. J., Kutzman, E. T., Maccoy, M. C., & Krakauer, R. (2009). Translating research into practice: Transitional care for older adults. *Journal of Evaluation in Clinical Practice, 15*(6), 1164–1170.

Naylor, M. D., Kurtz, E. T., & Pauly, M. (2009). Transitions of elders between long-term care and hospitals. *Policy, Politics, & Nursing Practice, 10*(3), 187–194.

Naylor, M. D., & Sochalski, J. (2010). Scaling up: Bringing the transitional care model into the mainstream. *The Commonwealth Fund*, Pub. 1453, 103.

Ouchida K., Lofaso, V. M., Capello, C. F., Ramsaroop, S., & Reed, M. C. (2009). Fast forward rounds: An effective method for teaching medical students to transition patients safely across care settings. *Journal of the American Geriatrics Society, 57,* 910–917.

Ouslander, J. G., Bonner, A., Herndon, L., & Shutes, J. (2014). The Interventions to Reduce Acute Care Transfers (INTERACT) quality improvement program: An overview for medical directors and primary care clinicians in long term care. *Journal of the American Medical Directors Association, 15*(3), 162–170. https://doi.org/10.1016/j.jamda.2013.12.005

Ouslander J. G., Lamb, G., Tappen, R., Herndon, L., Diaz, S., Roos, B. A., Grabowski, D. C., & Bonner, A. (2011). Interventions to reduce hospitalizations from nursing homes: Evaluation of the INTERACT II collaborative quality improvement project. *Journal of American Geriatric Society, 59*(4), 745–753. https://doi.org/10.1111/j.1532-5415.2011.03333.x

Project Boost (2010). Better outcomes for older adults through safe transitions: Implementation guide to improve care transitions, Society of Hospital Medicine. Philadelphia, PA.

Project RED. (n.d.). https://www.bu.edu/fammed/projectred

Sebelius, K. (2010, July 13). Meaningful use announcement. *Press Conference*. Speech.

Wu, S., & Green, A. (2000). Projection of chronic illness prevalence and cost Inflation. RAND Corporation.

Zander, K. (2001). Case management accountability for safe, smooth, and sustained transitions. *Professional Case Management, 15*(4), 188–199.

EXEMPLAR

CNL and Care Coordination

Gladis Mundakal

At the hospital's daily safety briefing, the difficulties regarding a patient who required multiple consultations before an ortho surgery that was scheduled for noon that day were communicated. This patient was a direct admit the day prior by the ortho surgeon. The CNL student anticipated many process breakdowns because of the direct admission process, the fact that a new hospitalist group had just started at this facility, and existing gaps in the current consultation process for pulmonary and cardiology.

The patient's surgery was originally scheduled for 7:30 a.m., which was already postponed to 12:30 p.m. due to pending consultations. The ortho surgeon indicated that if the consultations are not completed by noon, surgery would need to be postponed to the next day. The CNL student reviewed the medical record and then met with the patient and spouse. The CNL learned that the patient was oxygen dependent, which created the potential for ventilator management during the postoperative period. The CNL student talked to the hospitalist group, cardiologist on call, pulmonologist on call, and facilitated both consultations with many back and forth phone calls. The respiratory department did a spirometry test per the pulmonologist's request for surgery clearance. The CNL student reported those results directly to the pulmonologist to decrease the turnaround time in reporting.

The CNL was aware that there were problems with the medical record scanning, which could delay the consultation process and care. The CNL student continually communicated and partnered with the charge nurse to meet the patient's needs and communicate the progress in the plan of care for the day. By 10:30 a.m., all issues that were pending for surgery were cleared. The patient went to surgery as scheduled at 12:30 p.m. The patient remained free from complications during the post-op period and was weaned back to her baseline oxygen use. The patient was discharged home the next day.

In summary, the CNL student assisted in decreasing the length of stay by two days, increased patient satisfaction, and prevented a delay in care. The following core competencies were evident by: (1) facilitating collaborative, interprofessional approaches and strategies in the design, coordination, and evaluation of patient-centered care; (2) facilitating lateral integration of healthcare services across the continuum of care with the overall objective of influencing, achieving, and sustaining high-quality care; (3) promoting a culture of continuous quality improvement within a system; and (4) evaluating patient handoffs and transitions of care to improve outcomes.

EXEMPLAR

The CNL's Role in Optimizing Care

Brunella Neely

It is not every day one can change the course of a person's life with their profession. CNLs have a unique opportunity to orchestrate care for individuals that can have a profound and life-changing impact.

Ms. A, a 34-year-old patient, was transferred to the medical-surgical unit from an intensive care unit on hospital day 3. Her admitting diagnosis was acute respiratory distress and incapacitating weakness due to morbid obesity. She was 650 pounds, had a BMI of greater than 100, and she required assistance with all care because she was unable to even turn herself. On arrival to the unit, supervision of her clinical care was assigned to a CNL.

The CNL immediately began attempts at establishing a relationship; however, this was difficult at first because of the patient's depression and lack of trust in healthcare. With the CNL seeing the patient daily, a relationship was established, and Ms. A began sharing feelings of hopelessness surrounding her obesity and outlook for the future. She was tearful as the two discussed her care and projection for the future. It was her perception that the physicians assigned to her care were essentially avoiding her debilitating weight even though she knew it was the root of all her problems. The CNL not only had a comprehensive understanding of her clinical course and poor mortality with her current condition but was also acutely aware the patient would ultimately be the one to make the decisions regarding change. Together, Ms. A and the CNL discussed options and decided a consult with a bariatric surgeon while hospitalized would be a first step.

The CNL, while rounding with the hospitalist, discussed this plan. Obesity is not an acute medical problem, and consults of this nature are extremely rare. The CNL urged the hospitalist to consider the consult for this individual case because her current weight was a barrier to proper follow-up after discharge. As a result of her obesity, she was unable to walk and had not ridden in a car for at least six months. The hospitalist reluctantly agreed and made the referral to a bariatric surgeon; he also ordered twice daily physical therapy to assist with strengthening.

Care coordination became a crucial part of Ms. A's care. The CNL was the essential link between the patient, the direct care staff (both licensed and unlicensed), dietary staff (dietitian and meal delivery), the physical therapist team, the social worker/case manager, and the physicians. The CNL met with the patient daily and discussed care with each team member to assure continuity, bariatric sensitivity, and plan of care to prevent errors. On hospital day 18, Ms. A was able to stand on her own for a few seconds at a time, and two days later was able to ambulate 10 feet with a bariatric walker and standby assistance. On hospital day 21, Ms. A was discharged home with arrangements made for appropriate follow-up with a PCP (complete with appropriate transportation), follow-up with the bariatric surgeon, and home healthcare to continue her road to recovery.

Ms. A was motivated to make the necessary lifetime changes to turn her condition around, however, it was the consistency and the continuity of that one contact person (the CNL) that she states helped her to see that a brighter future was possible. Since discharge 18 months ago, Ms. A has undergone bariatric surgery and has lost approximately 300 pounds. She continues her weight loss journey and keeps in contact with the CNL she attributes to saving her life.

As noted previously, CNLs possess a variety of competencies resulting in quality and coordinated care. Through planned actions and effective collaboration and communication, patient outcomes are positive and patient-centric.

EXEMPLAR

The Role of the CNL in Care Coordination

Cassie Crauswell

A patient was transferred from an outside rural hospital within our hospital system for a neurological consult. Cervical legions were discovered on her MRI, and she was newly diagnosed with multiple sclerosis (MS) by the neurologist. The treatment plan was for the patient to complete five days of immunoglobulin therapy (IVIG) to assist with the MS exacerbation. The CNL identified early that the patient had no insurance, poor health literacy, and minimal resources in her rural county. The CNL began early with reinforcement of education about this degenerative neurological disorder and made sure the patient understood the course of the disease and the importance of follow-up care. This education was reinforced daily to improve the patient's understanding of health management after discharge and prevent readmission. The CNL coordinated care with the case manager, who linked the patient with medical care at a free county health clinic near her home.

The patient was discussed on day 4 of admission in the daily interdisciplinary meeting led by the CNL. The direct care RN brought up the excellent point that the patient was due to receive her last dose of IVIG at 2000 hours. The RN stated the estimated transition date should be extended by one day to finish the treatment. The CNL knew that an additional stay in the hospital would be costly not only for the unfunded patient but also for the hospital by affecting throughput. To avoid delay in discharge, the CNL contacted the pharmacist to determine a safe time adjustment for earlier administration time of the IVIG. The CNL then contacted the neurologist with the recommendation and received permission to move the IVIG dose 4 of 5 to 1800 and the final dose to 1600 the following day. While coordinating care with the neurologist, the CNL also addressed the need for neurology follow-up, since the patient was unfunded. The neurologist stated that he did not take unfunded patients in his clinic but wanted to ensure neurology follow-up was arranged prior to discharge. The neurologist gave the patient permission to discharge once the follow-up was established and the fifth dose of IVIG completed. The CNL performed a chart review from the prior hospital stay and identified the name of a local neurologist who accepted unfunded patients. The CNL connected the patient with this neurologist and assisted to arrange follow-up on an affordable payment schedule for the patient.

The following day, the CNL requested a discharge order from the attending physician when he rounded early that morning. The attending voiced concern that the patient was receiving the last dose of IVIG late in the afternoon and had not yet been cleared for discharge by the neurologist. The CNL had closed these gaps the previous day and was able to reassure the medicine physician that the IVIG dose had been safely moved to an earlier administration time. The CNL was also able to verbalize that neurology follow-up was secured and that the neurologist was okay with discharge after the last dose of IVIG was completed. Furthermore, the case manager had provided discount prescription cards and linked the patient with a free medical clinic. The attending was reassured and provided the discharge order. Due to the care coordination and daily discussions led by the CNL with the multidisciplinary team, a delay in discharge was prevented. The involvement of the CNL also improved the patient's understanding of health management and ensured she was provided with tools and resources to prevent future re-admission.

The CNL's actions demonstrate a number of competencies that include the following: (1) facilitate lateral integration of healthcare services across the continuum of care with the overall objective of influencing, achieving, and sustaining high-quality care; (2) assume a leadership role, in collaboration with other interprofessional team members to facilitate transitions across care settings to support patients and families and reduce avoidable recidivism to improve care outcomes; and (3) facilitate modification of nursing interventions based on risk anticipation and other evidence to improve healthcare outcomes.

EXEMPLAR

Reuniting Families Through Care Coordination

Lucila Duarte

Mrs. M, an 81-year-old female patient was admitted due to complaints of anemia and an altered mental status. Mrs. M was noted to have a left breast mass that she reported knowing about five years ago but had decided not to seek medical attention, which led to a palliative care consult being placed. During testing, the patient was noted to have had an acute stroke.

During the multidisciplinary briefings led by the CNL student, the nurse and charge nurse expressed concerns due to Mrs. M's husband having soiled himself, and the CNL student was asked to assist with encouraging Mr. M to go home. After the multidisciplinary briefings, the unit manager approached the CNL student, also asking if it was possible to encourage Mr. M to go home as there was a fear of Mr. M falling. Upon rounding on Mrs. M, the CNL student was able to speak with the palliative care nurse practitioner (PCNP) regarding Mrs. M. Per the PCNP, Mrs. M was alert and oriented and decided to be made DNR. The PCNP expressed concerns regarding the Mr. M, as Mr. M had not driven Mrs. M to the hospital as was previously understood—the couple had taken a cab, and Mrs. M was the primary caregiver for Mr. M who had dementia. When speaking with Mrs. and Mr. M, Mrs. M informed the CNL student the couple had two sons, one who was incarcerated and the other lived in Virginia. Mrs. M reported having the son's number in Virginia, but it was at home, and the couple had no family or friends in the area available to obtain the son's information.

Following the advice of the social worker (SW), the CNL student e-mailed the head of security to assist in finding Mrs. M's family contact information. The SW and CNL student knew Mr. M could not go home alone because he would likely harm himself. The CNL student relayed Mrs. M's living situation to the unit manager, primary RN, and charge RN. While waiting for security to respond, the CNL student bought Mr. M lunch because the CNL student knew he had probably had not eaten anything since the day before. Security was able to provide two family members' contact information: one who Mrs. M stated was her incarcerated son and a female in Delaware who Mrs. M identified as her incarcerated son's ex-wife and stated would likely have her other son's information. With the patient's permission, the CNL student called the ex-daughter-in-law in Delaware who stated she would find Mrs. M's son's contact information and call back. The CNL student received a call from Mrs. M's son 10 minutes later, who lived in Maryland. The son had no idea of his mother's illness, her hospitalization, or of his father's severe mental decline. The son thanked the CNL student multiple times for getting in touch with him and confirmed there was no family in the immediate area to look over his father. The son was going to work on flying in soon and was contacting family who might be able to arrive sooner than he could. Prior to leaving for the day, the CNL student went back to see Mrs. M and let her know her son would be contacting her soon and assured her Mr. M could stay at her side. The charge RN that night assured the CNL student that Mr. M would receive something for dinner.

During the next two days, the CNL student continued to provide breakfast, lunch, and dinner for Mr. M, and bought him fresh clothes as Mr. M had soiled the ones he had and was wearing paper scrubs. The CNL student updated Mrs. M on the plan of care and provided emotional support along with answering multiple calls from the patient's son and granddaughters, who Mrs. M had given permission to speak with regarding her care. Mrs. M's family was traveling from as far as Oregon to come and be with Mrs. M and her husband. One granddaughter was able to provide some history that helped explain why Mrs. M had decided not to seek treatment for her breast mass. Mrs. M's daughter had passed away of breast cancer seven years prior; Mrs. M had been the primary caregiver for her daughter until she passed. According to Mrs. M's son, the death of his sister had been "very traumatic" and "hard on the patient." While the family had kept in constant contact with Mrs. M and her husband, they could not convince them to move to Maryland to be closer to family; the son believed it was because Mrs. M did not want to be far from her incarcerated son. The information learned from Mrs. M's granddaughter and son was relayed to the treatment team, giving the doctors some insight on Mrs. M's decision to not seek medical treatment and providing the nurses reassurance that this couple was loved and simply chose to live away from family and not tell them of their struggles.

Mrs. M's son arrived from Maryland. He had not seen his parents in over five years due to financial difficulties of traveling, having four children at home, as well as his own medical problems. When the CNL student was able to meet Mrs. M's son, the son expressed happiness over being able to place a face to the person he had been speaking to multiple times during the last couple of days. During the CNL student's rounding with Mrs. M and her family, her son was sitting next to his father holding his hand the entire time. The CNL student was touched to see the change in Mrs. M's and her husband's face; there was a happiness that was not there before, and it grew as more family began arriving. On Friday Mrs. M was discharged home on hospice with plans for the son to fly Mrs. M and her husband to Maryland accompanied by their granddaughter.

It took a lot of time to get all the pieces together with Mrs. M to help the physicians in their plan of care for the patient. The CNL student was able to spend the time the SW, RN, or doctors could not spare. With the assistance of security, SW, and staff, the CNL student was able to help in providing a safe discharge for both Mrs. and Mr. M, before Mr. M suffered any consequences of not taking his own medications. The CNL student was able to assist in decreasing Mrs. M's length of stay, because had Mrs. M not discharged home with family, the SW would have had to have found a facility who would take not only Mrs. M but Mr. M as well.

Had the CNL student been the primary RN and not the CNL student helping with the coordination of care for Mrs. M, the CNL student would not have been able to spend the time finding and speaking with family or helping care for Mr. M. The constant gratitude the CNL student received from Mrs. M's son and family was overwhelming. The CNL student received a call from Mrs. M's son in Maryland a month later with an update that Mrs. M and her husband had been moved to Maryland and were "doing great" and enjoying being surrounded and doted on by their loved ones.

This is only one example of how CNLs coordinate care and engage treatment teams in the delivery of care. CNLs can coordinate care as they are not assigned to the direct care of multiple patients in today's healthcare environment. Effective communication, as noted in this example, is another asset of CNL practice.

EXEMPLAR

Collaborating for Complex Patients: Extending CNL Competencies to the Community

Lauran Hardin

Mercy Health Saint Mary's is in the urban core of Grand Rapids, Michigan, and serves many vulnerable populations, including patients experiencing homelessness, psychiatric illness, substance abuse, and complex social determinant of health issues. A complex care center, led by a CNL, was created to meet the needs of the population.

Analysis of the high-frequency patients was performed by the center and a surprising number of people were found who utilized Mercy Health for hospitalization but received their primary care from systems outside of our network, including our competitors. To achieve stabilization in patient care, we needed to reach outside the walls of the hospital and the traditional definition of our "partners" to build new bridges for healthcare delivery.

One agency with a large population of high-frequency patients was approached by the CNL to explore the potential for collaboration. We began by finding shared purpose. Improving outcomes for high-frequency patients is challenging work and often takes a team approach. The fragmentation in the healthcare delivery system is often a contributor to patient destabilization and the complexity faced by the patients was a motivator for our agencies to work together to solve difficult problems.

After identification and discussion of our mutual patients, we implemented interprofessional rounds every two weeks to develop and maintain shared plans of care. Like rounds in the unit-based microsystem, we applied this CNL practice to the community and held rounds at the clinic focused on outcomes and quality improvement in the delivery of care.

Our shared plans were integrated in the hospital through a tool called a complex care map embedded in the EMR with an alert that fires when a provider opens the medical record. The map identifies the cross-continuum team, and the emergency room staff and the inpatient team began to call the clinic directly to coordinate care for their patients and include them in conferences held at the hospital.

Collaboration resulted in improved outcomes for patients. One year after intervention, the first population of 18 patients experienced a 60% reduction in inpatient admissions and length of stay, a 17% reduction in emergency room visits, and a 42% reduction in uninsured visits. Financial outcomes included a reduction in expense per patient of 19% and operating margin improvement of $74,000. Working together saved time and expense for both agencies and most importantly strengthened the system of delivery around vulnerable patients to improve outcomes.

The project was undertaken as a clinical QI initiative at Mercy Health and as such was not formally supervised by the Mercy Health Institutional Review Board per their policies.

EXEMPLAR

A Nursing Initiative to Improve the Patient's Care Transition: A CNL Initiative to Improve the Patient's Experience with Care Transition in the Urology Oncology Surgical Unit by Bringing Interdisciplinary Rounds to the Bedside

Carla Johnson

As a new CNL to the urology oncology surgical team, part of my initial onboarding was to assess my cohort and identify opportunities to enhance the patient's experience. During the assessment phase an observation was made that patient/family engagement in interdisciplinary rounds was noted as an opportunity for improvement. Current interdisciplinary rounds were conducted in a conference room with the healthcare team but no patient family presence. This lack of partnership and patient/family participation resulted in fragmented communication and a disjointed care transition process.

The CNL conducted a literature review on initiatives to improve interdisciplinary rounds. The literature review highlighted successful initiatives that involved patient-centered bedside interdisciplinary rounds. The outcomes of bedside rounds included improving patient satisfaction, reducing errors, increasing efficiency, and decreasing length of stay. Patient-centeredness is also one of the "Aims for Improvement" in the IOM's 2001 report, *Crossing the Quality Chasm: A New Health System for the 21st Century*.

The CNL shared this evidence with the interdisciplinary team to gain support for an initiative to transition interdisciplinary to the bedside. The interdisciplinary team, which included the case manager, social worker, physical therapist, occupational therapy, provider, and chaplain, were very receptive and supportive of the initiative. Thus, a plan was implemented to transition interdisciplinary rounds from the conference room to the bedside. This plan includes conducting weekly rounds on Thursday from 10:00 a.m. to 11:00 a.m., placing a *next* to the patient name on a whiteboard to indicate bedside rounds, reminding nurses during brief of bedside rounds, preparing the patient for bedside rounds through patient education, and placing beside round date and time on the patient's communication board.

The entire team was educated on the new initiative. A PowerPoint presentation was used as the education tool. This PowerPoint included the benefits and outcomes of bedside rounds, as well as the new bedside rounding process. Education occurred over a one-week period starting February 2, 2015. Implementation occurred the week of February 9, 2015. The outcome measure used to support an improvement in patient experience was HCAPHS Domain Care Transition.

A year postimplementation has trended a gradual increase in the patient satisfaction for care transition. With the current HCAPHS Domain Care Transition data sustaining a 2% increase and 94th percentile ranking compared to the Press Ganey Database.

This process of identifying an opportunity to enhance the patient experience with care transition and implementing a nursing initiative for change by placing the patient/family at the center has improved patient/family engagement, partnership with patient/family in the discharge process and interdisciplinary team communication.

EXEMPLAR

Re-Admission Reduction Through Improved Care Transitions in Complex Patient Populations

Sheri Salas and Lisa Mestas

The Institute for Healthcare Improvement launched the State Action on Avoidable Rehospitalizations (STAAR) Initiative to reduce re-admissions by improving care

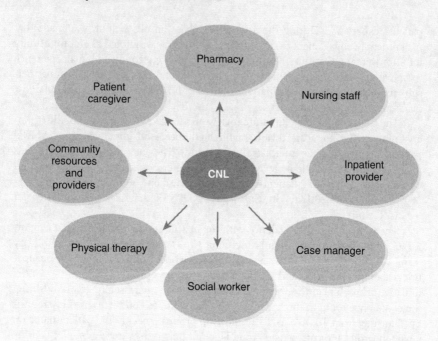

transitions (IHI, 2009). A medical surgical unit caring for a complex patient population, including those with multiple comorbidities and limited resources, was noted to have a re-admission rate of 16.04%, while the national benchmark for the organization is 15.2%. Patients frequently returned to the ED, had a low compliance rate of PCP visits after discharge from the hospital, and many did not obtain medications required to maintain chronic illnesses.

The patient data from six months of re-admissions were analyzed utilizing those that were admitted most frequently and those that had the re-admissions with the highest financial impact. The indicators that led to these re-admissions were used to develop a predictive tool specific to this population. If indicators raise a patient's score to a certain level on the re-admission risk tool (RRT), they are a high risk for re-admission and require focused attention to care transition actions throughout their hospitalization beyond those that the rest of the patient population receives. This led to the development of the CNL Transition of Care (TOC) protocol.

Patients that score high on the RRT are placed on the CNL TOC protocol. The protocol consists of the CNL on the unit coordinating the care transition for these patients as the facilitator along with the healthcare team to ensure a quality progression across the continuum and after discharge. Some of the actions involved in the protocol include: daily rounding, follow-up on indicated education, collaboration with Clinical Pharm D on the unit to ensure medication reconciliation/education/access, coordination with each member of the healthcare team daily, ensuring a follow-up appointment prior to discharge with PCP, involving patients and caregivers in transition plans, and making follow-up phone calls after discharge. The CNL began this effort by education sessions with staff and physicians, which has greatly improved the culture of care transitions. There has also been collaboration with community agencies in regard to how to better facilitate care transitions, which has created an environment in which they share data regarding patients discharged to their care.'

The TOC project was initiated mid-January 2015 when the CNL started in her role on the unit. The tool was modified once throughout the year when data showed that certain elements being monitored did not influence re-admission. At one point re-admissions were rising and the CNL team analyzing data drilled down on the indicators noting the trends and targeted those areas of need. It was found the issues were not related to the tool, but the data showed a subset of patients with a specific diagnosis in need of intervention. It also showed that the CNL needed to screen patients more often than upon admission. Patients were becoming high risk during their stay that were not high risk upon admission. The CNL met with the providers of the patients that needed intervention to develop a plan and began screening patients daily. This changed the outcomes of re-admission rates.

The baseline 30-day re-admission rate of 16.04% from the fourth quarter of 2014 has decreased to 14.14% as of the fourth quarter of 2015. The analysis of the high-risk patients screened with the tool has shown a decrease of 12% in that patient population with a cost avoidance of $310,560 in 2015. The TOC project was spread to the surgical trauma floor in July 2015, and the tool was modified specifically for that patient population. The team is hopeful that by continuing to utilize data to maintain the PDSA process, they will see further improvements in the outcomes of care transitions.

Reference

Institute for Healthcare Improvement. (2009). *IHI initiatives.* http://www.ihi.org/Engage/Initiatives/Completed/STAAR/Documents/STAAR%20State%20Based%20Strategy.pdf

EXEMPLAR

Improving Pain Management for the Neurosurgical Patient Population

Kristin S. Mast

Every month, the leadership team on the acuity adaptable neurosurgical and neuroscience inpatient unit monitors the monthly HCAHPS pain satisfaction scores. Different interventions have been implemented and attempted over the past several years. Scores improved over time but soon became inconsistent again, well below our target. We did an analysis of our unit HCAHPS scores to determine what areas drive the overall patient satisfaction. Pain management was our number-one driver for the overall experience. This time around, we decided to narrow our focus to a specific patient population: neurosurgical patients.

A CNL-led interdisciplinary team was formed to look at current practice, identify barriers, and develop a process improvement plan using LEAN principles. A root-cause analysis was done with input from staff nurses, the leadership team, and the outpatient spine office. We identified a breakdown in RN-to-RN communication at shift change regarding the patient's pain plan. We included pain plan talking points in the SBAR guide used during shift report. We collaborated with our palliative care service for evidence-based strategies for optimizing pain control in the spine population. We also consulted their expertise for patients with chronic pain, opiate-dependence, and any patient not achieving optimal pain control despite interventions.

Each day prior to patient rounds, the CNL reviews the documented pain scores and focuses on the scores above the patient-stated goal. As a mentor, the CNL assists the nurses with developing a pain plan and to ensure the patient is aware of the plan. Our CNL was instrumental in obtaining a single-patient-use cooling device that can be given to the spinal fusion patients for use in the hospital and continued at home upon discharge.

Since we started this initiative, staff nurses are regularly discussing the patient's pain plan with each other, during daily interdisciplinary rounds, and with the patient. After discharge, patients are stating their pain is better controlled and staff did everything they could to control their pain. Pain satisfaction scores are more consistent now, in the 75th to 90th percentiles, compared to below the 50th percentile when we started this initiative.

EXEMPLAR

The Need for Cross-Continuum Care

Elizabeth Triezenberg

The orthopedic program at Saint Mary's Health Care is a collaboration of a group of highly aligned surgeons not employed by Saint Mary's Health Care. Prior to the implementation of the CNL's role, there was limited communication among the office, surgeons, residents, and the staff nurses. Cross-continuum care was quickly identified as the root factor necessary for improving the orthopedic patient experience.

To define the cross-continuum, the CNL did a "gemba" walk of the orthopedic patient—starting in the outpatient surgeon's office and continuing through preadmission testing, surgical prep, surgery, recovery, inpatient unit, and returning to the office. Representatives from each of the areas were asked to participate in a short-term Lean project requiring weekly meetings.

The initial meeting was focused on identifying the experience of the patient undergoing a total joint replacement. It quickly became evident that the confusing, fractionated experience of the patient was a reflection of the team's knowledge of the system. Using Lean tools, the team decided to focus on preoperative patient education.

Structured weekly meetings were essential to the timely success of this work group. The group worked to identify, describe, and critique the patient experience. Barriers to care and communication were identified and addressed. Key information for each step of the system was defined and written into a preoperative patient education booklet, specific to our cross-continuum of care. The information the group felt was most important for the patient was summarized in a patient checklist in the front of the booklet.

The goal of the project was to improve the experience for the orthopedic patient by enhancing the cross-continuum of care. Once relationships were formed, the patient experience defined, and the patient preoperative booklet outlined, the group agreed to stop the weekly meetings. The remainder of the editing, marketing, and finalization of the book was done through small group meetings with e-mail updates. The Lean team representatives were responsible for sharing the information with their departments and having the booklets available for reference. As a result of the Lean team's work, the conversations throughout the system have switched from "if the patients only knew _____" to patients stating, "The book states _____ was going to happen." The established cross-continuum of orthopedic care has since created additional focus teams for short-term quality improvement projects.

EXEMPLAR

Pain and Complex Care

Lauran Hardin and Rebecca Valko

DL is a 36-year-old man with a devastating and rare neurological syndrome. Despite being wheelchair bound, he maintains as much independence as possible with a service dog, high-end wheelchair, and a strong spirit.

The illness started to take his body in pieces—a Harrington rod, a colostomy, a urostomy, and a feeding tube were all necessary procedures in the last few years.

DL has had the same PCP for many years, but as his physical status declined and he developed more complications, he added an array of specialists to his team, including urologists, gastroenterologists, hospitalists, pain physicians, and neurologists.

His admissions to the hospital escalated from once a year to six admissions within three months. Using the skills of systems analysis, CNLs looked at the root cause of these admissions to see if the outcomes of his care could be improved.

Several factors were identified, including fragmentation among the medical providers causing divergent plans of care, complex medical illness without framing it in the context of prognosis, fragmentation among the outpatient providers, lack of communication of plans of care between settings and EMRs, and lack of a proactive intervention plan to anticipate and react early to problems.

CNLs led a cross-continuum conference of interdisciplinary providers, inviting everyone to come together to creatively see if we could improve outcomes in his care. A complex care plan was created and shared across systems and EMRs to coordinate his care. Evidence-based stoplight tools were engaged with the patient, his family, and the home care and PCP staff to teach everyone how to anticipate the development of complications and intervene before his medical condition required hospitalization.

Creating a web of support among his providers with a clear plan resulted in DL being able to manage his condition at home, with his family and his dog by his side and no hospitalizations or emergency room visits for more than a year.

Communication and Handoff in the Emergency Department

Madalyn Frank-Cooper

The emergency department in our facility has a holding area for admitted patients. Because the two areas are within one department, the handoff between staff tended to be informal and inconsistent, which frequently has resulted in delays or omitted doses of medication. We asked the staff to identify flaws with the handoff process, with the goal of providing standardization and decreasing chances of error. We created a template for a report, which gave the nurses a regular reporting format. It also provided accountability for the report, as signatures were required. The challenge was not to teach staff how to give an accurate report, but to change the culture to become consistent in providing specific information during a handoff. Implementing a new tool and the expectation of staff compliance was a challenge, but the new procedure was incorporated into daily practice in conjunction with direct observation and positive reinforcement.

In the preimplementation period, 13 reports regarding medication/fluid error were reviewed. Of those reported, 7 were due to communication issues. In the post-implementation period, 10 reports were reviewed. Of those reported, 4 were due to communication issues. Not only was there a slight decrease in errors secondary to communication, there was also a slight decrease in total reported occurrences.

The CNL: Utilizing Effective Communication and Lateral Integration to Meet the Care Needs of a Dying Patient

Beth VanDam

It was a typical morning as I stepped onto the unit as a CNL. I reviewed the unit census to prioritize my day. Kim would be my first patient to meet as her story and plan of care were complicated and her physical condition was tenuous. Ensuring the newly assigned nurse had a clear understanding of Kim's plan of care would be essential to providing the best care. I had met Kim and her family the day before when she was admitted. I had listened carefully as she shared her journey with cancer. Kim, a 35-year-old mother of two young children, struggled with end-stage cancer, now requiring a hospital admission due to dehydration. Her request, as well as the wish of her family, was to remain a full code. She was alert and pleasant but obviously suffering with emotional distress. Physically she was extremely cachectic—unlike I had ever seen before.

As the events of the day transpired, there were many opportunities as a CNL to not only impact the patient/family care experience but also provide support for the nursing staff as Kim transitioned from being extremely ill to dying. First, I facilitated continuity of care by communicating Kim's cancer story and plan of care to changing caregivers. Kim's husband and both sets of parents were present; however, due to recent traumatic experiences, there were different levels of acceptance around the reality of Kim's rapidly changing condition. At times the nursing staff were also troubled by the physician orders and focus of care as Kim remained a full code although she became unresponsive and had mottling. Knowing the patient story, I was able to help connect the dots for the staff and share the plan of care along with the reasons why we were still providing some nonlife-sustaining treatments. Laterally integrating the team was essential to ensure a smooth transition of care took place for the patient/family as well as point-of-care support for the nursing staff.

Coordination of care became an increasing need throughout the day. As CNL, I evaluated and involved key members of the interdisciplinary team. Palliative care was called for assistance in managing changing symptoms; a cancer resource specialist was called for psychosocial support for the family, including the two young children; and ongoing clinical support for nurses regarding when and how to verbalize changing patient needs/conditions to the physician was provided. Kim remained a full code until a few minutes before dying. She remained comfortable in her room with family close by, as well as key members of the oncology interdisciplinary team who cared for her throughout her cancer journey.

My role continued after Kim expired. It was a very emotional time, not only for the family but also for the staff. Being a resource to ensure time and emotional support for the staff was instrumental to allowing the team to grieve appropriately. Supporting and encouraging the staff to take the time to grieve enabled them to carry on with once again providing excellent care to our other patients.

EXEMPLAR

Introducing the Buddy Break System to Strengthen Self-Care Among Nurses on a 26-Bed Gynecology and Radiation Oncology Unit

Kenia Latin and Patricia Davis

The aim of this quality improvement project was to implement a break buddy system on a 26-bed gynecology and radiation oncology unit where the nurses had another nurse cover patient assignment to be free of patients to take a meal break. Based on results from the NDNQI survey from 2013, direct observation by the leadership team, and recognition by the nurses that the practice of taking breaks, or doing so with interruptions on this unit was of minimal practice, the decision was made to develop an action plan to address the results and improve the way that nurses took meal breaks. The unit leadership expressed concerns and difficulty in having nurses take meal breaks due to the current culture practices of the nursing staff discouraging the practice of self-care, therefore, increasing the percentage of fatigue, burnout, and turnover rates of nurses leaving this unit. There is mounting evidence of the link between practitioner's personal resilience and well-being and the quality and safety of the care they provide patients (University of Virginia Alumni Association and School of Nursing, 2013). A decline in function because of fatigue and burnout leads to concern for practice and safety concerns for patients and for nurses alike (Witkowski & Dickson, 2010). Nurses provide direct patient care 24 hours a day. This implies working long hours with omitting meal and nonmeal breaks resulting in increased fatigue (Witkowski & Dickson, 2010). Increased nurse satisfaction is directly tied to improved patient outcomes and adverse outcomes of care (Stimpfel & Aiken, 2013). The methodology used was Deming's PDSA cycle, a model for continuous improvement. The needs assessment for this unit revealed that nurses would not consistently take meal breaks, and when they did, they were interrupted, not free of a patient assignment.

This caused dissatisfaction, verbalization of frustration, and burnout of the staff. Prior to the implementation date for this project, staff in-services were conducted to educate on the review of the literature supporting the importance of self-care, patient safety, and patient satisfaction, highlighting the institution's Quality Caring Model in which self-care is an essential factor within this framework that encompasses basic human needs and creating a healing environment. Additionally, posters were created and posted throughout the unit, unit break-buddy guidelines were written, and the assignment sheet was updated to include the name of the assigned break-buddy nurse per each shift. Unit leadership made frequent observations and supported the initiative to ensure it was being carried out. Post-intervention the percentage of nurses taking a meal break equal to or 30 minutes was at 65%, in comparison to the prior 31%. Most significantly, the percentage of nurses that were able to be free of patients went from 11 to 65%. Continued mentoring and coaching, team building, and rounds by the leadership team will be integral in the sustainability behaviors of self-care of the nursing staff.

As entrenched in the culture of nursing, the unit assessment performed identified that the nursing unit culture is that responsible nurses do not take a break or a lunch. As pointed out in the literature, the biggest resistance is for nurses to take meal and nonmeal breaks and give up control of the patient care to a colleague (Hendren, 2010; Smith, 2013).

References

Hendren, R. (2010). Nurses say they need a break; why leaders should listen. *Health Leaders Media,* 1. http://www.healthleadersmedia.com/page-1/NRS-256422/Nurses-Say-They-Need -A-Break-Why-Leadership-Should-Listen##

Smith, L. D. (2013). Reaching for cultural competence. *Nursing, 43*(6), 30–37.

Stimpfel, A. W., & Aiken, L. A. (2013, April–June). Hospital staff nurses' shifts length associated with safety and quality care. *Journal of Nursing Care Quality, 28*(2), 122–129. https://doi .org10.1097/NCQ.0bq013e3182725109

University of Virginia Alumni Association and School of Nursing. (2013). The architecture of compassion. *Virginia Legacy,* 8–12. http://uva.healthfoundation.virginia.edu/sites/healthfoundation. virginia.edu/files/publicatins/UVASON_VirginiaLegacy_F13.pdf

Witkowski, A., & Dickson, V. V. (2010). Hospital staff nurses; work hours, meal periods, and rest breaks: A review from an occupational health nurse perspective. *American Association of Occupational Health Nurses Journal, 58*(11), 489–497.

Postdischarge Calls in the ED: Improving Quality and Efficiency

Megan Pashnik

According to Huber (2006), a microsystem can be defined as "a small group of people who work together on a regular basis to provide care to discrete subpopulations of patients" (p. 5). Microsystems produce performance outcomes and are often embedded in larger organizations (Huber, 2006). The role of the CNL is to maximize the potential of the microsystem so that the larger healthcare organization can provide the best care possible.

Much like a CNL, the priority for a CNL student is microsystem assessment. This requires a variety of techniques, including interview, direct observation, and data collection. The student must determine the overall aim of the microsystem and identify key processes within the microsystem. Data on the microsystem's quality improvement indicators and quality and safety metrics must also be considered. To achieve this goal, every aspect of the microsystem must be observed, evaluated, analyzed, and reviewed with a focus on value and patient outcomes. Identifying and improving even one area of waste, one aspect of patient care that is not adding value, or one process that is inefficient can lead to safer, more effective, and more affordable care for patients.

In the context of this student's assessment, the microsystem is a 44-bed Level II trauma center ED embedded within a larger 378-bed acute care organization in the Midwest. Based on the observation processes within the ED microsystem and interviews with nursing staff, postdischarge follow-up calls were identified as an area for quality improvement and a dissatisfier for nursing staff. Improving, developing, and revising the process for follow-up calls will serve as a scholarly project for this CNL student.

Nursing staff in the ED have been placing follow-up phone calls to its patients for seven years. When the calls were first initiated, the nursing staff received some initial education regarding the calls; however, the process has received very little attention since. As a consequence, there is great disparity between the standard of work and how the process is actually implemented day-to-day. Additionally, these calls are time-consuming and inefficient.

Nurses placing follow-up calls while caring for patients in the busy ED setting cannot perform the task of follow-up calls efficiently. Because nurses are engaged with caring for the patients who are physically present in the ED, they experience frequent interruptions while placing follow-up calls. Data from call tracking logs indicate that nurses spend as much as three times the number of minutes addressing issues identified in the follow-up calls compared to the actual time spent speaking with patients on the phone. While follow-up calls may take a nurse 15 minutes, it is not uncommon for it to take the remainder of the hour to address the concerns brought forward. As such, the time spent making the calls is far less than the actual time spent addressing concerns that are brought forward. This "lost" time may lead to increased costs for the ED as nurses are not able to perform the task efficiently.

Modifying the process for follow-up calls may improve the quality of the calls and decrease the amount of time necessary for placing the calls. These changes may also increase nurses' satisfaction with the follow-up call process, which could lead to increased nurse retention and, ultimately, better outcomes for patients (Andrews & Dziegielewski, 2005; Newman & Maylor, 2002; Newman et al., 2002). The purpose of this student's evidenced-based practice protocol (scholarly project) is to revise the current standard of work in an effort to optimally and efficiently utilize nursing time, improve the quality of postdischarge calls, and improve job satisfaction for ED RN staff.

References

Andrews, D. R., & Dziegielewski, S. F. (2005). The nurse manager: Job satisfaction, the nursing shortage and retention. *Journal of Nursing Management, 13*(4), 286–295. https://doi .org/10.1111/j.1365-2934.2005.00567.x

Huber, T. P. (2006). *Micro-systems in health care: Essential building blocks for the successful delivery of health care in the 21st century* [PowerPoint slides]. https://www.google.com/url?sa=t&rct=j& q=&esrc=s&source=web&cd=5&ved=0ahUKEwj7gqCwi83JAhUE54MKHY0fB TIQFggzMAQ&url =http%3A%2F%2Fwww.dhcs.ca.gov%2Fprovgovpart%2Finitiatives%2F- nqi%2FDocuments%2FMicroSysHC.ppt&usg=AFQjCNEQlm4t4F3Wy3xtwB6ZSY_w7GX3T w&sig2=GcXwskPCEq7iiGEWqvYeyg&bvm =bv.109332125,d.amc&cad=rja

Mercy Health. (2015). *Mercy Health Saint Mary's campus, downtown Grand Rapids.* http://www.mercy healthsaintmarys.com/saint-marys

Newman, K., & Maylor, U. (2002). The NHS plan: Nurse satisfaction, commitment and retention strategies. *Health Services Management Research, 15*(2), 93–105. https://doi.org/10.1258 /0951484021912860

Newman, K., Maylor, U., & Chansarkar, B. (2002). The nurse satisfaction, service quality and nurse retention chain: Implications for management of recruitment and retention. *Journal of Management in Medicine, 16*(4/5), 271.

EXEMPLAR

Reducing Length of Stay for the Neurosurgical Patient Population via a Lean Management System

Sarah Price, Yarshika Barringer, Brandy Santana, and Janice Sills

Between 1994 and 2006, spinal stenosis diagnosis increased by 926%, and procedures for intervertebral disc disorders increased by 540%. In 2014, the AHRQ reported spinal fusion ranked fifth for costliest surgical procedure ($27,600 per hospital stay) and first for highest aggregate hospital cost ($12.8 billion). Unfortunately, this explosive growth in high-cost surgery is accompanied by poor levels of patient satisfaction and wide variations in length of stay, complication rates, postoperative pain, and postoperative functionality (Wainwright et al., 2016).

This problem was realized within our hospital system where data showed a predicted volume increase of 650 cases per year by 2022 as well as the opportunity to decrease length of stay in over half of the neurosurgery spine population.

Improvement Process

In response to this dual problem of capacity and quality, an interdisciplinary team specialized in the care of neurosurgical patients integrated a Lean management system (LMS) into unit culture. The cornerstone of this LMS was the development of surgical pathways that standardized care to improve patient outcomes and decrease hospital length of stay without increasing risk of re-admission or adverse events.

Pathways were designed to follow the patient through the continuum of care; so first, preoperative assessment was restructured by the clinic nurse to better identify risk factors that most impact patient recovery after spinal surgery. For each of these risk factors, an agreed on assessment or screening tool was used to gather pertinent patient information. Analysis of this comprehensive assessment was then used to determine categorization into a low, moderate, or high-complexity pathway. Next, details of the patient assessment and pathway assignment were sent to hospital nursing leadership where this information was used to tailor preoperative education at an in-person, CNL-led class. Once the patient was admitted for surgery, EMR templates triggered the appropriate pathway orders for inpatient care so that all preoperative preparation flowed seamlessly into hospitalization.

For inpatient care, all pathways included the same fundamental postoperative patient goals (early mobilization, adequate nutrition and hydration, drain management, return of bowel and bladder function, and pain management); however, the steps to achieve these goals and time frames for doing so varied depending on the pathway. To support these differences between pathways, orders within each respective EMR template matched the proposed goals and time frames, creating clear and meaningful orders that allowed the nurse to drive patient care. The design of these orders focused on using standardized language and built-in time frames. For example, an activity order that previously read, "out of bed with assistance," became, "out of bed within 2 hours of arrival to unit, ambulate, and out of bed with all meals." Additionally, an order for PRN IV Dilaudid that previously had a default duration of 14 days now defaulted to 24 hours.

Considering the measurable goals and clear communication regarding expected length of stay built within the pathways, the nurse became empowered to accelerate the discharge planning process through the concept of "checkout times." To supplement traditional care provided by clinical case management, this nurse-driven concept encouraged the curse to continuously assess the patient's progress toward their respective goals. As the patient approached meeting all goals, the nurse was triggered to initiate a discharge planning discussion with the patient and family. This discussion included review of the discharge plan, notification of expected discharge within 24 hours, confirmation of ride, and agreement on checkout time. This time was then shared with the interdisciplinary team, establishing a collective goal for all to ensure their respective responsibilities were completed within a timely manner.

To encourage accountability and sustainability without losing focus on existing quality priorities, tiered interdisciplinary buddies and visual management boards were created to track real-time compliance, identify gaps, and support staff.

Results/Outcomes

After implementation, improvements were realized in all targeted areas. Opportunity days for the spine population were reduced from 522 to 220, and opportunity days per patient were reduced from 1.60 to 1.12. All corresponding balancing measures also showed improvement. Patient experience scores improved from 60.7 to 67.3%. The re-admission rate reduced from 4.91 to 4.59%. Additionally, the CAUTI rate (per 1,000 catheter days) reduced from 1.72 to 0.95.

Reflection

In the project described previously, multiple CNLs were integral collaborators within the interdisciplinary team. From analyzing data and brainstorming ideas with administrators to performing patient care with frontline staff, CNLs were present at every step of the way. And it is within this balance of being a "thinker" and a "doer" that the CNL finds success personally and among peers. Many changes, process improvements, and evidence-based practice initiatives meet challenges and barriers because of conflict between nonclinical nurses who are creating new ideas and bedside nurses who must implement them. However, the CNL is in the unique position of experience and expertise to function as a leader, bringing understanding and cohesion between all members of the team.

Additionally, this project exemplifies the importance of the CNL to consistently validate the role with data outcomes. The more the CNL can provide objective evidence of positive results, the more they show worth, which is imperative to role sustainment in today's healthcare market. The CNL also needs to be mindful of and speak to corollary benefits that may indirectly result from CNL-led initiatives. While these may not be as easy to define or present statistically, they are valuable and worth noting. For example, during the time frame of the project mentioned previously, teammate engagement improved according to annual survey results, HCAPHS scores increased, and additional evidence-based practice initiatives for mobility and surgical site infection prevention were initiated. Leadership in the current healthcare environment calls for "big picture" or systems thinking to tackle the issues of today. And that is what the CNL brings to the table, an appreciation and understanding of how each proposed change is part of an integrated system driven by continuous improvement that maximizes the value of small wins.

References

Price, S., Smith, L., & Barringer, Y. (2019, February 21–22). *Optimizing the care of spinal surgery patients using lean methodology to develop surgical pathways* [Poster presentation]. 2019 Clinical Nurse Leader Summit, Tampa, FL.

Wainwright, T., Immins, T., & Middleton, R. (2016). Enhanced recovery after surgery and its applicability for major spine surgery. *Best Practice & Research Clinical Anaesthesiology, 30*(1), 91–102.

CHAPTER 16

The CNL's Role in Population Health and Management

Margaret Moore-Nadler, Linda A. Roussel, and Patricia L. Thomas

LEARNING OBJECTIVES

1. Define population health and the implication for communities and healthcare systems.
2. Provide an overview of health promotion and illness prevention.
3. Discuss the *Healthy People 2020* and *2030* indicators and how CNLs contribute to the achievement of healthcare goals.
4. Discuss the role of CNLs in promoting the foundational capabilities of population health.

KEY TERMS

Access
Advocacy
Change
Health promotion
Illness prevention
Innovation
Measuring and sustaining progress

Partnership
Patient engagement
Population health
Social determinants of health
Wellness
Patient engagement

CNL ROLES

Client advocate
Clinician
Educator

Outcomes manager
Lifelong learner
Team manager

CNL PROFESSIONAL VALUES

Accountability
Altruism
Human dignity

Integrity
Social justice

CNL CORE COMPETENCIES

Assessment

Communication

Design/Management/Coordination of care

Disease prevention

Health promotion

Healthcare systems and policy

Human diversity

Illness and disease management

Member of a profession

Provide and manage care

Population Health

In today's global society, the myriad of commonly diagnosed disease conditions brings the requirements for population-based rather than individual level attention to the forefront (Fawcett & Ellenbecker, 2015). Kindig and Stoddart's (2003) definition of population health as health outcomes of a group of individuals, including the distribution of these outcomes within the group, supports this idea. Outcomes imply the expressed focus within the group. As one component of the IHI, Berwick and colleagues (2008) identify improving the health of populations as one of the triple aims (the other two components focus on improving the individual experience of care and reducing the per capita costs of care for populations). Jacobson and Teutsch (2012) described a similar goal, using the term *total population health* defined by geographic areas. The CMS Innovation Center's mission also focused on better health as one of three elements to support healthier lifestyles in the entire population. Healthy lifestyles include an emphasis on increased physical activity, avoidance of behavioral risks, better nutrition, and a more expansive use of preventive care (CMS, 2020). The distinction between public health and population health offered by the CDC (2020) is that public health works to protect and improve health of communities through policy recommendations, education, outreach, and disease detection and injury prevention where population health provides the opportunity for healthcare systems, agencies, and organizations to work together to improve health outcomes of the communities they serve.

Stoto (2013) focused an organization's potential contributions and responsibility in advancing the evidence base for population health policy and practice describing a number of commonalities. Stoto purports that population health is more than the sum of individual parts or a cross-sectional perspective. Measurement of population involves upstream factors, not just health outcomes, and the goal of reducing disparities and inequities are included in this holistic perspective of population health.

Stoto (2013) further states that the population health perspective mandates that we are thoughtful about a broader set of health determinants than what is typical in either healthcare or public health. He focused on the work of Stiefel and Nolan (2012), which considers health promotion and disease prevention as well as on interventions focusing on upstream factors rather than solely on outcomes. These perspectives recognize the role of healthcare and personal prevention services as part of the population health production system.

Improving population health within systems and communities demands that partnerships are developed and nurtured beyond state and local public health agencies and healthcare delivery systems. Expanding partnerships necessitates that data is shared and a systems focus is adopted that outlines accountability for and measures contributions to population health outcomes (IOM, 1999, 2010, 2012; Stoto, 2013).

With renewed emphasis on health and well-being of communities and systems, the literature suggests that population health is instrumental as a means to improving the healthcare system rather than the end goal. Through the actions and intervention of CNLs using skills in advocacy, understanding health delivery, and team leadership, promoting active involvement in the health of citizens and population health is an essential focus.

Health Promotion and Illness Prevention: Overview

Health promotion is not just a healthcare system or healthcare provider responsibility. Promoting health and preventing disease require collaboration with both governmental and nongovernmental agencies (Interprofessional Education Collaborative Expert Panel, 2011, 2016). Health promotion encompasses the interactions between individuals, care providers, community agencies, technology, and health literacy.

Governments, businesses, and the healthcare system collaborating and developing partnerships can promote health effectively and efficiently by linking social and health determinates that endorse a health promotion infrastructure focused on the whole individual (DeSalvo et al., 2016; Jia et al., 2009; Kjellstrom et al., 2007). Political and business leaders (local, national, and international) must recognize that the social determinants of poverty, education, employment, and environment strongly impact physical and mental health (DeSalvo et al., 2016; Jia et al., 2009; Kjellstrom et al., 2007). Acknowledging and correcting the social determinants reduces morbidity and mortality rates for all humanity (Kjellstrom et al., 2007). CNLs—educated in an understanding and historical perspective of health promotion and illness prevention locally, nationally, internationally, and globally—are well prepared to intervene in positive ways that will have sustainable outcomes. Additionally, CNLs appreciate how to navigate complexity across different sectors necessary to bring teams and collaborators together to define shared goals and purposes.

Understanding the Larger Perspective Through the Lens of *Healthy People 2020* and *2030*

During the past three decades, the *Healthy People* initiative, managed by the US Department of Health and Human Services and the Office of Disease Prevention and Health Promotion, has encouraged a national agenda to improve the health status of US residents. *Healthy People* strives to improve the health of the nation, as well as to educate and support individuals in choosing healthy lifestyles. According to *Healthy People 2020*, applying the concepts of social and physical environments, health services, individual behaviors, and biology and genetics will improve national health outcomes (US Department of Health and Human Services, 2012a, 2020a).

Healthy People 2020 measures national health improvement by 12 leading health indicator topics:

1. Access to health services
2. Clinical preventive services
3. Environmental quality
4. Injury and violence
5. Maternal, infant, and child health
6. Mental health
7. Nutrition, physical activity, and obesity
8. Oral health
9. Reproductive and sexual health
10. Social determinants
11. Substance abuse
12. Tobacco

Each topic has one or more measureable outcomes. Moreover, *Healthy People 2020* provides individuals and communities with evidence-based strategies for implementing health promotion and prevention (US Department of Health and Human Services, 2012a).

The *Healthy People 2030* goals represent the fifth iteration of *Healthy People* work and updates past work to streamline the 2020 goals from over 1,000 to 355 core objectives centered on public health priorities through eliminating redundancy and clarifying purpose. For the first time in history, there is a focus on individual and organizational health literacy. Personal health literacy is defined as the ability for individuals to find, understand, and use information and services to inform health-related decisions and actions where organizational health literacy centers on the equity in enabling individuals to enact their health literacy (US Department of Health and Human Services, 2020c).

Like the predecessor, *Healthy People 2030* includes a framework, objectives specific to topics, and a set of priority measures known as Leading Health Indicators (LHIs). Thirty-four LHIs are structured by 12 themes specific to the framework. Each of the LHIs includes health, equity, and well-being. Fewer health conditions are identified in *Healthy People 2030* and focus more on the causes of poor health. The LHIs are to a lesser degree linked to a healthcare system's capabilities and metrics. More emphasis is evident in how people live life and shaped by a broader content of policies, systems, social structures, and economic forces. Finally, the LHIs' intent is to balance those operating and measured at an individual level (National Academies of Sciences, Engineering, and Medicine, 2020).

Context for Public Health and Health of Communities: Policy and Action

Protecting the health of US citizens began in the formative years of the country's independence. In 1798, the federal government enacted a bill to provide healthcare to sick and disabled sailors. A marine hospital network was established, and over the next hundred years it evolved into the Public Health Department. In 1887, the federal government began researching disease, which resulted in the NIH. In 1902, the United States established the International Sanitary Bureau in Washington, DC (WHO, 2012).

Throughout the 20th century, the federal government has implemented a variety of agencies designed to protect and provide services for all residents regardless of race, creed, age, or gender in the United States (US Department of Health & Human Services, 2012b, 2020b). The health of the nation has improved because epidemiologists stepped into unknown paths to find the causes of infectious diseases and discovered methods to prevent reoccurrences of disabling and deadly infections (Frieden & Garfield, 2012). Health has improved significantly in the United States during the 20th century (Altman, 2012). New and improved treatments and therapies have reduced mortality and disability and improved the quality of life for people suffering from cancer or heart disease (DeVol & Bedroussian, 2007).

The lead agency for public health in the United States is the CDC in Atlanta, Georgia. The CDC's role is to provide leadership in public health that protects the health of a diverse population and to educate healthcare professionals to promote healthy lifestyles (Communicable Disease Center, 2018). Public health in the United States has made great strides over the past 100 years with reducing preventable injuries, illness, and premature deaths and increasing life expectancy throughout the country (IOM, 2002; OECD, 2019).

In recent years, the US healthcare system has come under great scrutiny, with the high cost of healthcare and patients being harmed by the system that is designed to help and protect them (Altman, 2012; IOM, 1999). Current reports on the public health system indicate that it lacks adequate funding, and there is inadequate collaboration within communities to support public health (Majette, 2011). Recommendations to improve public health have been presented to Congress, including redesigning local public health departments so that they become proactive and lead their communities in promoting and protecting health, as well as develop collaborations within the community to promote healthy lifestyles (IOM, 2002).

Public health experts testified to Congress about the significant impact of creating a framework based on health promotion, prevention, and wellness in the US healthcare system and improving public health. The national debate resulted in Congress supporting the recommendations for a healthcare act that became the Patient Protection and Affordable Care Act (PPACA). President Obama signed this legislation into law on March 23, 2011 (Majette, 2011). Now the national agenda in healthcare requires a focus on health promotion and wellness, as opposed to a system focused on sick care or cure. Implementing a new healthcare agenda will require partnerships with public and private sectors working together to overhaul the healthcare system (National Prevention Council, 2011, NIH, 2020).

The CDC will lead health promotion, prevention, and preparedness efforts in the United States. The public health system has developed a new framework to strengthen public health infrastructure, develop partnerships, improve communication, use evidence to support actions, develop accountability systems, and address multiple determinants of health for communities (IOM, 2002).

To become effective and efficient, the CDC has identified five strategic areas for improvement:

1. Supporting state and local health departments
2. Improving global health
3. Implementing measures to decrease leading causes of death
4. Strengthening surveillance and epidemiology
5. Reforming health policies (Communicable Disease Center, 2018)

Indeed, the CNL plays a vital role in understanding and using the priority measures of *Healthy People 2030* and its predecessor. The roles of manager of care, coordination of care, and outcomes manager provide opportunities related to the achievement of healthcare goals. Population health perspectives recognize the role of healthcare personnel as part of the population health production system. Improving population health within all systems and communities demands establishment and nurturance of partnerships that go beyond state and local public health agencies and healthcare delivery systems. The upstream analogy, according to James (2020), is a moral and financial obligation to improve education, income, financial and housing stability, and access to food and healthcare, and reduce violence. Contributions and responsibility are multifactorial that includes public policy and healthcare practice changes. Stoto (2013) suggests that population health is more than the sum of individual parts or a cross-sectional perspective. Population health involves upstream factors and measuring what happens within that population or community and not just health outcomes. The goal of reducing disparities and inequities is included in this holistic perspective of population health.

Expanding partnerships necessitates data sharing and systems that outline accountability to measure contributions to population health outcomes (IOM, 1999, 2010, 2012; Stoto, 2013). With renewed emphasis on health and well-being of communities and stakeholders, the literature suggests that population health is instrumental to improving the healthcare system rather than the end goal. Given this, the CNL can lead and contribute to the promotion of health by partnering, implementing evidence-based health promotion strategies, leading interprofessional teams, and measuring outcomes to improve the health of individuals, groups, and populations.

Promoting the Foundational Capabilities of Population Health

Improving any understanding or the subsequent improvement dimensions that follow is foundational to population health. Population health management and the well-being of communities are central to positive outcomes. This requires that care is accessible and affordable, and agents of change exchange knowledge that is innovative and thought provoking. As such, populations must be understood, which includes culture, norms, rituals, and the interactions among individuals and groups. Based on this understanding, actions and new strategies can be identified by healthcare systems that culminate in ways to measure outcomes and maintain their sustainability. Action-oriented and sustainable partnerships among the population, healthcare providers, and administrators will be the cornerstone and function as the

North Star for the nation's population health efforts and contir (American Hospital Association, 2020; National Academies c ing, and Medicine, 2020).

CNLs will play an important role in promoting the foun population health through the use of leadership skills, leadir and evidence-based information to guide actions. At no other time in out has this been evident than during the COVID-19 pandemic. CNLs have been called on in a variety of ways to lead emergency planning, protocol development, transition of care management, and development of team members.

Being socially responsible, as a professional, will guide how the social determinants of health can reduce preventable diseases of populations. The zone of complexity is great; however, multiple opportunities await the dedication of CNLs who understand microsystem complexity and change that lend support to a healthy population.

Summary

- Population health has emerged from unmet needs.
- Access to care remains a concern despite the passing of the Affordable Care Act.
- There are still disparities in health outcomes, and addressing health will require the engagement, collaboration, and shared goals of providers, policy makers, and organizations to improve health outcomes in communities and the country.
- While policy and regulatory influences are a starting point, heath outcomes require health literacy that extends beyond the confines of the provider's office or hospital well into the fabric of communities centered on health promotion, access, and lifestyle.
- CNLs are well positioned with knowledge and skill to innovate, collaborate, and measure indicators relevant to population health outcomes.

Reflection Questions

1. Watch the local news and count the number of times a reference is made to a topic related to the 12 *Healthy People 2020* focus areas. How many references did you hear? Were you surprised? Why or why not?
2. Select one of the reference topics from question 1 and identify three ways a CNL could bring awareness to this issue through conversations with family and neighbors.
3. What are the top three population health initiatives in your organization? Do they have formal action plans? Is there a population health goal for your microsystem? If not, why not and what would you recommend?

References

Altman, D. (2012). Pulling it together: Reflections on this year's four percent premium increase. *Henry Kaiser Family Foundation*. http://www.kff.org/pullingittogether/altman_premium_increase.cfm

American Hospital Association. (2020). *AHA population health framework*. https://www.ihi.org/Topics/Population-Health/Documents/PathwaystoPopulationHealth_ Framework.pdf

Berwick, D. M., Nolan, T. W., & Whittington, J. (2008). The triple aim: Care, health, and cost. *Health Affairs (Millwood)*, 27(3), 759–769.

ers for Disease Control and Prevention. (2020). *What is population health?* https://www.cdc.gov/pophealthtraining/whatis.html

Centers for Medicare and Medicaid Services. (2020). *About the Innovation Center: Our Mission.* https://innovation.cms.gov/about/our-mission#:~:text=The%20CMS%20Innovation%20Center%20fosters,through%20improvement%20for%20all%20Americans.

Communicable Disease Center. (2018). *About CDC: Our history our story.* https://www.cdc.gov/about/history/index.html#:~:text=On%20July%201%2C%201946%20the,from%20spreading%20across%20the%20nation.

DeSalvo K., O'Carroll, P., Koo, D., Auerbach, J., & Monroe, J. (2016). Public health 3.0: Time for an upgrade. *American Journal of Public Health, 106*(4), 621–622.

DeVol, R., & Bedroussian, A. (2007). *An unhealthy America: The economic burden of chronic disease—Charting a new course to save lives and increase productivity and economic growth.* Milken Institute.

Fawcett, J., & Ellenbecker, C. H. (2015). A proposed conceptual model of nursing and population. *Nursing Outlook, 63*(3), 288–298. https://doi.org/10.1016/j.outlook.2015.01.009

Frieden, T. R., & Garfield, R. M. (2012). The cover. *Journal American Medical Association, 307*(19), 2005–2006.

Institute of Healthcare Improvement. (n.d.). *The IHI triple aim.* http://www.ihi.org/Engage/Initiatives/TripleAim/Pages/default.aspx

Institute of Medicine. (1999). *To err is human: Building a safer health system.* National Academies Press. http://www.iom.edu/~/media/Files/Report%20Files/1999/To-Err-is-Human/To%20Err%20is%20Human%201999%20%20report%20brief.ashx

Institute of Medicine. (2002). *The future of the public's health in the 21st century.* National Academies Press. http://www.iom.edu/~/media/Files/Report%20Files/2002/The-Future-of-the-Publics-Health-in-the-21st-Century/Future%20of%20Publics%20Health%202002%20Report%20Brief.pdf

Institute of Medicine. (2010). *Integrating primary care and public health.* National Academies Press.

Institute of Medicine. (2012). *Improving health in the community: A role for performance monitoring.* National Academies Press.

Interprofessional Education Collaborative Expert Panel. (2011). *Core competencies for interprofessional collaborative practice: Report of an expert panel.* Interprofessional Education Collaborative.

Interprofessional Education Collaborative Expert Panel. (2016). *Core competencies for interprofessional collaborative practice: Report of an expert panel: 2016 update.* https://hsc.unm.edu/ipe/resources/ipec-2016-core-competencies.pdf

Jacobson, D. M., & Teutsch, S. (2012). *An environmental scan of integrated approaches for defining and measuring total population health by the clinical care system, the government public health system, and stakeholder organizations.* National Quality Forum.

James, T. (2020). *What is upstream healthcare?.* HealthCity. https://www.bmc.org/healthcity/population-health/upstream-healthcare-sdoh-root-causes#:~:text=Upstream%20healthcare%20is%20any%20health,people%20floating%20down%2C%20nearly%20drowning.

Jia, H., Moriarty, D. G., & Kanarek, N. (2009). County-level social environment determinants of health-related quality of life among US adults: A multilevel analysis. *Journal of Community Health, 34,* 430–439.

Kindig, D., & Stoddart, G. (2003). What is population health? *American journal of public health, 93*(3), 380–383. https://doi.org/10.2105/ajph.93.3.380

Kjellstrom, T., Friel, S., Dixon, J., Corvalan, C., Rehfuess, E., Campbell-Lendrum, D., Gore, F., & Bartram, J. (2007). Urban environmental health hazards and health equity. *Journal of Urban Health: Bulletin of the New York Academy of Medicine, 84*(1).

Majette, G. R. (2011). PPACA and public health: Creating a framework to focus on prevention and wellness and improve the public's health. *Journal of Law, Medicine & Ethics, 39*(3), 366–379. https://doi.org/10.1111/j.1748-720X.2011.00606.x

National Academies of Sciences, Engineering, Medicine. (2020). *Leading health indicators 2030: Advancing health, equity, and well-being.* National Academies Press. https://doi.org/10.17226/25682

National Center for Interprofessional Practice and Education. (2011). *About interprofessional practice and education.* https://nexusipe.org/informing/about-ipe

National Institute of Health Office of Disease Prevention. (2020). Mind the Gap: The national prevention strategy: prioritizing prevention to improve the nation's health. https://prevention.nih.gov/education-training/methods-mind-gap/national-prevention-strategy-prioritizing-prevention-improve-nations-health

National Prevention Council. (2011). *National prevention strategy*. US Department of Health and Human Services, Office of the Surgeon General.

Organization for Economic Cooperation and Development. (2019). *Health at a glance: OECD Indicators*. http://www.oecd.org/health/health-systems/health-at-a-glance-19991312.htm

Stiefel, M., & Nolan, K. (2012). *A guide to measuring the triple aim: Population health, experience of care, and per capita cost* [White paper]. IHI Innovation Series. Institute for Healthcare Improvement.

Stoto, M. A. (2013). Population health in the Affordable Care Act era. *Academy Health*. https://www.academyhealth.org/files/AH2013pophealth.pdf

US Department of Health and Human Services. (2012a). *Healthy people 2020: Leading health indicators, 2012*. http://www.healthypeople.gov/2020/LHI/default.aspx

US Department of Health and Human Services. (2012b). *Historical highlights*. http://www.hhs.gov/about/hhshist.html

US Department of Health and Human Services. (2020a). 2020 Leading health indicators. *Healthy People 2020*. https://www.healthypeople.gov/2020/leading-health-indicators/2020-LHI-Topics

US Department of Health and Human Services. (2020b). About *Healthy People 2030*. https://health.gov/our-work/healthy-people-2030/about-healthy-people-2030

US Department of Health and Human Services. (2020c). Health Literacy in Healthy People. https://health.gov/our-work/healthy-people-2030/about-healthy-people-2030/health-literacy-healthy-people

World Health Organization. (2012). *Origin and development of health cooperation*. http://www.who.int/global_health_histories/background/en/index.html

EXEMPLAR

Evidence-Based Project: Early Referral to Palliative Care Using a Trigger Tool

Bridget Graham

Nationally, chronic illnesses and symptom management associated with advanced age make early palliative care consultation an important service for patients. Our senior adult unit believed that we were underutilizing the services of our palliative care team. Palliative care is used to prevent and relieve suffering, as well as to support the best quality of life for patients and their families, regardless of the stage of the disease or the need for the therapies. Multiple studies have demonstrated the benefits of palliative care, including its ability to decrease patients' symptom burden as well as increase the likelihood that patient's end-of-life care will align with their preferences.

The trigger tool was created with the goal of increasing the overall number of palliative care consults and to also obtain the consults earlier in the patients' admission. Our trigger tool was created by an interdisciplinary team. This team was led by a CNL, palliative care physician, palliative care RN coordinator, palliative care RN, and the medical director of the senior adult unit. The tool we created included triggers that were pulled from discrete fields in our EHR. The categories on the trigger report included: patient name, age, LOS, admit date, insurance, reason for visit, Morse Fall score, Braden Skin score, advance directive status, albumin level, orientation memory concentration test, IV morphine given, ejection fraction, speech consult, nephrology consult, pulmonary consult, and code status. The trigger report was run daily on all 32 patients on our unit and then e-mailed automatically to the CNL and palliative care RN. The patients that had four or more triggers were recommended to have a palliative care consult. The physician was asked for an order, and if they agreed, an order was placed for a palliative care consult. Our tool went live on March 1, 2014.

Pre- and post-data were compared for the trigger tool. The comparison extended over a six-month time frame from March 1, 2013, to August 31, 2013 (before the tool went live), and a six-month time frame from March 1, 2014, to August 31, 2014 (after the tool went live). The total number of patients evaluated is 461. Outcomes were as follows:

1. Number of consults: 35% increase in the number of palliative care consults.
2. Consults to palliative care were ordered 14% sooner in the admission than prior to the use of the tool. Average day of admission consult was ordered before tool was 2.38, after was 2.04.
3. Patients seen by palliative care had 50% fewer re-admissions six months after the consult was completed compared with six months prior to the consult being done.
4. LOS: 4% increase in LOS (not an expected finding but had a number of patients with high LOS during this time).
5. Disposition code summary: Top four discharge locations included SNF, home with hospice, home, and home with HC. Prior to initiation of the tool, these locations represented 63% of the total discharges. After initiation of the tool, these locations represented 66% of the total discharges. This was a relatively stable increase.
6. Reason for consult summary: Top three reasons for palliative care consult remained the same prior to and after the initiation of the tool.
   a. End of life
   b. Goals of care
   c. Pain

We believe this trigger tool has proven to be a useful means in getting early referral to palliative care services for our patients. We plan to replicate this process on another unit.

EXEMPLAR

Quality, Core Indicators, and Vaccine Rates

Rebecca Valko

Vaccination rates for influenza and pneumococcus were a challenge on my acuity-adaptable/cardiac/medical/renal floor. I educated the staff several times regarding the importance and value of vaccinations for hospital patients. Even though we had improved since the implementation of the CNL's role on the unit, the vaccination rates were still not meeting standards. With the mentoring of staff to assist in audits and a process change whereby vaccines were given at admission, not at discharge, our unit vaccination rates are now between 95% and 98%. The CNL must look at process steps that make it easier for the staff to do the right thing.

Patient Satisfaction with Pain Management

Maureen Tait

In an effort to increase patient satisfaction in the pain management arena, a few CNLs decided to host a competition. We had been working within our units on a daily basis, educating staff about establishing a pain goal with their patients and developing a plan to meet it. The metrics that were used were the Press Ganey survey results, along with monthly unit audits. These measurements showed that further work was needed.

Working within a microsystem at times can give you tunnel vision. We individually knew that organizational goals were set at a high level, and we strived to achieve them. But we were still falling short. What could we do to improve them? What were other units doing?

The CNLs who joined together on this project all work on surgical floors where pain management is a strong component of quality patient care. We decided that for a period of one week each of us would audit our units for pain goal documentation. Setting a pain goal with patients establishes a sense of trust and safety. It shows a concentrated effort to include patients in their plan of care. The results were posted on each unit's huddle board. The anticipation and interest in these numbers were beyond our expectations. On the one hand, staff would clap and cheer when their numbers were greater than the others. On the other hand, staff would challenge each other to improve if they were not number one. At the end of the week a blue ribbon was presented to the winning unit. It is proudly displayed on its huddle board. Since then, when we have been challenged in a quality improvement project, the suggestion for a competition comes up frequently!

Population of Complex Care

Lauran Hardin

Friday afternoon at 3 p.m. the classic complex call came in over the pager: "There's a patient here with multiple admissions who has no insurance, needs a new heart valve, is schizophrenic, homeless, and is discharging in two hours—can you take care of this?" It would take a village to resolve this situation in two hours.

After reading the patient's chart and assessing the root cause of her readmissions, it was clear that there were cross-continuum issues that needed to be addressed. The patient needed a safe place to live and a PCP to lead her team. She needed insurance to get access to the complex medical care she required. She needed help to stop smoking crack. She needed to learn how to take critical medicines to prevent her from being overcome by heart failure. She needed transportation, and so much more.

Engaging the CNL core competencies of healthcare systems coordinator of care and facilitator of interprofessional teams, the CNL called the hospitalist, the master's prepared social worker (MSW), the case manager, the new PCP, and the PCP's lead nurse. A collaborative complex care conference was organized in the patient's room within the hour. After hearing a summary by the CNL of key issues that needed to be solved, each discipline stepped up to the plate to offer its best. The hospitalist was linked with the new PCP to give direct patient reports, decreasing fragmentation in care. A Medicaid application was completed, housing obtained, and bus tickets provided by the MSW. The case manager obtained the medications gratis. The staff nurse set up the medication box and provided teaching. The CNL coordinated the team and set up a joint care conference with the patient, the PCP, and the lead nurse on the following Monday to transfer the plan of care and link the patient with her new physician. A focus on solutions, combined with the facilitation to make it happen, allowed the patient to leave in two hours, with everything she needed to start over again.

EXEMPLAR

CNL in Public Health Practice

Sallie Shipman

Background Information

A microsystem organizational assessment was conducted within the Alabama Department of Public Health's pandemic influenza planning efforts or more specifically the 72-element template for pandemic influenza (PI; Shipman et al., 2013). The CNL's role was used to provide evaluation while promoting progress and improvement of planning efforts within the PI planning microsystem. AACN determined that the role would vary across the various levels of healthcare. However, application of the CNL's role within public health has been limited. Gaps and recommendations for improvement of PI planning efforts were identified by the CNL in an organizational assessment, which led to the development of a strategic plan. The strategic plan was the basis of the master's level CNL clinical immersion project.

Outcome Data and Description of Methods

The strategic plan's goal was to provide a standardized mutually acceptable approach for the areas and the state regarding PI planning. This goal was accomplished through the CNL by improvement of the 72-element template used for county PI planning while progressing toward the inclusion of all hazards. Two main objectives were incorporated to complete the stated goal. The first objective was to improve communications, provide education, and elicit input for improvement and progress. Second, input from all 11 public health areas was needed to incorporate best practices. These input derived ideas for improvement and documented lessons learned were shared with the entire PI planning team by the CNL.

A primary quantitative planning score was calculated by a Center for Emergency Preparedness (CEP) analyst. This score was compared to a score calculated after the implementation of the strategic plan providing measurable data for evaluation of the improvements. The qualitative assessments conducted by the CNL revealed that significant changes to the 72-element template would need to be made for progression to continue. Also, during this time, updated guidance from the CDC was received combining general medical emergency preparedness planning with PI. This CDC recommendation combined planning efforts from a single focus on PI to an all-hazards/pandemic perspective. In light of these significant occurrences, upper management agreed to the rewriting of the 72-element template to include several important measures: all-hazards planning, best practices incorporation, explanations of requirements, and input from area core team staff. Improvement measures were a direct result from the data that was collected from the root-cause analysis.

The process of compiling best practices from each area was continuous throughout this project. Each area had different strengths and weakness. The CNL facilitated sharing of strengths from the areas that helped to reach the overall goal of creation of a standardized mutually acceptable approach for the state regarding PI planning while progressing toward all hazards. Collaboration on all levels of planning is essential to ensure success in process improvement projects. The process of emergency planning is never ending, and there is always room for improvement. This process improvement project demonstrated the use of the CNL as an outcome's measurement specialist and a leader in problem solving for public health emergency medical planning.

References

American Association of Colleges of Nursing. (2013). *Competencies and curricular expectations for Clinical Nurse Leader education and practice.* http://www.aacn.nche.edu/cnl/CNL-Competencies-October-2013.pdf

Shipman, S., Stanton, M., Hankins, J., & Odom-Bartel, R. (2013). Incorporation of the clinical nurse leader in public health practice. *Journal of Professional Nursing, 29*(1), 4–10. https://doi.org/10.1016/j.profnurs.2012.04.004

EXEMPLAR

Leading the Change in Insulin Delivery: Leading Groups/Moving Forward with Ideas Not in the Mainstream

Mary Harnish

Education of a CNL includes courses in quality improvement of microsystems and microsystem leadership. Our clinical facility/healthcare system challenged us as students to lead change projects identified by the clinical service directors and the chief nursing officer. These projects needed clinical leadership to be implemented. With years of experience in diabetes, I was selected to oversee implementing mainstream basal-bolus insulin as a hospital protocol.

I brought together a multidisciplinary team with key stakeholders, including nursing staff, physicians, pharmacists, nutrition services, informatics, and administration. Clinical practice guidelines and literature reviews illuminated EBP in this area, from which the team worked. The team met weekly, employing the Lean process to move this project forward.

Collaboration with nutrition services resulted in listing carbohydrate content of all foods on patient menus and on each meal ticket on the patients' food trays. The implementation of a standardized order set was accomplished by working with the pharmacy and information systems. The protocol was presented to the pharmacy and therapeutics, which, after reviewing the EBP literature, approved the protocol.

The biggest challenge was changing physician practice, especially the hospitalists group, who were responsible for the majority of insulin orders in the hospital. I presented the protocol and order sets to the hospitalists and residents and provided guidebooks on how to use the order sets.

Nursing staff education included a CD learning module and an instructional manual. I provided point-of-care education with multiple scenarios, color-coded dosing cards, and wall charts for reference material.

Months of work went into the challenge of changing clinical practice. Now, four years later, basal-bolus insulin is not the new way of ordering and administering subcutaneous insulin—it is the only way! Rates of severe hyperglycemia improved from a rate of 1.22% to 0.48%. Severe hypoglycemia with blood glucose < 50 mg/dL decreased from 1.5% to 0.48%.

EXEMPLAR

Health Literacy-Language Barrier

Christina Lupo

A Spanish-speaking patient was admitted to the neurological ICU for DKA/seizures and was intubated in the ED. He was extubated a few days later and the CNL met with him and the Spanish translator to discuss his diabetic health management. From reading all the physician's notes, it appeared that he was a very noncompliant diabetic who was not taking his medication because of cost. The diabetic educator came to see him and offered him a discount drug card and a referral to the social worker.

The CNL noticed that there were not any diabetic medications listed on his home medications. The CNL called the patient's pharmacy and confirmed that he does take metformin and glipizide, and that he is compliant with them. The pharmacist explained that the patient had recently tried to pick up his metformin, but it was "too soon" for him to get it refilled, so it was placed on hold.

The pieces were not adding up, so the CNL met with the patient and translator again. The patient was insistent that his insurance was "no good" and "would not cover" his medication. After a few more questions, the puzzle pieces came together.

His PCP recently doubled his dose of metformin, so the patient started doubling up on his current supply of medication. When he ran out, he tried to get it refilled, but the pharmacy told him his insurance wouldn't approve it (because it was too soon, but he didn't understand that). All he understood was that insurance would not pay for it. The CNL called his pharmacist back and explained that his PCP changed the dose. The pharmacist sheepishly said that it was a misunderstanding and if they had known there was a dosage change, they could have called the insurance company and explained that, and his medication would have been approved.

Unfortunately, from the patient's perspective, he thought his insurance was bad and that he no longer had access to his medication. He stopped taking it (once he ran out), and ended up in the ICU. The pharmacist called the CNL back a few minutes later and confirmed that his medication would be ready for him to pick up once he discharged from the hospital.

In summary, the patient was challenged by a language barrier and a lack of understanding of how his insurance plan worked. He was labeled as a noncompliant patient, and his real problem was overlooked. A communication problem as simple as not clarifying the dosage change with his pharmacist resulted in him not having access to medication, and spending three days in an ICU, critically ill.

CNLs are in pivotal positions to be advocates for patients and families to assure that quality and safe care is delivered. Communication is another key skill of CNLs and interfacing daily with interprofessional teams.

EXEMPLAR

Transformation and Quality Improvement in the Delivery Model

Elizabeth Triezenberg and Lauran Hardin

HCAHPS pain satisfaction scores for orthopedics were in the 50th percentile and identified as a first priority for intervention.

The orthopedic CNL and the pain management CNL collaborated to uncover the root cause of pain dissatisfaction. Rounding with surgeons, staff, and patients revealed gaps in education and communication. Pain was managed using a reactive approach with little communication among surgeon, nurse, and patient.

Using the systems analyst role of the CNL, pain satisfaction was looked at across the continuum of care—from the orthopedic surgeon's office to care at home after surgery. Initial intervention focused on education. The preoperative total joint class was redesigned to better prepare patients to partner in managing their pain. A multidisciplinary collaborative process was engaged with the surgeon's office, pre-admission testing, surgery, and inpatient staff to redesign patient education, screening, and pain management on discharge.

An evidence-based process was created to assess and treat pain during hospitalization. The orthopedic CNL rounded on patients daily and mentored staff in how to create a plan for pain management. Mentoring and modeling best practice care in the moment resulted in nurses rapidly developing the skills to differentiate types of pain and the appropriate medication, partner with patients for a pain plan, and communicate the plan across disciplines.

Patients who have had a total joint replacement are now able to verbalize their need for pain medications as well as the plan they are using to manage pain during hospitalization and at discharge. Staff nurses are discussing the patients' pain plans not only with the patients but with the other nurses and the surgeon. Most importantly, patients are stating their pain is better controlled and that staff are doing what they can to control their pain. HCAHPS scores improved from the 50th percentile to the 90th percentile.

Health Promotion in an Acute Care Setting: A Quality and Process Improvement Initiative

Laurie Sayer and Kristin Mast

Influenza and pneumonia are major causes of hospitalization and death in the United States. As a clinician, the CNL promotes better health for populations by creating awareness, knowledge, and system changes to increase the adult inpatient immunization rate. This ensures improved compliance with the CMS quality-of-care measures and accountable care and will have a financial impact related to pay-for-performance standards. A higher immunization rate also aligns with the *Healthy People 2020* goal of increasing immunization levels and reducing preventable infectious diseases.

Our organization was not consistently meeting established benchmarks for pneumonia's quality core measures. In addition, a baseline audit undertaken October to December 2010 indicated that only 51% of patients actually received their ordered Pneumovax 23 (pneumococcal polysaccharides [PPSV]) vaccine and 41.7% their ordered influenza vaccine prior to discharge.

A CNL-led interdisciplinary task force was formed to look at current practice, analyze data, identify barriers, and develop a process improvement plan using Lean principles. At a system-wide and microsystem level, CNLs support immunization processes through both formal and informal education, mentoring, system changes, data awareness, and accountability.

A root-cause analysis was performed with essential input from staff nurses to identify issues affecting immunization compliance. The team recognized several problems related to the immunization process and sought input from staff nurses to identify barriers to vaccine administration. Based on feedback from staff on all inpatient units, the team identified three main focus areas: education, accountability, and continual awareness of vaccine compliance.

CNLs were champions of the quality initiative. As outcome managers, unit CNLs received daily and monthly reports to monitor compliance and trends, and to evaluate gaps for unit-specific improvement options. Inpatient CNLs were instrumental in obtaining accurate patient immunization history. This created an increased awareness and actions to take. Data were monitored to ensure quality and safety and following the first quarter of using the CII protocol, glycemic control was achieved.

CHAPTER 17

Achieving Excellence in CNL Practice

James L. Harris, Linda A. Roussel, and Patricia L. Thomas

LEARNING OBJECTIVES

1. Describe innovation as critical to the CNL's role.
2. Discuss the need for clinical nurse leadership.
3. Identify the core skills necessary to lead change in a microsystem.
4. Discuss contemporary leadership theories and the relation to leading and achieving excellence.
5. Describe the impact of skillful partnerships and leadership through the lens of team science, giving examples of CNLs in action.

KEY TERMS

Chaos

Clinical leadership

Complexity

Evidence-based practice

Innovation

Outcomes

CNL ROLES

Communicator

Lifelong learner

Outcomes manager advocate

CNL PROFESSIONAL VALUES

Accountability

Integrity

CNL CORE COMPETENCIES

Collaboration

Communication

Education

Facilitating

Innovation

Leadership

Lifelong learning

Introduction

Achieving excellence in CNL practice requires blending a strong foundation of evidence-based practices as well as innovative thinking. According to
BusinessDictionary.com, *innovation* implies an idea be usable at an economical cost
and address a specific need. Innovation requires deliberate application of information, imagination, and initiative in getting greater or different values from resources,
including new idea generation developed into meaningful products. Innovation often results when one applies new ways to further satisfy the needs and expectations
of the patients and stakeholders. Being creative and innovative are challenging as
one's brain is wired to maintain life and "business as usual." Quick fixes, to remain
comfortable and safe, resort to a level of thinking that addresses issues related to
the problem's creation. Purposely moving from the known to the unknown requires
new skill sets such as asking probing questions, seeking counsel from others who
think and act differently, and accepting new ideas and methods through creativity.
Ways to enhance creative thinking and innovation include mindful meditation and
yoga, which unlock spatial areas of the brain, thereby generating new ideas and
more creative thought processes. These practices assist in quieting the judgmental
and analytical brain, which often limits free-flowing and imaginative ideas. While
daydreaming, doodling, playing, making free word association, and using art may
seem lighthearted, through exploration of the creative brain, breakthrough innovations are realized and actualized. Creating space involves complexity and chaos
thinking as innovative ideas are aligned, merged, and reinvented that provide superior quality and new forms of evidence that will inform thought and connection
building (Weberg & Davidson, 2019).

Science of Innovation

Gutsche (2015), in *Exploiting Chaos*, provides ideas and examples to spark creative
thinking, and innovation focusing on meeting unmet needs and opportunities. Gutsche purports that innovation is only successful if it addresses an unmet need. Understanding the need, making sense of the chaos and information overload, moving
away from success, and rethinking strategies are a few ideas that are presented by
Gutsche. Gutsche proposes an exploiting chaos framework, which includes *culture
of revolution, trend hunting, adaptive innovation*, and *infectious messaging*. Using this
model, Gutsche describes the culture of revolution noting that it is more important than strategy. Culture underlies an organization's ability to adapt, and in times
of dramatic change magnifies this importance. Despite knowing that adapting to
change is crucial, uncertainty and resistance often immobilize innovation. Creating
an organizational culture of revolution can generate a new paradigm for creative
change.

A culture of revolution includes identifying four areas for the implementation of change and includes: perspective, experimental failure, customer obsession, and intentional destruction. Gutsche (2015) provides countless ideas and
examples to test. Perspective is defined as the way one views practice, a project,
or gap. One's perspective is a destiny. It asks the question, What are you really
trying to accomplish? Ways to think about perspective include avoiding same-
ness, looking beyond the failures of others, exploring uncertainty, avoiding the

desire to return to a comfort zone, questioning rational thought, understanding the pattern of destruction, and exploiting crisis to accelerate change. Gutsche outlines the top enemies of innovation as lengthy development, lack of coordination, a risk-aversive culture, and limited customer insight. CNLs are prepared and positioned to deal with making sense of the perspective for interprofessional teams and patients.

Experimental failure means being open and willing to test even if failure may be the result of your efforts. Knowing one's strengths is important, however, it may create a sense of complacency within the organization. Gutsche offers some excellent ways to think about experimental failure such as breaking down confidences, creating a gambling fund so that new ideas can be tested without knowing the success of the project, celebrating the efforts to "get to the next big idea," and not only the win. Notably, this would be the place many quality improvement initiatives stall. CNLs often assist teams in moving through this stage when faced with PDSA cycles that do not achieve a desired result or a quality improvement project that does not accomplish an intended outcome.

Customer obsession requires knowing patients, stakeholders, and interprofessional team qualities. Customer obsession means having a deep understanding of individual engagement, and it is only with this wisdom one truly has breakthrough ideas and disruptive innovation. Customer obsession includes creating an emotional and cultural connection with patients, but also with stakeholders. Inspiring stakeholders to champion a product or idea is possible by having an understanding of the mission, values, and goals. Ways to facilitate customer obsession is to be an attentive observer where care is happening, hearing, and seeking authenticity. Being mindful of preconceived notions of what patients want before seeking to understand will be essential to innovation within any system.

Intentional destruction relates to breaking down the structure and hierarchy to see what changes need to be made. Exploring processes and observing as an outsider can facilitate intentional destruction. It is resisting the urge to tell others what to do and to build creative work environments. Hiring people who think and embrace difference and are willing to let reason triumph over hierarchy may be a great facilitator of such. Creative work environments can be facilitated by intentionally eliminating barriers to seek opportunities for engagement and the assimilation of ideas. It is important to actively seek inspiration, which requires time and attention. Moving away from rigid schedules and rituals that often add little or no value except to put checkmarks that signal the task was completed. This may seem to be a sign of success as the activity was completed, but it may often be singular it its focus and not connected to a larger vision. There are many traditions in nursing practice that are not evidence-based, yet continue. This is a space CNLs can help team members unlearn or release traditions and practices to attain desired outcomes. Reviewing the best ways to inspire and connect with others will often lead to improving work togetherness and achieve stronger outcomes.

Trend hunting involves knowing that innovation and strategic advantage depend on the ability to anticipate trends and seek out the next big idea. What are clusters of opportunity that exist that were "invisible" because one failed to look at the possible patterns being created?

Adaptive innovation is described as using other strategies from various industries. Examples would include engineering and information technology to apply possible solutions to a system's gaps.

Infectious messages refer to what one is communicating about an organization, system, and projects, which have the potential to go viral. Not all messages are memorable or will stick. Knowing what "makes it stick," such as timing, clear and simple wording, possibly rhyming, can enhance the ability to "supercharge" messages (Pink, 2010). Well-packaged messages can travel at rapid-fire speed given the many ways information pushes out. This can work well for an innovation, however, may get lost in the deluge of information. Being intentional in being infectious affords opportunities for ideas to resonate and spring forward to greater connectivity, thus creating more ways to think about work. As a leader, the CNL is responsible for taking charge, leading change, and building innovation from a foundation of evidence-based practice. Innovation is the force that propels evidence creation where CNLs evolve and infuse energy to catalyze change (Weberg & Davidson, 2019).

CNLs engage in clinical leadership, but also must adapt to change. This suggests potential innovations for change in the leadership role competently. Clinical leadership is about clinicians informing the quality and safety of care through innovation and improvement—both in their organizational processes and in individual care practices. CNLs have advanced knowledge in quality improvement, measurement, systems, leadership strategies, and care delivery, and are well positioned to evaluate quality and guide improvement. CNLs function in multiple areas of healthcare systems, as clinical leaders, and critically appraise care processes with respect to outcomes. Bleich (2012) notes in a discussion on leadership responses to the IOM's report, *The Future of Nursing: Leading Change, Advancing Health* (2010), that there are too few nurses at the table as models of accountable care, and this, he asserts, is serious. Nurse leaders must influence others to give voice and perform the unique roles of nursing.

The AACN (2007) posits that CNL education provides the skill set necessary to assume horizontal leadership positions within the healthcare team. With the revision of the CNL competencies there is greater emphasis on leadership and change management (AACN, 2013). Horizontal organizations are described as having decentralized power and/or control, at least within specific departments, and support greater flow of communication and collaboration. With the revision of the CNL competencies, there is greater emphasis on leadership and change management (AACN, 2013). In horizontal leadership a number of individuals can assume leadership of a team or teams in the attempt to achieve a common goal. Vertical leadership, in contrast, has one leader, often with centralized control. As a clinical leader in a horizontal organization, the CNL has the opportunity and responsibility of bringing individuals together, giving them a voice, and creating an environment that is safe for communication and feedback. As such, understanding and applying leadership theories are important aspects of the CNL's role to demonstrate strong, effective clinical leadership (Woo, 2013).

The Need for Clinical Leadership

There is need for a more programmatic, strategic approach to clinical leadership, because the ailing US healthcare system is in urgent need of reform. Although many believe that the responsibilities of the clinician and of an administrator are completely separate, the distinction between clinical leadership and administrative leadership is often blurred. This requires individuals from different disciplines to contribute their expertise in order to achieve outcomes that are central to the interplay of factors associated with health and healthcare (Bruzzese et al., 2020). This chapter suggests while there are unique elements within each of these roles, there is far greater commonality than what is typically described in the literature. Beyond the scope of formal or informal leadership, bridging this false dichotomy with CNLs offers a transition point to support the transformation and transitions of care delivery across the continuum (Agomoh et al., 2020).

Porter-O'Grady (1997, 1999) proposed a new way of thinking about leadership, describing how the changing healthcare system necessitates new leadership characteristics and roles. Porter-O'Grady noted that knowledge of technology has changed the traditional hierarchy of leadership. That is, nursing knowledge rose vertically as the nurse moved up the chain of command. Historically, as the knowledge base increased, so did the demands and responsibilities that nurses experienced in many positions. Leadership and the knowledge associated with demands have consistently shifted. The CNL has a complex role in the dissemination of information as an outcomes manager and through the use of technology in taking the lead as the lateral integrator.

The success of the US healthcare system in treating infectious disease, the changing social and economic environment, modern lifestyles, and an aging population have dramatically shifted the burden of care from acute conditions to chronic disease. Chronic conditions such as some cancers, diabetes, cardiovascular disease, and asthma now account for some 80% of the total burden of disease (National Health Priority Action Council, 2006). CNLs are prepared to assume leadership for coordinating care and collaborating with interdisciplinary teams necessary for management of chronic conditions. CNLs share these processes with patients, stakeholders, and providers.

Clinical Leadership Behaviors

Clinicians can lead in many ways, both formal and informal, as part of an organizational position and/or through collegial relationships. There are many ways to function as a clinical leader, including:

- *Developing personal qualities:* qualities such as self-awareness, self-reflection, self-management, professionalism, and self-development
- *Working with others:* developing networks, building and maintaining relationships, team building, developing others, engaging with clients and consumers, and collaborating with other service providers
- *Improving services:* ensuring patient safety, critically evaluating, encouraging innovation, evaluating services, improving healthcare processes, and developing new services and roles
- *Managing services:* planning; managing resources, people, and performance
- *Setting direction:* identifying opportunities for change, applying knowledge and evidence, making decisions, and evaluating outcomes.

CNLs are well positioned to lead safety and quality improvement initiatives, and, at a practical level. This translates into a range of activities, including the knowledge and skills to initiate and guide safety and quality activities at a professional and team level.

Additional tasks of CNLs include the following:

- Translating high-level organizational strategy into operational improvement activities
- Leading systems development, planning, implementation, evaluation of quality, and openly communicating safety and quality issues and adverse events while developing solutions
- Adhering to policies and procedures for preventing, reporting, and disclosing adverse events, ensuring that care and services are delivered according to the best available evidence, health service protocols, and policies
- Ensuring that safety and quality risks are proactively identified and managed through effective systems, delegation of accountabilities, and properly trained and credentialed staff
- Developing a partnership approach with patients and caregivers in individual episodes of care as well as the prevention, treatment, and discussion of adverse events, leading a team approach to patient care, quality improvement, and problem solving, and ensuring that this adds to participants' organizational and professional status
- Fostering a culture that does not blame, but rather seeks to solve problems and learn from them while supporting staff in the process
- Empowering and holding staff accountable at all levels involved in monitoring and improving care and services
- Recognizing the importance of effective team communication in patient care, and supporting staff training and development
- Improving systems to support and share best practices concerning individual patient care, modeling a professional and evidence-based approach in the delivery of care

Information Management, Technology, and Analysis: A Core Skill to Lead Change

Healthcare information technology initiatives are more successful when a collaborative redesign approach is taken, in which clinicians are intimately involved in all aspects of the change process. Clinical engagement is a well-documented determinant for the success of new initiatives and their sustainability (Boonstra & Broekhuis, 2010; Davidson et al., 2017; Diamond et al., 2010; Yackanicz et al., 2010). A lack of clinical engagement is a commonly cited reason for failure (Westbrook et al., 2007). Garling (2008) notes that non-clinicians have limited opportunities to effect change in clinical practice. CNLs bridge the gap that often exists in organizations between those who understand clinical processes and those who understand information systems. The CNL has the knowledge and language to narrow the space between what have historically been isolated decision-making bodies.

Engagement, Teams, Satisfaction, and Outcomes Necessary to Lead

The key to achieving successful clinical outcomes is to develop a clinical engagement model where representative CNLs can have an equivalent position at the executive level to engage in strategic planning for initiatives that have an impact on care delivery. Subsequently, CNLs can promote clinical engagement by driving awareness of change initiatives within clinical communities. This clinical executive role can work to heal the divide between clinicians and management, facilitating successful change. New and innovative pathways eliminate lost opportunities, and a culture that mobilizes and synchronizes systematic change emerges.

By including members of the interdisciplinary team in the creation of a change, the CNL emphasizes the shared goals, shared commitments, and shared successes in leveraging the strengths of the team members. As a facilitator of the team, the CNL manages the group dynamics, ensures participation of all team members, and fosters trust and respect. Major challenges in leading teams are to ensure that meetings start and end on time and that multiple means of gathering data (including observation of different processes) are built into the team interactions.

Several studies on the CNL have demonstrated increased patient satisfaction (Bender et al., 2012; Hix et al., 2009), as well as staff satisfaction in qualitative examination (Hartranft et al., 2007). Studies on teams, staff satisfaction, and engagement demonstrate that healthy work environments are developed when strategies to enhance communication and promote interdependence of team members are established (Amos et al., 2005). The investment of CNL time in leading interdisciplinary teams creates improved satisfaction and supports healthier environments.

Contemporary Leadership Theories

Understanding contemporary leadership theories is foundational to the CNL assuming an effective leadership role. The following section offers a brief overview of principles of a variety of useful leadership theories. While no individual can embody every element of the tenets in a leadership theory, it is suggested that all nurses should have a sound leadership theoretical base. Depending on the situation, nurses change behaviors to address needs, underscoring flexibility that is principle based, exemplified in theory, and deliberate with evidence-based practice.

Servant Leadership

Greenleaf (1977) describes servant leaders as there to serve those they lead, implying that the employees are an end in themselves, rather than a means to an end (bottom line). Servant leadership can be an alternative to a command and control style, with a greater focus on how others can be served and their needs.

Greenleaf (1977) offers 10 principles of servant leadership: listening, empathy, healing, awareness, persuasion, conceptualization, foresight, stewardship, commitment to the growth of people, and building community.

Listening

Servant leaders make a deep commitment to listening intently to others, seeking to identify and clarify the needs of the group. Servant leaders are receptive to what is being said (and nonverbal cues of what is not being said), are self-aware, and seek to have a greater understanding of the connection of body, mind, and spirit communicated through self.

Empathy

The servant leader accepts and recognizes the uniqueness of those being led. Servant leaders assume the good intentions of coworkers and the acceptance of others.

Healing

Healing denotes a powerful force that transforms and integrates teams. This is considered one of the greatest strengths of the servant leader. According to Greenleaf (1977), "There is something subtle communicated to one who is being served and led, if implicit in the compact between the servant-leader and led is the understanding that the search for wholeness is something that they have" (p. 345).

Awareness

Self-awareness is the foundation of the servant leader's awareness of their own strengths and abilities to provide healing and a supportive environment. Developing inner security is paramount to the success of a servant leader.

Persuasion

Persuasion is described as influence. The servant leader focuses on persuading the process rather than using positional authority in making decisions. Rather than being coercive, the servant leader seeks consensus. This is a distinguishing feature from a more traditional authoritarian model.

Conceptualization

Helping those being led to focus on the big picture is particularly important to the servant leader. The skill of looking at an issue (problem) from a conceptualizing view requires a focus beyond the day-to-day operations. This requires a balance between vision and real-world thinking.

Foresight

Using this principle, the servant leader assists others to understand lessons learned from past experiences, put into perspective the realities of the present, and consider implications of future decisions. This principle is grounded in self-knowledge, being intuitive, and trusting one's voice.

Stewardship

Transcending the self to consider the greater good of the organization defines stewardship. Being a good steward of the resources of time, humanity, and spirit requires dedication to each of the principles described.

Commitment to the Growth of People

Growing others means believing that the people who the servant leader assists have an intrinsic value beyond their "job worth" as workers. Servant leaders are deeply committed to the personal and professional growth of individuals in the organization.

Building Community

Servant leaders have a keen awareness that becoming a large institution may create feelings of loss for community and connectedness for those they serve. Servant leaders, in building community, seek ways to bring people together for the good of individuals and the organization (Greenleaf, 1977). CNLs, as strong and effective clinical leaders, have the ability to use servant leader principles to enhance the effectiveness of patient outcomes through collaborative teams.

Transactional and Transformational Leadership

Transactional leadership is based on transactions or exchanges between the leader and the led where rewards and benefits are offered to subordinates if they fulfill agreements and contribute to the achievement of goals (Avolio & Bass, 2002; Bass, 1990; Nielson et al., 2009). While transactional leaders tend to be caretakers, they often have little vision or few overtly shared values with followers (Avolio & Bass, 2002; Barker et al., 2006). Transactional leaders focus on the completion of tasks or assignments and consider how to modify processes to incrementally improve and maintain the quality of performance, how to substitute one goal for another, and how to reduce resistance to a particular action and implement decisions (Avolio & Bass, 2002). The transactional leader strives to carry out decisions with little disruption or conversation (Klainberg & Dirschel, 2010). This can be effective for groups under stress, providing satisfaction through immediate solutions; however, long-term effectiveness is not often an outcome of transactional processes (Tomey, 2010). Transactional leadership is often displayed in healthcare organizations where immediate or unpredictable patient care needs necessitate immediate responses or actions. It is also congruent with traditional definitions of management that include goal setting, establishing priorities, developing an action plan, and delegating (Barker et al., 2006; Tomey, 2010). Northouse (2015) suggests that the transformational leader assists followers to transcend and become members of extraordinary teams.

As an extension of transactional leadership, transformational leadership includes a change or transformation of both the leader and the follower (Avolio &

Bass, 2002; Barker et al., 2006; Tomey, 2010). Bass (1990) describes transformational leadership as a superior form of leadership that occurs when leaders act as agents of change influencing others through the change process. Transformational leaders expand the sphere of influence of their employees by increasing awareness and engagement of the aims and mission of the community of practice. Transformational leaders are instrumental in coaching employees to transcend their own self-interest thereby providing a means to think beyond what is their current reality.

Transformational leaders motivate followers to perform beyond normal expectations through a transformation of thoughts and attitudes and by enlisting vital support of the vision while striving for its fulfillment. Avolio and Bass (2002) and Tomey (2010) summarized the behaviors associated with transformational leadership, including attributed charisma (modeling behaviors), inspirational motivation (creating a vision for the future), intellectual stimulation (questioning assumptions and reframing problems from a new perspective), and individualized consideration (delegating work that attends to individual needs, abilities, and aspirations). Transformational leadership is a visionary leadership style that has a long-term focus. As a result, change focuses on the systems and culture of an organization. Transformational leaders act as agents of change for both the leader and the follower. They arouse strong positive emotion and influence the beliefs, behaviors, attitudes, and perceptions of others. Changes that occur using this leadership style have longer-lasting effects because they change patterns of thinking, beliefs, and values through the interaction between the leaders and followers (Avolio & Bass, 2002; Bass, 1990; Tomey, 2010).

Transformational leadership has been defined as a superior form of leadership that occurs when leaders bring awareness to the shared or common desires of leaders and followers. This awareness, commitment, and acceptance of the purposes and mission of the group or organization are the motivating factors followers embrace as they look beyond self-interest and embrace change for the good of the group (Klainberg & Dirschel, 2010; Tomey, 2010). These goals are accomplished by using transformational leadership behaviors, including the aforementioned: attributed charisma or modeling behaviors that gain admiration and trust, inspirational motivation or the ability to envision and articulate a future, intellectual stimulation involving questioning assumptions and reframing problems from a new perspective, and individualized consideration by delegation and empowering groups while attending to individual needs, abilities, and aspirations (Klainberg & Dirschel, 2010; Marquis & Huston, 2006; Tomey, 2010). This contributes to increased satisfaction and meaningfulness in one's work (Marquis & Huston, 2006; Tomey, 2010).

The theory of transformational leadership suggests that people need a sense of mission that extends beyond transactions and interpersonal relationships (Avolio & Bass, 2002; Barker et al., 2006; Marquis & Huston, 2006; Tomey, 2010). This is especially true in the CNL's role, where the commitment is made to remain at the point of care and service to lead efforts in improving quality and safety. Nurses often choose the profession as a means to display and convey a commitment to the greater good for humankind. Transformational leadership behaviors create unity, wholeness, and collective purpose though the use of a common vision and inspiration focused on a larger purpose that is fundamental to the CNL's role (Barker et al., 2006; Tomey, 2010).

Microsystem Partnerships and Clinical Leadership Through Team Science

Implied in clinical leadership is the integration and collaborative partnership between the CNL and all members of a team within a microsystem. The IOM (2003), in *Health Professions Education: A Bridge to Quality,* identified interprofessional collaboration and communication as needs of 21st-century healthcare delivery systems. The literature describes individual choices and individual professional development as cornerstones of this change imperative.

Depending on the care delivery system, organizational structures, and organizational cultures, CNLs can have a significant impact on teams, particularly interdisciplinary teams whose aim is to improve clinical outcomes between departments or locations of care. Given the CNL's attention to evidence-based practice and commitment to safety and quality improvement, CNLs leading interdisciplinary teams within a microsystem can facilitate improved outcomes through team-determined metrics.

In *The Science of Improvement*, the IHI (2011) highlights characteristics of effective teams representing different kinds of expertise and leadership within the organization, within a system, holding technical expertise, and in day-to-day leadership. Critical to the success of a team are a clinical leader with the authority to test and implement change, a technical expert who knows the subject of change intimately and understands the processes of care and quality improvement tools and strategies, and a day-to-day leader to drive and oversee the change project and facilitate changes in the system. CNLs consistently engage in each of these activities.

CNLs in Action

As clinical leaders, CNLs are action oriented, connecting mission and purpose to outcomes with impact. CNLs function as leaders for the greater good of the microsystem. Collaborating with an interprofessional team, CNLs translate evidence into quality practice. CNLs lead with conviction; influence processes through deliberate, thoughtful inquiry; and use tools such as appreciative inquiry (AI), transformational leadership, and change strategies. Positive communication strategies and relationship-based care are modeled by CNLs who are sensitive to the nuances at the intersection of the patient, system, and provider. Exemplars of outstanding leadership are provided throughout this text, including reducing pressure ulcers and falls with harm, improving patients' abilities to self-manage their chronic illnesses, and improving lifestyles. The future actions of CNLs will be predicted on using resilience, steadfastness to the role, and professional actions.

Conclusion

Clinical leadership is about CNLs informing the quality and safety of care through innovation and improvement—both in organizational processes and individual care practices. It is based on the premise CNLs deliver care and possess the abilities to evaluate quality and guide improvement using the expertise of clinical teams and collaborative partnerships. Clinical leadership can be assumed by any direct provider of patient care, including physicians, nurses, allied health professionals, clinical pharmacists, and paramedics.

Summary

- CNLs are leaders in innovation and evidence-based care.
- CNLs are in a key position to influence healthcare delivery models and outcomes.
- CNLs use a variety of leadership strategies to influence microsystems, resulting in positive outcomes.
- CNLs demonstrate a number of clinical leadership behaviors in the execution of their various role functions.
- CNLs consider a variety of change theories in leading innovation.
- CNLs engage stakeholders in understanding the improvement process.
- CNLs use improvement and team science to create interdisciplinary teams to foster greater coordination and collaboration.

Reflection Questions

1. Think deeply about a task or activity you do every day. How does this connect to the mission, vision, and values of your organization? Are there other ways to think about this activity? If you were told to stop doing the activity, what would change? Use some of the innovative strategies outlined in this chapter to guide your thinking differently about your routines and rituals.
2. Consider a typical day from your experiences as a CNL student, graduate, and then in the role. Identify at least one example in which you demonstrated clinical leadership. Were you intentional in your communication with others? How would you rate yourself? Would you respond differently now that you have had time to reflect on your actions, how individuals responded to you, etc.? Then reflect on an interaction you observed in the last week in which leadership was critical to the outcome of decisions made during the interaction (meeting, task force, etc.). Were you able to recognize a particular leadership style? What constituted leadership in this example?
3. Assess your leadership style using any number of leadership appraisal tools. What are your areas of strength? What are the areas that need improvement? Share your assessment with your mentor as you develop an action plan for future growth.

Learning Activities

1. Consider a clinical situation on your unit where you have not been able to sustain a change. What elements of leadership were present? What elements of leadership were missing?
2. Examine the clinical indicators on your unit/microsystem. Select an indicator that could benefit from clinical leadership and propose how you would establish a team to address it. Who would be on the team? What tools would you use in planning the change? What evidence is available to support the change?
3. Consider a process that impacts your unit and the clinical outcomes that are possible. Is there clinical leadership of the initiative? An interdisciplinary team

or task force responsible for the outcome? What do you attribute to the success or failure of this clinical intervention?

4. Describe the attributes of a clinical leader versus an administrative leader. What do they hold in common? What distinguishes them from one another? Using any number of self-appraisal leadership tools, assess your leadership abilities, developing an action plan to address areas that you would like to further develop. Have your mentor work with you to monitor your progress.

References

Agomoh, C. J., Brisbois, M. D., & Chin, E. (2020). A mapping review of Clinical Nurse Leader and nurse educator transitional care skills and competencies. *Nursing Outlook, 68*, 504–516. https://doi.org/10.1016/j.outlook.2020.02.003

American Association of Colleges of Nursing. (2007). *White paper on the role of the clinical nurse leader*. http://www.aacn.nche.edu/publications/white-papers/cnl

American Association of Colleges of Nursing. (2013). *Competencies and curricular expectations for clinical nurse leader education and practice*. http://www.aacn.nche.edu/cnl/CNL-Competencies-October-2013.pdf

Amos, M. A., Hu, J., & Herrick, C. A. (2005). The impact of team building on communication and job satisfaction of nursing staff. *Journal of Nurses Staff Development, 21*(1), 10–18.

Avolio, B., & Bass, B. (2002). *Developing potential across a full range of leadership: Cases on transactional and transformational leadership*. Lawrence Erlbaum Associates.

Barker, A., Sullivan, D., & Emery, M. (2006). *Leadership competencies for clinical managers: The renaissance of transformational leadership*. Jones & Bartlett Learning.

Bass, B. (1990). *Bass & Stogdill's handbook of leadership: Theory, research, & managerial applications* (3rd ed.). The Free Press.

Bender, M., Connelly, C. D., Glaser, D., & Brown, C. (2012). Clinical Nurse Leader impact on microsystem care quality. *Nursing Research, 61*(5), 326–332. https://doi.org/10.1097/NNR .0b013e318265a5b6

Bleich, M. R. (2012). Leadership responses to the future of nursing: Leading change, advancing health IOM report. *Journal of Nursing Administration, 42*(4), 183–184. https://doi.org/10.1097 /NNA.0b013e31824ccc6b

Boonstra, A., & Broekhuis, M. (2010). Barriers to the acceptance of electronic medical records by physicians from systematic review to taxonomy and interventions. *BMC Health Services Research, 10*, 231. https://doi.org/10.1186/1472-6963-10-231

Bruzzese, J., Usseglio, J., Goldberg, J., Begg, M. D., & Larson, E. (2020). Professional development outcomes associated with interdisciplinary research: An integrative review. *Nursing Outlook, 68*, 449–458. https://doi.org/10.1016/j.outlook.2020.03.006

Davidson, S., Weberg, D., Porter-O'Grady, T., & Malloch, K. (2017). *Leadership for evidence-based innovation in nursing and health professions*. Jones & Bartlett Learning.

Diamond, E., French, K., Gronkiewicz, C., & Borkgren, M. (2010). Electronic medical records: A practitioner's perspective on evaluation and implementation. *Chest, 138*(3), 716–723.

French, W., & Bell, C. (1994). *Organization development: Behavioral science interventions for organization improvement* (5th ed.). Prentice Hall.

Garling, P. (Ed.). (2008). *Final report of the Special Commission of Enquiry. Acute care services in NSW public hospitals*. http://www.lawlink.nsw.gov.au/lawlink/Corporate/ll_corporate.nsf/pages /attorney_generals_department_acsinquiry

Greenleaf, P. (1977). *Servant leadership: A journey into the nature of legitimate power and greatness*. Paulist Press.

Gutsche, J. (2015). *Exploiting chaos: 150 ways to spark innovation*. Penguin Random House.

Hartranft, S. R., Garcia, T., & Adams, N. (2007). Realizing the anticipated effects of the clinical nurse leader. *Journal of Nursing Administration, 37*(6), 261–263.

Hix, C., McKeon, L., & Walters, S. (2009). Clinical Nurse Leader impact on clinical microsystems outcomes. *Journal of Nursing Administration, 39*(2), 71–76.

Hubbard, B. M. (1998). *Conscious evolution: Awakening the power of our social potential*. New World Library.

Institute for Healthcare Improvement. (2011, April 24). *Science of improvement: Forming the team*. http://www.ihi.org/knowledge/Pages/HowtoImprove/ScienceofImprovementFormingtheTeam.aspx

Institute of Medicine. (2003). *Health professions education: A bridge to quality*. National Academies Press.

Institute of Medicine. (2010). *The future of nursing: Leading change, advancing health*. http://www.iom.edu/Reports/2010/The-Future-of-Nursing-Leading-Change-Advancing-Health.aspx

Klainberg, M. K., & Dirschel, K. M. (2010). *Today's nursing leader: Managing, succeeding, excelling*. Jones & Bartlett Learning.

Lewin, K. (1951). *Field theory in social science: Selected theoretical papers*. In K. Lewin & D. Cartwright (Eds.), *MIT Research Center for Group Dynamics*. Harper and Brothers Publishers.

Lippitt, R., Watson, J., & Westley, B. (1958). *The dynamics of planned change*. Harcourt, Brace and World.

Marquis, B., & Huston, C. J. (2006). *Leadership roles and management functions in nursing: Theory and application*. Lippincott Williams & Wilkins.

National Health Priority Action Council. (2006). National chronic disease strategy. *Australian Government, Department of Health and Ageing, Canberra*. http://www.health.gov.au/internet/main/publishing.nsf/content/7E7E9140A3D3A3BCCA257140007AB32B/$File/stratal3.pdf

Nielsen, K., Yarker, J., Randall, R., & Munir, F. (2019). The mediating effects of team and self-efficacy on the relationship between transformational leadership, and job satisfaction and psychological well-being in healthcare professionals. A cross-sectional survey. *International Journal of Nursing Studies, 49*(9), 1236–1244.

Northouse, P. G. (2015). *Leadership: Theory and practice*. Sage.

Pink, D. (2010). *To sell is human: The surprising truth about moving others*. Penguin Random House.

Porter-O'Grady, T. (1997). Quantum mechanics and the future of healthcare leadership. *Journal of Nursing Administration, 27*(1), 15–20.

Porter-O'Grady, T. (1999). Quantum leadership: New roles for a new age. *Journal of Nursing Administration, 29*(10), 37–42.

Schein, E. (1999). Kurt Lewin's change theory in the field and in the classroom: Notes toward a model of managed learning. *Reflections: The SOL Journal, 1*(1), 59–74.

Tomey, A. (2010). *Guide to nursing management and leadership* (8th ed.). Mosby-Elsevier.

Weberg, D., & Davidson, S. (2019). *Leadership for evidence-based innovation in nursing and health professions* (2nd ed.). Jones & Bartlett Learning.

Westbrook, I., Braithwaite, J., Georgiou, A., Ampt, A., Creswick, N., Coiera, E., & Iedema, R. (2007). Multimethod evaluation of information and communication technologies in health in the context of wicked problems and sociotechnical theory. *Journal of American Medical Information Association, 14*, 746–755. https//:doi:10.1197/jamia.M2462"10.1197/jamia.M2462

Woo, T. (2013). Horizontal leadership. In C. King & G. O'Toole (Eds.), *Clinical Nurse Leader certification review*. Springer.

Yackanicz, L., Kerr, R., & Levick, D. (2010). Physician buy-in for EMRs. *Journal of Healthcare Information Management: Journal of Health Management, 24*(2), 41–44.

EXEMPLAR

Enhancing Continuity of Patient Care Through Improved Multidisciplinary Communication

Toby Meyers

The CNLs at an NCI-designated comprehensive cancer center observed that standing ICCs were poorly attended. The CNLs felt that coordination of patient care was suffering in part due to the lack of attendance at these regularly scheduled meetings between team members. The CNLs undertook an effort to improve attendance at the ICCs.

A work group of CNLs collaborated with interprofessional colleagues to identify barriers to attendance and developed a plan establishing consistent and regularly scheduled ICCs. The primary aim of this work group was to improve interprofessional attendance at the ICCs. A secondary aim was to improve communication, coordination, and collaboration among the team members to promote continuity and quality of patient care as a result of this collaboration.

Prior to practice change, the interprofessional work group reviewed the current unit process and required criteria for ICCs. According to the CMS guidelines, the meetings should at minimum involve representatives of two unique disciplines. To meet the group's aim and the CMS criteria, the CNLs proposed a more inclusive ICC that consists of case managers, social workers, nutritionists, chaplains, physical and occupational therapists, and RNs.

The CNLs met and discussed the proposal with the different disciplines to solicit their support in implementing the change. Additional changes discussed and approved included establishing a standard schedule for weekly ICCs, facilitating the ICCs for each of the three nursing pods on the unit, and utilizing a standardized form to document pertinent patient data after discussing patient care needs with the bedside RN in preparation for the ICC. The CNLs facilitated all ICCs to ensure consistency with the format.

After one year of participation in the new plan, attendance audits showed about 90% attendance from all disciplines. An informal survey of participants indicated that interdisciplinary team members find the new standardized ICCs improve communication and facilitate timely identification of needs and coordination of patient care. The CNLs monitored and trended Press Ganey and HCAHPS scores and observed a steady increase in patient-reported outcomes, specifically in the domains of discharge information and care transitions.

The ICC is a contributor to quality improvement, particularly in relation to developing individualized care planning for patients and timely, successful transitions of care. ICCs also reflect a core component of the CNL's role in coordinating interprofessional care at the microsystem level.

EXEMPLAR

A CNL-Led Initiative to Advance the Nursing Profession on a Medical-Surgical Unit

Veronica Rankin, Heidi Chappell, Kasia Qutermous, and Katrina Lindsay

Nursing has been charged by various organizations with the responsibility to help promote the advancement of the profession and healthcare outcomes. Roles such as the master's prepared CNL serve as guardians of the nursing profession and a modern-day solution designed to develop and empower direct care nurses.

Since 2010, four CNLs using a 12-bed microsystem model have worked tirelessly to transform the culture of a 36-bed telemetry medical-surgical unit in order to help advance and empower the nursing staff. The CNLs were integrated into the medical-surgical unit in 2010 as CNL students to begin their internship. As part of their 5 Ps assessment, they identified deficits in unit rewards and recognition, staff certification, clinical ladder advancement, and overall nursing pride. The CNLs encouraged clinical advancement by teaming up with high-performing nurses and offering clinical ladder project ideas as well as assistance with organizing the plan, required documents, and presentation for advancement. They planned and implemented annual "end-of-year" celebrations, which included awards for the management team, review of unit metrics, and patient/staff satisfaction scores as well as recognition of certifications and clinical ladder and academic advancements.

The CNLs also identified an opportunity to gain recognition for the various specialized populations cared for on the unit such as patients and families dealing with end-of-life challenges. They led the 3T team in completing education and leadership training programs in order to gain specialized training and designation in the care of the elderly through the NICHE program.

Finally, to boost staff pride on the unit, CNLs also spearheaded the tedious task of writing up internal and external award nominations for the unit to recognize the hard work, commitment, and integrity of the 3T team. Numerous awards were and continue to be presented to staff as a result of the culture fostered by the CNLs and the outcomes the unit has achieved. This includes the prestigious PRISM award given by the Academy of Medical-Surgical Nurses (AMSN) and the Medical-Surgical Nursing Certification Board (MSNCB).

Since initiation of the CNL's role on the unit in 2010, the unit has held a Tier I status in teammate engagement as measured by Press Ganey from 2011 until 2014, only dropping two points below the threshold in 2015. Physician satisfaction scores have also continued to rise by more than 6% annually above the hospital's average. From 2009 to 2013 the unit noticed marked positive increases in PRC patient satisfaction scores in the areas of Overall Quality of Care and Likelihood to Recommend, and aggregate patient satisfaction scores continue to improve.

Efficiency and effectiveness have also been positively impacted. The average length of stay for patients on the unit dropped from a steady upward trend of 6.88 in 2012, 7.04 in 2013, and 7.11 in 2014 to 6.30 in 2015, currently holding a record-breaking low of 5.46 for 2016. The fall rate on the unit dropped from 8.05 in 2009 prior to initiation of the CNL's role to 3.77 as of 2015. Many other examples exist that can highlight the impact of the CNL's role on quality of care on this unit, but the loudest testament to this impact is heard from the staff. When asked by the chief nurse officer and assistant vice president of the CNL program, the staff of the unit unanimously agreed that CNLs added great value to the unit's quality of care and that they did not want the role to leave their unit. Staff on the unit described CNLs as "priceless," "irreplaceable," and "necessary to be able to complete our jobs." One nurse who has just been accepted into a CNL program shared that her previous hospital would have greatly benefited from the role. She shared that she "applied to this hospital because I knew CNLs were here" and that "CNLs make me feel like someone is always there to have my back and help me when I need them."

CNLs at Carolinas Medical Center in Charlotte, North Carolina, continue to strive for excellence, top-quality patient care provision, and the improvement of patient outcomes. We know that this cannot be achieved without empowered and confident nursing colleagues at the front line. Our major takeaway from this initiative is that the CNL must support, empower, and help to develop nursing staff in order to advance healthcare.

EXEMPLAR

Implementing the CNL's Role in an Ambulatory Heart Failure Clinic for the Underserved

Erica Arnold

Background

The current state of the nation's healthcare delivery system requires urgent attention focusing on quality, safety, and cost of delivering effective and equitable care. Thus, the purpose of this exemplar is to describe how the University of Alabama at Birmingham (UAB) hospital (UABH) and the UAB School of Nursing partnered to implement a grant-funded interprofessional collaborative practice (IPCP) model to address the healthcare needs of an underserved HF patient population with goals to reduce 30-day hospital readmissions and improve patient outcomes. Utilizing a nurse-led clinic with the triple aim as a framework, the clinic's goals were to: (1) improve the patient experience, (2) improve the health of populations, and (3) reduce the cost of healthcare in an underserved heart failure population. As a key team member, the CNL acts as a lateral integrator of care and patient advocate along the care continuum, serving as an information manager to the multiple disciplines on the IPCP team.

Methods

Within the IPCP model, the CNL contributed care coordination expertise across the healthcare continuum making daily rounds on all HF panel patients hospitalized at UABH. The CNL executed the role coordinating a postdischarge follow-up visit within seven days prior to patient hospital discharge, making follow-up phone calls on all patients, confirming clinic visits, arranging home visits for new patients, and leading IPCP team morning huddles and postclinic conference meetings on clinic days. Huddles and conferences focused on improving communication among professionals and ensuring customized and coordinated care based on individual patient needs.

Outcomes

Patient care delivery in the grant-funded HF clinic began in late December 2014. Considering objectives of the triple aim and using data from the first eight months of clinic operations, desirable outcomes were achieved: (1) The clinic has exhibited impressive patient satisfaction scores, reflecting optimal patient experiences. Of 124 patient responses, 95% rate responsiveness of staff as very good/excellent, 92% feel providers always listen, and 96% feel providers always treat them with respect. (2)

Thirty-nine percent of established patients ($n = 29$) had a clinical improvement in their HF classification. (3) In a short time, there has been a trend toward lower 30-day re-admission rates compared to a national average readmission rate of 22.7%, which highlights the clinic's effectiveness in improving patient outcomes and decreasing healthcare costs.

Conclusion/Recommendations

Delivering care that is safe, timely, effective, equitable, efficient, and patient-centered is the primary focus of the CNL. Utilizing the CNL's role in an ambulatory HF clinic and implementing an IPCP model around transitional care coordination has demonstrated outstanding achievement in all three dimensions of the triple aim. Our findings affirm the value of the CNL's contribution and suggest the CNL's skill set has applicability beyond the acute care environment. Therefore, it is recommended that the CNL's role be integrated into care environments beyond the in-hospital setting to better address the continuum of care.

EXEMPLAR

A Practice Innovation to Reduce Unit-Acquired Ear Pressure Ulcers on a Medical Specialty Unit

Beverly Phillips, Jennifer Kareivis, Michelle Sheets, and the nursing staff of 3 West Medical Specialty Unit

Background

An increase in unit-acquired pressure ulcers on a medical specialty unit was found to be device related, specifically to methods of oxygen delivery. The firm oxygen tubing and elastic strap from the face mask/tent were identified as factors contributing to ear pressure ulcers for patients unable to communicate needs, including stating pain/discomfort related to oxygen via nasal cannula or face mask/tent. Prior attempts to reduce ear pressure ulcers with alternative means failed. Data were presented by Certified Wound and Ostomy Care Nurse (CWOCN) at a unit meeting. The CNLs championed solving this problem.

Aim

To prevent device-related ear pressure ulcers in patients wearing oxygen cannula or face mask/tent.

Methods/Programs/Practices

Nasal oxygen cannula was changed to softer tubing for any patients requiring supplementation. The CWOCN designed an alternative to the face mask/tent strap, replacing it with a soft trach strap. The Braden scale sensory perception subscale identified patients at risk, with scores of three or below indicating that the patient might be unable to feel/communicate discomfort related to oxygen devices. Staff were educated and given visible protocol sheets and prepared supplies. The CNLs facilitated communication and education about the protocol. The CWOCN was the resource person/data collector. If the patient required face mask/tent and had a Braden scale sensory perception score of three or below the strap was replaced per protocol. Ear skin assessment was done every shift. Changes were reported to the CWOCN.

Outcome Data

In 2010, preintervention, nine patients developed ear pressure ulcers. Postintervention, one patient in 2011 had an ear pressure ulcer related to oxygen face mask/face tent. Unit-acquired ear pressure ulcers were reduced by 100% related to the oxygen tubing.

Conclusion

Collaboration between the CWOCN and CNLs led to a practice innovation that decreased unit-acquired ear pressure ulcers. The CNLs were integral in educating staff, improving quality care, and identifying patients at risk.

EXEMPLAR

CNL and Microsystem Assessment on a Trauma Unit

Tiffany Tscherne

Critical Thinking

The TPM is responsible for assessing the microsystem of the trauma patient to find out why poor outcomes have been obtained, and/or why evidence-based guidelines are not being adhered to. Through application of the chosen quality improvement model (PDCA), how it can be corrected is created by the TPM and the CNL student in consultation with the trauma medical director or multidisciplinary trauma operations committee.

The microsystem assessment can be as simple as interviews or as complex as workflow diagrams and retrospective analysis of charts and data from the trauma registry. Upon completion of the assessment through the CNL's clinical immersion experience, the CNL completed a new design for the corrections process and selected the outcome metrics, based on regulatory guidelines such as the American College of Surgeons or the state of Michigan, in concert with evidence-based practice.

Communication

In addition to e-mail, the CNL student must master both business and clinical venues of communication. The CNL student in the TPM role is responsible for developing high-level reports to senior leadership utilizing the A3 and other standard formats. Identifying the route of communication with the direct-care-level provider is necessary for program operations. So, familiarity with marketing tools throughout the hospital as well as the staff communication venues allows the TPM (CNL student) to share everything from "kudos" to classes to educational tools.

Assessment

The CNL student's assessment focused on identification of the primary trauma population for the area served by the hospital. In my case, falls in those over the age of 55, with orthopedic injury are my primary population of interest. The information on falls was obtained through chart reviews, usage trends, the Michigan Hospital Association MIDAS database, and the hospital's central data warehouse.

Why is this knowledge so important? It allows us to focus on our injury prevention activities to the community that we serve. While handing out bicycle helmets to children is a noble cause, it doesn't help the seniors who are falling due to poor knowledge of fall risks. Anticipating the risk allows us to decrease the high mortality rates that often follow falls in those considered to be in their golden years.

Assessment of the microsystem, especially when poor outcomes or regulatory standards are not being met, is a primary job role of the TPM. Whether through the 5 Ps, (purpose, patients, professionals, processes, and patterns), or a fishbone chart, the TPM utilizes tools to answer why this issue or outcome is occurring. This microsystem assessment, when done correctly, will yield valuable information and data to improve fall reduction outcomes for the elder population.

Health Promotion, Risk Reduction, and Disease Prevention

Injury prevention activities are a mandate for a trauma center according to the American College of Surgeons. As discussed, after an assessment of the primary trauma risks to the community, the CNL student evaluates EBP to develop a plan that best addresses the risk. The CNL student develops the outcome matrix tool, gathers the relevant data from the trauma registry, and then reports the findings to the trauma operations committee. No change in outcomes? Back into the PDCA it goes!

So who is responsible for delivering the programming? The CNL serves as the primary creator and the educator as well by going out into the community to give lectures, provide health fairs, and to also serve on committees throughout the community. This level of community involvement lends the CNL expertise to shape policy for health promotion, risk reduction, and disease prevention.

Illness and Disease Management

The CNL student served as the case manager for the trauma patient throughout the care spectrum. Yes, the CNL student served as one of the primary authors of the process, but she will also be the de facto case manager for the trauma patient through daily rounding, participating in multidisciplinary care planning, and applying both EBP and regulatory guidelines in order to shape a positive patient outcome.

Information and Healthcare Technologies

In addition to being a clinical care force, the TPM is responsible for the trauma registry. The trauma registry serves as a clinical repository for trauma patient care data on a myriad of data points ranging from demographics to procedures and even comorbidities. The CNL student is responsible for the operations of the data collection, creating the data collection process, data integrity, and the management of the trauma registry.

Healthcare Systems and Policy

Writing policy, managing all aspects of trauma center operations including staff and budget, are part of the CNL student's role expectations. A CNL student managed a team of two or more and assumed responsibility for office operations. The CNL student is responsible for the trauma services budget, which can include not only paper clips but on-call fees for physicians, as well as staff trauma training for an entire hospital.

The CNL student writes policy that affects not only trauma service, but the operations of the entire multidisciplinary team in regard to the trauma patient. Trauma policy must remain valid and applicable as the patient moves from the ED to diagnostic testing, to the inpatient realm, and upon discharge and transfer. Policies on trauma activations, transfer criteria, and even trauma education are crafted under the guidance of the CNL student.

Designer/Manager/Coordinator of Care

The CNL student bears the responsibility for the cornerstone of the trauma program for any hospital, of any size or designation: the PIPS program. The PIPS program consists of daily activities, through trauma rounding and chart review, up to committee action by a physician peer review or the multidisciplinary operations committee. Whether a patient care failure or process failure, the issue moves through one of three levels of review, guided by the CNL student. The CNL student serves as the chief researcher, facilitator, and even outcomes manager for the issue in order to ensure loop closure.

EXEMPLAR

"Let's Get Moving" from the Microsystem to the Macrosystem: System-wide Implementation of a Mobility Program into 62 Microsystems

Darla Banks and Danell Stengem

CNLs on one microsystem within our large healthcare system successfully implemented a mobility project where improved HCAHPS scores, decreased LOS, reduction of HAPUs and decreased re-admission rates were realized. A CNL at another entity within the same healthcare system implemented a mobilization project where patient mobilization was ingrained into the culture of the unit. The outcomes of these projects were recognized as best practices across the healthcare system.

CNL leadership at the system level was sought to incorporate the successful mobility projects performed at the microsystem level and in turn to operationalize and standardize them utilizing the CNL team across 62 microsystems in a 14-entity healthcare system. Two existing best practice mobility projects were assimilated into a mobility program. Interdisciplinary feedback and support were critical components during development and implementation of the mobility program. CNL leadership developed and refined the processes for implementation prior to rollout.

A presentation and panel discussion was developed to provide guidance for implementation of this system-wide mobility project at the microsystem level. This presentation was televised via a videoconference training session to all entities on three separate dates. Entity chief nurse officers were communicated to regarding the program and their support was obtained. Nurse managers, CNLs, physical therapists, nursing supervisors, and charge nurses were asked to attend. Mobility program flyers and training materials were provided to all attendees via e-mail.

A push/pull methodology was employed with this project. Nurse managers were asked to "push" the mobility program to their staff while the CNLs were asked to "pull" the process down the hall by providing real-time point-of-care mobility education and support. CNLs worked to collaborate on the implementation process in conjunction with the nurse managers.

CNL leadership provided a progress report to the nurse executive team on the stages of implementation at their facilities during the first six months of this project. Monthly updates on each unit's progress with implementation stage, planning stage, or no plan to implement the mobility program were provided to CNL leadership by each microsystem's CNL.

One month after the go-live date of this mobility project, 63% of the units were implemented, 19% were in the planning stage, and 18% had no plan. Two months after implementation, 80% of the units were implemented, 17% were in the planning stage, and 3% had no plan. Three months after implementation, 82% of the units were implemented, 15% remained in the planning stage, and 3% had no plan to implement.

CNL leadership collaborated with EHR engineers to create an activity dashboard with the intent of providing data to measure the compliance with the mobility program at the microsystem level. CNLs across the healthcare system were then trained by the CNL leadership on how to access and run unit-specific reports that measured the documented activity (ambulating or out of bed for meals) of their patients. The reports also allow the user to deep-dive to individual patients in order to determine if the nursing documentation of activity was adequate or inadequate.

Ten months after the initiation of this project, all 123 CNLs across 68 microsystems in 14 separate entities are utilizing the data from the reports to continue pulling this project down the halls of their microsystem. The mobility data for each unit is recorded monthly on each individual unit's Microsystem Dashboard in order to track progress in meeting mobility goals.

Successful projects performed at the microsystem level often stay within that microsystem. CNL leadership at the system level of a large healthcare organization can provide awareness of these successes at the highest organizational level and work to move these successful projects from the microsystem throughout the macrosystem. CNLs placed on the unit at the point of care have the greatest influence on the culture and outcomes of the unit especially when initiatives are brought forth from the system level.

CHAPTER 18

The CNL Engagement in Health Policy

James L. Harris, Linda A. Roussel, and Patricia L. Thomas

LEARNING OBJECTIVES

1. Identify the importance of CNL engagement in health policy.
2. Discuss how health policy influences CNL practice, organizational effectiveness, and the well-being of citizens.
3. Recognize how health policies result in unintended consequences and opportunities that occur for CNL policy engagement.
4. Identify how CNLs can eliminate and/or reduce unintended consequences imposed by health policies.
5. Discuss trends and impact(s) of health policy on the health of individuals and society.

KEY TERMS

Advocacy
Change
Emotional intelligence
Engagement
Evidence-based practice

Health policy
Interprofessional teams
Microsystem
Social determinants of health
Unintended consequences

CNL ROLES

Advocate
Collaborator
Coordinator

Engager
Health promoter

CNL PROFESSIONAL VALUES

Advocacy
Integrity

Social justice

CNL COMPETENCIES

Advocacy	Emotional intelligence
Change agent	Health promotion
Collaboration	

Introduction

Health policy provides insights into clinical decisions that culminate in quantifiable quality outcomes. As a key influencer, health policy has implications for individuals, healthcare systems, and global populations (Teitelbaum & Wilensky, 2013). Engagement and advocacy by clinicians and healthcare administrators are central to health policies that promote the well-being of society. Health policy has historically informed clinical decisions and methods used to improve services, funding, and evidence-based practice. As health policies are developed and endorsed, CNLs are critical to informing, creating, and changing practice within microsystems. As practice is changed within any micro-, meso-, or macrosystem, opportunities to change practice throughout an organization emerge. CNLs who engage in the development and advocacy for health policy shape the emergence of new models of evidence-based care and the fidelity of social, political, and economic views dominant. Unintended consequences and adverse events decline, and quality practice prevails.

Throughout this chapter, influences of health policy, engagement, and advocacy are the central themes. An overview of how CNL health policy engagement and advocacy creates environments for evidence-based policy interventions is provided. The result is strategies aligned to create quality, safe, and value-based care delivery.

Health Policy, Engagement, and Advocacy Defined

To provide context for this chapter, health policy, engagement, and advocacy are defined. WHO broadly defines health policy as actions initiated by governments—local, state, and national—to advance and achieve healthcare goals of the public (WHO, 2015). Health policy is a series of regulatory and legislative initiatives framed around the healthcare goals of a society. The regulatory and legislative initiatives are the components of health policy that focus on any organization, the finances, and provision of healthcare services—a proviso grounded in the US Constitution.

Health policy achieves multiple outcomes. Being fully inspired with the belief that all ideas have value creates roadmaps for CNLs to leverage social change and meet the intent of a system's mission and assist in the development of public and private policies (Carthon et al., 2016). Encompassed in the belief are practical consequences and philosophical underpinnings. While health policy, at times, has been iterative rather than transformative, the series of evidence-based activities, short- and long-term priorities set the stage for sustainable change (Maddox et al., 2019). Ultimately, interprofessional teams become engaged and are influential advocates for policy implementation aimed at effecting change in strategies to meet the social determinants of health, a culture of trust, accountability, and diversity (Burrows, 2019). Priorities are met and measureable outcomes are evident. What started within a microsystem by a CNL advances to the creation of a community of health policy engagers and advocates.

Merriam-Webster (n.d.) defines "engagement" as an agreement to do something at a fixed time. CNLs who engage in health policy development and implementation are mindful of the needs and preferences of healthcare consumers and effective microsystem functions. In the current national healthcare landscape, patient engagement is essential. Through purposeful actions, CNLs engage in organized strategies to delineate population interests, interventions related to the population, comparisons of practices, and outcomes within the microsystem. A perfect storm of forces to understand how health policies effectively guides practice, improves abilities to anticipate risks associated with implementing policies, and engages care teams to use evidence-based policies as the full potential of an improvement team is achieved (Melnyk & Fineout-Overholt, 2015).

For purposes of this chapter, definitions of *advocacy* are provided. An advocate is one who summons to give evidence (Gates, 1995). Advocacy is to act, speak for, plead for, or defend or to inform, advise, or counsel (Gadow, 1980, 1989; Kohnke, 1982; Mitchell & Bournes, 2000).

Advocacy means many things to people, and there is no universally accepted health policy advocacy model. That does not mean that health policy advocacy is absent. "Advocacy is a concept that conceals more than it reveals" (Mitchell & Bournes, 2000, p. 209).

Advocacy is a social mandate for nurses. The social context in which nurses practice is foundational to the essence of nursing. This underscores the notion that CNLs must be advocates for health policies that are representative of needs and preferences, and policies uniquely accountable to society. *Nursing's Social Policy Statement* informs other health professionals, legislators, regulators, funding agencies, and the public about nursing's social responsibility, accountability, autonomy, and contribution to the health and well-being of individuals (American Nurses Association, 2010). Actions to ensure the clinical perspective is included in organizational decisions, and nurses being actively involved in decisions that affect practice, is central to CNLs fulfilling an advocacy role.

As advocates and agents of social change, CNLs use social change theory to plan for the implementation of microsystem change. Through a microsystem assessment, CNLs gain valuable information regarding how the microsystem functions, how others perform respective roles, and how an organization meets the needs of individuals. This information provides a deeper understanding into the discovery of simplicity on the other side of complexity. It functions as observational maps to assist CNLs in navigating the processes associated with change. As a result, organizations and teams gain insight into what really matters, and that change can be beneficial.

CNLs function as change agents. CNLs incorporate social change theory and the knowledge of complex adaptive systems to assist others through the change process. CNLs adopt an orientation of simple cause-and-effect thinking according to the needs that have been identified in the microsystem assessment. Interventions are developed based on one of three kinds of change: (1) emergent, (2) transformative, or (3) projectable (Coser, 1971; Olny, 2005; Plsek & Greenhalgh, 2001; Reeler, 2007).

Emergent change focuses on future emerging conditions or processes related to approaches where productive relationships are formed and issues of leadership and power are largely resolved. Balanced change follows and is beneficial to the whole. An action-learning cycle and horizontal learning approaches that include learning networks are formed as collaborative actions to guide the change process (Reeler, 2004/2005).

In contrast, transformative change is not characterized by learning, but by unlearning, processes immobilize individuals and organizations that are stuck in a revolving cycle of crisis. Releasing this cycle opens doors for new approaches toward positive change (Kotter, 1995).

Projectable change includes processes supported by planning and implementation. Care is provided to mobilize teams to be innovative and support the vision associated with the change. Through creative forms of organization and practice, powerful relationships are formed and change is accepted and cultivated. Comfort among others ensues, and a deeper sense of reality and insights are shared. Decisions about organizations, changes, and policies are developed and patient-centric.

CNLs are a catalyst for change. Change is not engineered, but cultivated. Processes associated with emergent, transformative, or projectable change are present regardless of the organization. CNLs assist others to adopt a culture that is respectful and inclusive. Skillful mastery of working through processes yields changes that are sustainable and creates measurable results. Adoption by others transpires, and this information becomes valuable as teams led by CNLs advocate for policy development and change within microsystems and across meso- and macrosystems.

Staff involved in the change process create conditions whereby patients receive the care that is desired. Care becomes a service rather than a commodity (Lundin & Lundin, 1993). Opportunities for new and improved structures flourish, and health connections among teams and patient advocacy receive primary consideration (Porter-O'Grady & Malloch, 2015). A notable example of healthy connections between providers and patients is the medical home model implemented in several healthcare systems. Medical home models focus care where the patient is, at the center of decisions, and actions that follow.

CNLs are also health promotion advocates. Through actions and collaboration with teams, CNLs maximize the health of individuals to capitalize on individual experiences and attributes. Recognizing and including patients and support systems in plans of care becomes a central part of CNL practice as a lateral integrator of care. This allows individuals to attain the highest level of health including physical, mental, social, and spiritual determinants and factors (Pender, 1982; US Department of Health and Human Services, 2010).

The pressure to improve quality and contain costs offers another venue for CNL advocacy and action. Through CNL led collaborative interventions, the goal for 20 percent of payments being value-oriented by 2020 will be realized (US Department of Health and Human Services, 2011). In the past decade, significant changes to payor and care delivery models have resulted in value-based care expectations that require transparency using quantifiable and reportable metrics. Across care settings, CNLs are in positions to proactively assist in value-based purchasing and incentives that connect to performance. CNLs are prepared to provide patients with education and information that support decisions and choices. As a result, higher quality, more efficient providers, safety, and financially sound care options have occurred.

Through continued actions toward patient engagement, change, health promotion, quality, and cost containment, CNLs can model behaviors that assist others to engage in open dialogue and engagement necessary for advancing advocacy. This parallels with the belief that advocating is learned when good is achieved and examined (Benner, 1991). Through a process of role modeling and mentoring by CNLs, others gain the confidence required to advocate for patients (Foley et al., 2002a). A confident and engaged CNL is equal to security that equals emotional intelligence and performance (Schwartz et al., 2011). As CNLs model behaviors and engage with teams, a competitive edge is created that benefits patients and communities of interest. Interprofessional team engagement signifies emotional connectedness to an organization, purpose (quality and safe patient care), and teams who are cognitively vigilant. Belasco and Stayer (1993) best described engagement by discussing the 10 Cs of employment engagement as follows.

1. *Connect:* Connecting leaders and employees results in initiatives that have measureable outcomes.
2. *Career:* Engaging in meaningful work and career advancement fosters development.
3. *Clarity:* Communicating a clear vision creates avenues toward success and engagement to the common goal.
4. *Convey:* Clarifying expectations creates small improvements that are spread.
5. *Congratulate:* Providing immediate feedback results in ownership and more engagement.
6. *Contribute:* Informing others about positive contributions stimulates additional action and common purpose.
7. *Control:* Involving creates opportunities for greatness that are central to feelings of control over situations.
8. *Collaborate:* Learning from others fosters collaborative activities with measurable results.
9. *Credibility:* Maintaining standards and ethical decisions foster engagement.
10. *Confidence:* Exemplifying high ethical and performance standards engages others.

Unintended Consequences of Health Policy: CNLs Respond

Unintended consequences of health policy exist. Opportunities for CNL action are present, especially if the IOM's 2020 goal that 90% of clinical decisions are evidence-based (McClellan et al., 2007). CNLs extend evidence-based practice in microsystems and engage other team members to incorporate evidence in decisions. As the number of CNLs has increased, practices and team decisions are being based on current evidence and used throughout healthcare systems.

One cannot dismiss that as health policies are endorsed throughout practice, unintended consequences occur. If one dismisses this reality, a disconnect will prevail and the intent of any policy is diminished. The intent of the health policy will be unmet or void, distractions dominate actions, and a paucity of theoretical and evidence acumen is diminished.

Historical context is one example of an unintended consequence of health policy. The idea that health policy should be based on the previous ways that care has been provided is a misconception. Learning from history offers options to revisit prior failures and contribute to future prosperity. Healthcare continues to be fragmented, and costs continue to escalate. While history plays a valuable role and cannot be diminished, evidence and new models of care delivery and reimbursement must be included in health policy decisions. Otherwise, fragmentation and costly care will prevail regardless of the environment.

Time is another unintended consequence of health policy. From the time a bill is introduced and progresses to vote and passage, the initial intent of the policy is often lost or diminished. For example, opportunities to access childcare in rural areas may have changed due to new regulations and evidence. This affords CNLs another opportunity to remain current on regulations, evidence-based practice, and political action in order to educate policy makers on current needs, regulations, and other available evidence.

The absence of including communities in health policy development is another unintended consequence. The exclusion of the community needs, preferences, and resources limits scope and future policy adoption in certain communities. This validates the need for CNLs to assess community preferences, needs, and resources. Using their knowledge of microsystem assessment and sharing this information with health policy makers is pivotal to a culture of inclusivity.

CNLs also collaborate with health services researchers to conduct small demonstration projects that will provide quantifiable evidence and support for policy development. As data repositories are created, evidence is sustenance for funding larger projects. This assists in promoting science and limiting the influence and politics from various lobbyists. Health policies are formulated and based on data and scientific rigor.

Thoughtful hesitation from the immediacy of situations is required as health policies are developed. This allows reflection versus reaction. CNLs are key players in researching and providing evidence to policy makers. Evidence must underpin health policy content and decisions. CNLs must give voice to policy development in order to avoid unintended and catastrophic consequences.

Trends and Impacts of Health Policy

Evidence-based health policies will have considerable solidarity on a global level. Conceivably, other nations will observe outcomes as evidence-based health policies are authorized and implemented. As a result of the positive outcomes, universal endorsement of the health policies occur and actions follow resulting in healthy communities and populations.

The critical health policy currently in the United States is sustaining the Patient Protection and Affordable Care Act (CMS, 2010). What has followed since the passage of the healthcare reform act are ongoing debates on its efficacy, more insured individuals, increased demands for care, new ways of care delivery, technological advances, changes for preventive services, new payment incentives, and its replacement. Multiple opportunities for CNL engagement and advocacy are available to ensure all Americans are insured with equal distribution.

CNLs must seize the moment and continue to engage themselves and others in actions that align with the changes in healthcare delivery based on the Affordable Care Act. The US healthcare system is dependent on informed nurses to lead and be advocates of quality improvement. CNLs are key players in this endeavor and understand what works and what does not. CNLs can assist others to contribute to effective solutions that avert unsafe conditions while improving quality and creating measurable outcomes. For example, the findings reported with the publication of the 2014 *National Healthcare Quality and Disparities Report* (QDR) provides opportunities to examine how the Affordable Care Act impacts care access and the immediacy to frame interventions that reduce access issues and strengthen quality and safety indices.

As noted in the QDR, major disparities in quality and safety of care persist (AHRQ, 2015). Therein lie opportunities for CNLs to implement quality projects that align with the six priorities that form the foundation for the National Quality Safety (NQS; Robert Wood Johnson Foundation, 2012). The six foundational priorities of the NQS include the following.

1. Making care safer by reducing harm caused in the delivery of care
2. Ensuring that each person and family is engaged as partners in their care
3. Promoting effective communication and coordination of care
4. Promoting the most effective prevention and treatment practices for leading causes of mortality, starting with cardiovascular disease
5. Working with communities to promote wide use of best practices to enable healthy living
6. Making quality care more affordable for individuals, families, employers, and governments by developing and spreading new healthcare delivery models.

"The NQS was created to align efforts on a set of public and private sector, consensus-based national priorities and goals" (Agency for Health and Human Services, 2014; Ricciardi et al., 2016, p. 10).

CNLs are prepared to impact resource utilization through engagement and advocacy, especially in ways that the social determinants of health will be met. Mechanisms such as value-based purchasing, bundled payments to providers, and payment reductions for poor clinical outcomes remain present. Value-based purchasing provides rewards to healthcare systems that provide high-quality care. Payments are based on quality of care, not the volume of services. Five measures guide the process to include the following:

1. Structure measures (characteristics of physician and healthcare facilities)
2. Process measures (components of encounters between providers and patients)
3. Outcome measures (descriptions of subsequent health status)
4. Patient experience (patient satisfaction, healthcare team member communication, discharge information, and pain management)
5. Efficiency

There were 24 measures for 2016 and 27 identified for 2017 with additions in subsequent years. Various percentages for measurement achievement change each year (CMS, 2010; US Department Health and Human Services, 2011).

Bundled payments to all providers, along the continuum of care to share, are the current norm and will continue in subsequent years. In this payment environment, all providers, regardless of the location of care, share reimbursement for the care provided. Healthcare organizations that manage costs and care coordination more efficiently will experience longevity (Penner, 2013). As care delivery and reimbursement changes progress, organizations must adapt and adopt a culture of quality and efficiency for ongoing survival. CNLs are actively involved in the process throughout the nation. For example, one CNL was selected by the American Academy of Nursing as an Edge Runner recipient for working with complex care and patient advocacy.

The trend toward increased technological innovation has affected how policies are developed and implemented. We live in a society that is informed, and one that demands information. Information guides the healthcare decisions of individuals today more than in the past. As partnerships evolve between patients and providers, the patient becomes the center of the interchanges. Quality outcomes and efficiency further guide technological advances and information that will be available to society. It is incumbent on providers to use this information and advocate for funds that will strengthen technology and the ongoing development of evidence-based health policies.

Achieving equilibrium between financial stability, patient preferences, and protection of society will influence future trends in healthcare and health policy development. This equilibrium is leverage for CNLs to engage in innovative care delivery and be advocates for the health policies that ensure the well-being of society. CNLs must be involved because nursing is directly impacted. As actions by state coalitions are initiated to meet the IOM's *Future of Nursing* recommendations, the impact of CNL practice and their relevancy across populations will strengthen (IOM, 2011).

Working collaboratively with other stakeholders to shape health policy cannot be overemphasized. Individuals and nations learn from one another. This creates greater certainty for future care delivery, finance, and efficiency. As CNLs engage and are advocates for the adoption of a culture that values evidence and includes others, the future landscape of well-developed health policies will follow.

Summary

- Health policy provides valuable insights into clinical decisions that yield quantifiable practice outcomes.
- CNL engagement and advocacy are pivotal to health policies that promote the health and well-being of society.
- Advocacy is a social mandate for nurses as evidenced by the social context in which nurses practice.
- CNLs are change agents that incorporate social change theory, knowledge of complex adaptive systems, and meeting the social determinants of health as change occurs.
- Models of care delivery highlight the value of CNLs in connecting teams with the immediate needs of patients.
- As health promoters, CNLs assist populations toward attainment of positive health outcomes.
- Collaborative team actions directed by CNLs result in health policy development and mandates for quality, safety, and value-based care.
- While there are unintended consequences of health policy, CNLs are responding to lessen such effects and contribute to future prosperity.
- History plays a valuable role in healthcare policy development and adherence.
- CNLs have the knowledge to effect change and engage in evidence-based inquiry that supports policy development and subsequent strategies to ensure all Americans are insured.
- The components of the Affordable Care Act offer venues for CNL engagement and advocacy for quality, safety, and resource utilization improvements.
- As technology advances, CNLs must remain involved in ways that advance care delivery in cost-effective ways to achieve equilibrium.

Reflection Questions

1. What distinctions can be made between CNL engagement and advocacy as related to health policy?
2. How can CNLs mitigate unintended consequences imposed by health policies?
3. What actions may CNLs take to influence health policy development, implementation, and evaluation?

Learning Activities

1. Consider a healthcare issue that is impacting the delivery of quality and safe patient care. Develop an action plan for advocating for change in a local, regional, or national policy.
2. Develop a letter to a congressperson in your local district for change of a national healthcare policy.

References

Agency for Health and Human Services. (2014). *Working for quality: Achieving better health and health care for all Americans.* Author.

Agency for Healthcare Research and Quality. (2015). *2014 national healthcare quality and disparities report.* Author.https://www.ahrq.gov/research/findings/nhqrdr/chartbooks/personcentered/pfcc.html

American Nurses Association. (2010). *Nursing's social policy statement. The essence of the profession.* Author.

Belasco, J. A., & Stayer, R. C. (1993). *Fight of the buffalo: Soaring to excellence, learning to let employees lead.* Warner Books.

Benner, P. (1991). The role of experience, narrative and community in skilled ethical comportment. *Advances in Nursing Science, 14*(2), 1.

Burrows, K. H. (2019). Health policy, laws, and regulatory issues. In C. R. King, S. O. Gerard, & C. G. Rapp(Eds.), *Essential knowledge for CNL and APRN nurse leaders* (pp. 139–149). Springer.

Carthon, J. M.B., Nicely, K. W., Sarik, D. A., & Fairman, J. (2016). *Policy Politics Nursing Practice, 17*(2), 99–109.

Centers for Medicare and Medicaid Services. (2010). *Affordable Care Act update: Improving Medicare cost savings.* http://www.cms.gov/apps/docs/aca-update-implementing-medicare-costs-savings.pdf

Coser, L. A. (1971). *Masters of sociological thought.* Harcourt Brace Jovanovich.

Egencer, B. E., Mason, D. J., McDonald, W. J., Okun, S., Gaines, M. E., Fleming, D. A., Rosof, B. M., Gullen, D., & Anderson, M. L. (2017). The charter on professionalism for health care organizations. *Academic Medicine, 92*(8), 1091–1099.

Foley, B. J., Minick, M. P., & Kee, C. C. (2002). How nurses learn advocacy. *Journal of Nursing Scholarship, 34*(2), 181–187.

Gadow, S. (1980). Existential advocacy: Philosophical foundation of nursing. In S. F. Spicker & S. Gadow (Eds.), *Nursing: Images and ideas* (p. 79). Springer.

Gadow, S. (1989). Clinical subjectivity: Advocacy for silent patients. *Nursing Clinics of North America, 24*(2), 535–541.

Gates, B. (1995). Whose best interest? *Nursing Times, 91*(4), 31–32.

Institute of Medicine. (2011). *The Future of nursing. Leading change, advancing health.* National Academies Press.

Kohnke, M. F. (1982). *Advocacy: Risk and reality.* Mosby.

Kotter, J. (1995, March/April). Leading change: Why transformational efforts fail. *Harvard Business Review* (Reprint 95204).

Lundin, W., & Lundin, K. (1993). *The healing manager: How to build quality relationships and productive cultures at work.* Berrett-Koehler.

Maddox, K. E, J., Bauchner, H., & Fontanarosa, P. B. (2019). US health policy—2020 and beyond. *JAMA, 321*(17), 1670–1672. https://doi.org/10.1001/jama.2019.3451

McClellan, M. B., McGinnis, M., Nabel, E. G., & Olsen, L. M. (2007). *Evidence-based medicine and the changing nature of health care.* National Academies Press.

Melnyk, B. M., & Fineout-Overholt, E. (2015). *Evidence-based practice in nursing and healthcare: A guide to best practice* (3rd ed.). Lippincott Williams & Wilkins.

Mitchell, G., & Bournes, D. (2000). Nurse as patient advocate? In search of straight thinking. *Nursing Science Quarterly, 13*(3), 204–209. https://doi.org/10.1177%2F089431840001300307

Olny, C. (2005). Using evaluation to adapt health information to the complex environment of community-based organization. *Journal of Medical Library Association, 93*(Suppl. 1), S57–S67.

Pender, N. (1982). *Health promotion in nursing practice.* Appleton & Lange.

Penner, S. (2013). *Economics and financial management for nurses and nurse leaders* (2nd ed.). Springer.

Plsek, P. E., & Greenhalgh, T. (2001). Complexity science: The challenge of complexity in health care. *British Medical Journal, 323,* 625–628.

Porter-O'Grady, T., & Malloch, K. (2015). Toxic organizations and people: The leader as transformer. In T. Porter-O'Grady and K. Malloch, *Quantum leadership: Building better partnerships for sustainable health* (4th ed.). Jones & Bartlett Learning.

Reeler, D. (2007). *A three-fold theory of social change.* Community Development Resource Association.

Reeler, D. (2004/2005). *Engaging freedom's possibilities: CDRA annual report.* http://www.dcra.org.za

Ricciardi, R., Moy, E., & Wilson, N. J. (2016). Finding the true north. Lessons from the National Healthcare Quality and Disparities Report. *Journal of Nursing Care Quality, 31*(1), 9–12. https://doi.org/10.1097/NCQ.000000000000016

Robert Wood Johnson Foundation. (2012). *What is the national quality strategy?* Author.

Schwartz, T., Comes, J., & McCarthy, C. (2011). *Be excellent at anything: The four keys to transforming the way we work and live.* Simon & Schuster.

Teitelbaum, J. B., & Wilensky, S. E. (2013). *Essentials of health policy and law.* Jones & Bartlett Learning.

US Department of Health and Human Services. (2010). *Healthy people 2020: MAP-IT.* http://healthypeople.gove/2020/Implementing/Default.aspx

US Department of Health and Human Services. (2011). *Hospital value-based purchasing program.* http://www.cms.gov/Outrearch-and-Education/Medicare-Learning-Network-MLN/MLNProducts/downloads/Hospital_VBPurchasing_Fact_Sheet_ICN907664.pdf

World Health Organization. (2015). *Health Policy.* http://www.who.int/topics/health_policy/en

EXEMPLAR

Health Policy Engagement and Advocacy

Mary Harnish

The Joint Commission certification for Advanced Inpatient Diabetes Care has been awarded to only 86 hospitals across the United States. This certification is designed to help hospital organizations provide safe, high-quality care to patients with diabetes. Mercy Health Saint Mary's initially received this certification in 2011 and has maintained it for five years.

The role of the CNL for diabetes was implemented at Mercy Health Saint Mary's in 2010. This CNL's cohort of patients consists of those with complex needs in regard to their diabetes and comorbidities. The processes around care and safety of the diabetes population are the CNL's concern as well.

The CNL for diabetes assesses outcomes related to diabetes care required by The Joint Commission including patient education about self-management and patients being informed of their A1C results. Safety issues, including insulin errors and the timely treating and rechecking of hypoglycemia, are assessed through reports from the information systems (IS) department. These outcomes are shared with the nursing staff through "just-in-time education" and ongoing reports.

Nursing and medical staff are supported in the care of the patient with diabetes by the CNL, who is seen as the expert that can assist with complicated patients' needs. New diabetes teaching material, computerized patient assessments, and insulin dosing software are promoted by the CNL to improve patient care at the bedside and across the system.

To enlist the bedside nurse to take an active role in diabetes care, the CNL for diabetes is developing diabetes champions on each of the nursing units. These champions will have additional training and act as a resource to other staff while educating and promoting best practices for their diabetes patients.

CHAPTER 19

CNL Certification and Professional Development

Linda A. Roussel, James L. Harris, and Patricia L. Thomas

LEARING OBJECTIVES

1. Discuss the value of residency programs, certification, and professionalism to advance CNLs.
2. Understand the importance of CNL residency programs for transition to practice.
3. Identify the process for preparing and attaining CNL certification.
4. Describe how the Clinical Nurse Leader Association (CNLA) advances CNLs.

KEY TERMS

Attitude
Certification
Character
Clinical Nurse Leader Association
Competency

Conduct
Lateral integration
Professional membership
Residency program

CNL ROLES

Advocate
Collaborator
Leader

Lifelong learner
Outcomes and environment manager
Team member

CNL PROFESSIONAL VALUES

Accountability
Diversity
Integrity

Honesty
Professionalism
Trust

CNL CORE COMPETENCIES

Facilitation	Lifelong learner
Leadership	Professional maturity

Introduction

Unprecedented changes in the healthcare market are having profound impacts in all practice settings. The changes provide a greater voice and image for nurses and the profession. To capitalize on opportunities, it is essential for nurses to advocate on behalf of colleagues and the profession. Active professional membership, specialty certification, and professionalism are three venues that will guide the profession's desired future (Tomajan, 2012).

CNLs are prepared to meet the challenges inherent in contemporary healthcare and influence others to embrace change. Influencing others is built on competence, credibility, trust, professionalism, and leadership. CNLs are socialized to address gaps in care and improve the quality, safety, and value-based disparities within a fragmented healthcare system. Through lateral integration, CNLs bring teams together toward a common goal. CNLs collaborate and exchange information while forming partnerships that ultimately reduces service redundancy. As redundancy is reduced, services become more patient-centric. Timely, effective, efficient, and safe care ensues (IOM, 2001).

This chapter highlights the value of professionalism as CNLs transition from students into practice settings, attain certification, and become active in professional organizations. While the content is not all-inclusive, the foundation for ongoing CNL success and development is discussed.

CNL Certification

Certification contributes to achieving desired health outcomes of society, advancing nursing, and validates an individual's qualifications for practice. More CNLs are being prepared, becoming certified, and accepting roles in nontraditional settings. The CNL mark of excellence promotes safe, quality care delivery through its ongoing requirements for lifelong learning and professional advancement (Commission on Nurse Certification, 2016). CNL certification is based on a national standard of required knowledge and experiences, which provides employers, the public, and members of the health professions criteria in the assessment of a CNL.

According to the AACN (n.d.), a certified CNL is a master's educated nurse, prepared for practice across the continuum of care within any healthcare setting in a constantly changing healthcare system. CNLs provide leadership for care coordination, engage in direct patient care in complex situations, work with interdisciplinary teams to place evidence-based practice in motion, make certain that patients benefit from the latest innovations in care delivery, assess patient outcomes, and evaluate cohort risk through decision-making authority plans of care plans. As a leader and active member of the interdisciplinary healthcare team, the CNL is instrumental in innovative changes in care across the continuum. The CNL's role may vary dependent on the care setting (AACN, n.d.).

The CNL Certification Program is managed by the CNC, an autonomous arm of AACN, and governed by the CNC Board of Commissioners. As such, CNC recognizes individuals who have demonstrated professional standards and knowledge through CNL certification. The CNC Board of Commissioners and staff are solely responsible for the policies and administration of the CNL Certification Program (AACN, n.d.). CNL students can access the CNC's CNL 2016 *Job Analysis Summary Survey and Certification Examination Blueprint* for greater details on the certification domains, and subdomains (CNC, 2016). Recently, the blueprint has been updated to reflect the dynamics associated with CNL practice and the healthcare environment.

CNL certification is an exceptional credential that recognizes graduates of master's and post-master's CNL education programs that have demonstrated exceptional standards of practice. Certification emphasizes leadership by collaboration with teams, leadership, and spreading evidence. A variety of resources are available to assist CNL graduates prepare for the examination and may be accessed at www.aacn.nche.edu/cnl.

Professionalism

Complementing the work by CNLs and role advancement are five attributes of professionalism. They include character, attitude, excellence, competency, and conduct (Ball, 2005).

1. *Character:* Character encompasses integrity based on trust. Honesty, trustworthiness, and being forthright are cornerstones of trust. Through deliberate actions, character is built. This includes being diligent and responsive through lifelong learning to elevate oneself.
2. *Attitude:* Professionals provide care in a positive manner with confidence and quality. When setbacks occur, they can regroup and initiate a different strategy. Professionals are responsible and accountable for actions and assume responsibility for coaching and mentoring others.
3. *Excellence:* Professionals seek excellence in all endeavors. High standards are set and they lead others to achieve maximum outcomes. Quality and quantity of work products are central to success.
4. *Competency:* Professionals are experts in their discipline and constantly seek opportunities to improve. They recognize that the real measure of success is results. New skills and knowledge are sought to meet goals.
5. *Conduct:* Professional maturity is a standard of conduct underpinned by well-developed social skills, practical approaches, and sensitivity toward others. Balancing work and leisure time are key to remaining grounded.

As noted in each of the five attributes of professionalism, blending and integrating each of them results in excellence as individuals communicate effectively, find ways to be more productive, and improve workplace situations. Today's workplace is constantly evolving as one generation retires and another assumes its place. The workplace may have a mix of baby boomers, Gen Xers, and millennials. In addition to generational differences are variances in education, social norms, and values. This variety of perspectives benefits and strengthens organizations and sets a new standard for professionalism. Part of understanding professionalism is figuring out how individual actions impact the work of others. Teamwork is an essential element of professionalism because it fosters development.

CNLs work in several teams across care settings, facilitate positive outcomes, and effect change, further demonstrating professionalism. The dynamic of complex teamwork necessitates various approaches to innovating healthcare. As more CNLs enter the workforce, innovative environments will be created that offer new opportunities where teams function at their highest potential and add sustainable value in the delivery of care.

CNL Transition to Practice

The challenge of assuming a new role can be daunting especially if the position is new to an organization. This requires the CNL to clearly articulate the role definition to all stakeholders for a smooth transition to practice. Major threads outlined in the CNL curriculum framework (**Figure 19-1**) provide the foundation for successful practice integration (AACN, 2007, p. 32, 2013).

The curriculum framework encompasses three foci: nursing leadership, clinical outcomes management, and care environment management. Ten threads are integrated throughout didactic and clinical immersions. These provide structure

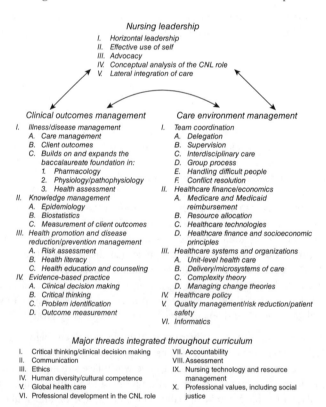

Nursing leadership

   I. Horizontal leadership
   II. Effective use of self
   III. Advocacy
   IV. Conceptual analysis of the CNL role
   V. Lateral integration of care

Clinical outcomes management

I. Illness/disease management
   A. Care management
   B. Client outcomes
   C. Builds on and expands the
      baccalaureate foundation in:
      1. Pharmacology
      2. Physiology/pathophysiology
      3. Health assessment
II. Knowledge management
   A. Epidemiology
   B. Biostatistics
   C. Measurement of client outcomes
III. Health promotion and disease
   reduction/prevention management
   A. Risk assessment
   B. Health literacy
   C. Health education and counseling
IV. Evidence-based practice
   A. Clinical decision making
   B. Critical thinking
   C. Problem identification
   D. Outcome measurement

Care environment management

I. Team coordination
   A. Delegation
   B. Supervision
   C. Interdisciplinary care
   D. Group process
   E. Handling difficult people
   F. Conflict resolution
II. Healthcare finance/economics
   A. Medicare and Medicaid
      reimbursement
   B. Resource allocation
   C. Healthcare technologies
   D. Healthcare finance and socioeconomic
      principles
III. Healthcare systems and organizations
   A. Unit-level health care
   B. Delivery/microsystems of care
   C. Complexity theory
   D. Managing change theories
IV. Healthcare policy
V. Quality management/risk reduction/patient
   safety
VI. Informatics

Major threads integrated throughout curriculum

I. Critical thinking/clinical decision making	VII. Accountability
II. Communication	VIII.Assessment
III. Ethics	IX. Nursing technology and resource
IV. Human diversity/cultural competence	management
V. Global health care	X. Professional values, including social
VI. Professional development in the CNL role	justice

Figure 19-1 CNL curriculum framework

that prepares the graduate to master identified competencies to fully use the unique skills and knowledge in a variety of practice settings (Stanley, 2014).

Five curriculum models for graduate CNL education programs are present. The five models are described in **Table 19-1**.

Regardless of the setting for CNL practice, a shared vision, understanding, and expectations for the role is required by all stakeholders for success. This provides a strategic approach to embedding the role in a setting that is both meaningful and consistent with CNL educational preparation. The value of this approach is driven by the need to ensure that CNLs entering practice are sufficiently prepared to provide efficient care with sufficient self-assurance that supports role satisfaction. This, in turn, provides a shared vision and set of expectations, acknowledges the new CNL as a novice in a new role, and provides a supportive structure and network within which transition is effective at the point of care (Avolio & Williams, 2014).

Several healthcare systems have developed and implemented a CNL transition to practice program with success. Transition to practice programs may also be considered a type of nurse residency program. For example, the AACN with Vizient have offered such a program whose overall purpose is to transition new nurses to their role within healthcare systems. Overall, residency programs purport to increase decision-making competence and confidence, improve professional commitment and satisfaction, and enable consistent evidence-based practice uptake. Nurse residency programs also can build stronger clinical nursing leadership and critical-thinking skills, and develop individual development plans for nurses' new roles (AACN, 2019).

An example of a CNL transition program is the Veterans Health Administration, an early adopter of CNLs. Five core elements of CNL transition to practice provide the blueprint for the program. The elements include: (1) theoretical framework; (2) curriculum development; (3) curriculum content, format, and learning activities; (4) program structure; and (5) evaluation framework. The curriculum is organized under domains of learning that represent critical components of CNL practice. **Table 19-2** illustrates the curriculum framework.

Table 19-1 CNL Curriculum Models

Model	Program Description
Model A	Program designed for BSN graduates
Model B	Program designed for BSN graduates; includes a post-BSN residency that awards master's credit toward the CNL degree
Model C	Program for individuals with a baccalaureate degree in another discipline; also known as a second-degree or generic master's
Model D	Program designed for ADN graduates; also known as an RN-MSN program
Model E	Post-master's certificate program

BSN, bachelor's of nursing science; ADN, associate's degree in nursing; RN-MS, registered nurse with a master's of science in nursing
Modified from American Association of Colleges of Nursing. (2014). *Clinical nurse leader education models being implemented by schools of nursing.* http://www.aacn.nche.edu/cnl/CNLEdModels.pdf

Table 19-2 The VHA ONS CNL Transition to Practice Curriculum Framework

Learning Domain	Content Module	Learning Objectives
Role differentiation	ONS CNL strategic initiative and spread plan overview	Describe the ONS strategic vision for the CNL's role. Identify how the ONS vision is consistent with the AACN's CNL white paper. Define individual CNL roles within the context of the ONS's vision. Determine how the microsystem supports the organizational strategic plan.
	Establishing and sustaining interprofessional, collaborative relationships	Identify key collaborative relationships for the microsystem. Understand the value of professional communication, leadership, and facilitation skills in establishing collaborative relationships. Identify resources to help develop collaborative skills.
	Role differentiation	Be able to differentiate the CNL's role from other nursing roles. Describe how implementing the CNL's role brings added value. Identify resources to help differentiate the CNL's role.
	Microsystems needs assessment and role establishment	Identify members of the team who will complete the clinical microsystem assessment. Using the clinical microsystems workbook that is appropriate for your microsystem, begin an assessment, diagnosis, and treatment that focuses on patients, purpose, professionals, processes, and patterns (5 Ps). Identify resources needed to complete the workbook.
	Owning your practice	Describe who you are as a professional. Develop a professional portfolio. Disseminate information about your CNL's role. Identify the elements of a culture of professional ownership.
Clinical outcomes management	Care coordination	Describe transitions of care. Identify a continuum of care collaborative team. Describe elements of safe and effective handoffs. Identify resources to facilitate seamless care transitions.

	Patient/Family education	Outline the principles and expectations of patient- and family-centered care. Identify the skills needed to achieve patient- and family-centered care outcomes through education. Identify resources to support patient- and family-centered care.
	Staff education and learning environment	Identify competencies needed to achieve optimal outcomes in the microsystem. Describe strategies for developing and maintaining competencies. Identify resources to develop staff skills and create continuous learning environments.
	Products/ Technology	Identify the products and technologies that impact the microsystem. Identify strategies to improve resource management. Identify resources to support and optimize efficiency and effectiveness.
	Patient-driven care protocols	Identify opportunities to improve management of clinical outcomes. Define processes and structures that impact clinical practice outcomes. Identify resources available to achieve optimal outcomes.
	Health promotion and disease prevention (HPDP)	Describe how HPDP is integrated in all aspects of care across the care continuum. Identify the performance measures related to the microsystem. Identify HPDP internal and external resources related to the microsystem.
Care environment management	Team coordination	Identify the team structures within the microsystem. Assess the communication pathways and patterns of team structures. Identify resources that support team function.
	Accreditation readiness	Describe the accreditation processes for the microsystem. Identify strategies to promote team ownership of readiness. Identify accreditation resources.
	Performance improvement, safety, risk aversion	Describe the elements that contribute to risks in the microsystem. Identify unique risks for obtaining optimal outcomes in the microsystem. Describe risk anticipation strategies. Identify resources to support performance safety and risk aversion.

(continues)

Table 19-2 The VHA ONS CNL Transition to Practice Curriculum
Framework *(continued)*

Learning Domain	Content Module	Learning Objectives
	Change	Identify conceptual models and theories of change. Identify a variety of strategies to approach and manage change. Identify resources to support change management.
	Shared governance/ high-reliability organizations	Define shared governance. Define high-reliability organizations. Identify strategies for leveraging microsystem governance structures. Identify resources for supporting shared governance and the development of high-reliability organizations.
Data management	Data—general considerations	Identify sources of useful and appropriate data. Describe elements of data collection strategies. Describe considerations for protecting data.
	Data management	Identify available systems for organizing data. Describe considerations related to ownership and accountability of data.
	Data analysis/ interpretation	Describe strategies for analyzing and interpreting data. Identify the appropriate audience for different types of data reporting.
	Dissemination	Describe considerations when determining dissemination methods. Identify suitable opportunities and venues for dissemination. Identify levels of review and approval required for dissemination.
Using evidence to guide practice	Using the EBP curriculum: transition to practice program	Define EBP. Identify how EBP can improve patient safety and quality patient care.

While this is one example, the CNL's entry into practice varies as well as the length and depth of orientation.

Professional Development

As the CNL transitions into practice and better understand the role, professional development is important to career planning and lifelong learning. Professional development takes a multifaced approach and includes such strategies as portfolio development, serving on boards, political involvement, educational advancement, and mentoring the next generation of healthcare providers. Engaging in one strategy flows into other career opportunities for the CNL. For example, serving on boards may begin with involvement at the local level as a member, and possibly serving on a committee. This could include professional as well as community-based organizations. Taking small steps can offer opportunities to learn more about the mission, purpose, and operations of the organization. This would serve as a bridge to taking on greater responsibility in the organization, thus preparing for regional, national, and international involvement. This also exposes the CNL to the "politics" of the organization, and the connection to policy making within the system and beyond (Sadler, 2019).

The CNL builds a portfolio through intentional engagement in directed professional development activities. Cope and Murray (2018) describe a portfolio as a means of helping nurses to store and manage their revalidation and certification documents in one place that can be updated and produced when required, for example, in performance reviews and job applications. Tracking and building on continuing professional development activities are essential to maintaining, updating, and improving knowledge and practice. A portfolio serves to document these activities, and useful in tracking progress, as well as identifying possible gaps in professional development and career planning. According to Cope and Murray (2018), creating and maintaining a portfolio can inform nurses of their strengths and learning needs, and to develop a learning plan to address these future needs for advancement.

Mentoring is also an important professional development strategy. Identifying mentors, as well as serving as a mentor for novice nurses can enhance career advancement. According to Hunt (2019), the goal of mentoring is to help another human being recognize and cultivate their strengths that may be different from your own. Mentoring "happens" through listening, discussing options, and guiding solutions. This allows the mentor and the mentee to grow and to experience the reward of learning how another individual critically thinks through problems. The mentoring relationship is a win-win for all engaged in the process. The portfolio can serve as a means to review the various professional activities documented, and to identify next steps toward career development.

The CNLA

Professional organizations provide opportunities to connect with peers, share practices, and learn new information. Individuals share information and collaboratively find solutions to issues that face nursing through professional engagement. Care is advanced as networks of individuals collectively interact. The CNLA is an example of a professional organization where a forum is provided for members across practice settings to collaborate, collect, and publish information, while maintaining a professional presence. The mission of the CNLA is realized as patient outcomes are improved. This is accomplished by focusing on safety and quality outcomes and implementation of EBP (CNLA, 2016).

The history of the CNLA dates to 2008 when a group of CNLs proposed the establishment of an organization. As the CNLA has matured, a steering committee was formed, bylaws developed, elections occurred, a partnership with the AACN was formed, a 501(c) established, and membership continues to grow as regional chapters are being formed. Ongoing educational presentations are common. An online community of members is available to share outcomes, learn from one another, and network in support of sustaining the role (CNLA, 2016).

Summary

- Active professional membership, certification, and professionalism are three venues that guide the profession's desired future.
- CNLs are socialized to address gaps in care and improve disparities in a fragmented healthcare system.
- Through lateral integration, CNLs bring teams together toward a common goal.
- Five attributes of professionalism include character, attitude, excellence, competency, and conduct.
- The face of the workplace is constantly changing, and CNLs must be prepared to manage successfully in such dynamic environments.
- Major threads outlined in the CNL curriculum framework are foundational for practice.
- Three foci encompass the curriculum framework: nursing leadership, clinical outcomes management, and care environment management.
- Certification contributes to achieving desired outcomes and advancing nursing.
- CNL certification is a unique credential that recognizes program graduates by continuously advancing the role and acceptance by the profession.
- Professional organizations, such as the CNLA, provide opportunities to share practices and advance the profession of nursing.
- The CNLA, dating to 2008, has continuously defined its mission by improved patient outcomes across the continuum of care.

Reflection Questions

1. What attributes do you bring to the table to advance the CNL's role?
2. How did the three foci of the CNL curriculum framework prepare you for entry into practice?
3. What steps are required to CNL certification and recertification?

References

Avolio, A. E., & Williams, M. D. (2014). Toward achieving desired outcomes: The clinical nurse leader's transition to practice. In J. L. Harris, L. Roussel, & P. L. Thomas (Eds.), *Initiating and sustaining the clinical nurse leader role. A practical guide* (2nd ed.). Jones & Bartlett Learning.

American Association of Colleges of Nursing. (n.d.). *Clinical Nurse Leader (CNL) certification.* https://www.aacnnursing.org/cnl-certification

American Association of Colleges of Nursing. (2007). *White paper on the role of the clinical nurse leader.* Author. https://nursing.uiowa.edu/sites/default/files/documents/academic-programs/graduate/msn-cnl/CNL_White_Paper.pdf

American Association of Colleges of Nursing. (2019). *Vizient/AACN nurse residency program.* https://www.aacnnursing.org/Portals/42/AcademicNursing/NRP/Nurse-Residency-Program.pdf

American Association of Colleges of Nursing. (2013). *Competencies and curricular expectations for clinical nurse leader education and practice* [White paper]. https://www.aacnnursing.org/Portals/42/News/White-Papers/CNL-Competencies-October-2013.pdf

American Association of Colleges of Nursing. (2014). *Clinical nurse leader education models being implemented by schools of nursing.* http://www.aacn.nche.edu/cnl/CNLEdModels.pdf

Ball, J. (2005). *Professionalism is for everyone. Five keys to help a professional.* Goals Institute.

Clinical Nurse Leader Association. (2016). *Mission and vision.* http://cnlassociation.org

Commission on Nurse Certification. (2016). *Transform. Lead. Experience. Clinical Nurse Leader certification.* http://www.aacn.nche.edu/CNL

Commission on Nurse Certification. (2016). *Job analysis summary and certification examination blueprint.* https://www.aacnnursing.org/Portals/42/CNL/CNL-Exam-Content-Outline-2017.pdf

Cope, V., & Murray, M. (2018). Use of professional portfolios in nursing. *Nursing Standards. 32*(30), 55–63. https//doi.org/10.7748/ns.2018.e10985

Hunt, P. (2019). The mentoring relationship. *Nursing Management, 50*(10), 5–6. https://doi.org/10.1097/01.NUMA.0000580616.68498.67

Institute of Medicine. (2001). *Crossing the quality chasm: A new health system for the 21st century.* National Academies Press.

Sadler, F. (2019). *Three critical components of nursing professional development across the care continuum.* https://www.relias.com/blog/3-components-of-professional-development-for-nurses

Stanley, J. (2014). Introducing the Clinical Nurse Leader: Past, present, and future. In J. L. Harris, L. Roussel, & P. L. Thomas (Eds.), *Initiating and sustaining the clinical nurse leader role. A practical guide* (2nd ed.). Jones & Bartlett Learning.

Tomajan, K. (2012). Advocating for nurses and nursing. *The Online Journal of Issues in Nursing, 17*(1), Manuscript 4.

EXEMPLAR

Nurse Empowerment Through CNL-Facilitated Certification Prep

Toy Bartley

In July 2015, a CNL new to the hospital system assessed the need for increased education in the ICUs. Increased turnover of nurses resulted in a decreased number of experienced nurses. The CNL presented the idea of a two-day review class to the nurses.

Utilizing resources and books from the AACN, the CNL created a two-day review class for the nurses. The CNL then met with the unit manager and the education coordinator (EC) to plan for the class. The EC took care of the room reservations and processed the contact hours. The unit manager provided breakfast, lunch, and snacks for the two-day class. PowerPoint materials were provided to each participant as part of the class material to keep for reference. Following the completion of each organ system, to assess the efficacy of the training, the CNL used scenario-based multiple-choice test questions in an informal discussion.

During unit downtime hours, the CNL provided, "5–10 min bedside in-services" discussing disease processes currently seen on the unit. These short reviews reinforced the materials from the class. At times, physician residents also participated in bedside in-services.

Prior to each staff's CCRN testing date, the CNL met with each of the staff to ensure staff understood the components of the exam and shared test-taking strategies. From July 2015 to December 2015, the CNL was able to provide four sets of two-day CCRN review classes.

Within six months of the staff taking the CCRN review class, 15 critical care nurses took the CCRN exam and successfully passed on their first attempt! Due to the number of staff who passed, registration for future review classes increased significantly.

The nurses who became CCRN certified were observed to be more involved in the care of the patients. They participated and felt empowered to speak and give their opinions during interdisciplinary rounds. The CCRN certified nurses were also observed to be more willing to teach the novice nurses in the intensive care unit.

The whole process of participating in the two-day review class, the camaraderie, and the support they provide to one another as each prepares to take the exam, significantly improved the way nurses care for their patients and one another.

CHAPTER 20

Creating a Culture of Health and Wellness: A Catalyst for Sustaining the CNL's Role

Linda A. Roussel, James L. Harris, and Patricia L. Thomas

LEARNING OBJECTIVES

1. Describe a culture of health and wellness.
2. Outline strategies for creating a joyful workplace.
3. Identify major work and initiatives of national and international organizations focused on sustaining healthy work environments.
4. Describe assessment tools for better understanding joy in the workplace.
5. Provide system and local level measures of resilience that can be tracked in identifying areas for improvement over time.
6. Describe the CNL's role in coaching for resiliency and facilitating joyful workplaces.

KEY TERMS

Advocacy
Authentic leadership
Autonomy
Coaching
Collaboration
Fairness and equity
Healthy work environments
Mindfulness

Networking
Nurses Bill of Rights
Peer Support
Physical and psychological safety
Recognition and rewards
Resilience
Team building

CNL ROLES

Clinician
Educator

Lifelong learner
Member of the profession

CNL PROFESSIONAL VALUES

Accountability   Integrity
Genuineness

CNL CORE COMPETENCIES

Communication   Health promotion
Ethics   Risk reduction

Introduction

Health and well being are important to joyful workplaces and healthy work environments. Toxic worksites lead to burnout, depression, compassion fatigue, and secondary stress influencing positive patient care outcomes and has an impact on our healthcare system (Chau et al., 2015). Frontline nurses hold an essential role in the quality and safety of patient outcomes (Chau et al., 2015). Nurses are at high risk for and experience high levels of burnout and sickness-related absenteeism. Nurse leaders, healthcare systems, and educational entities are concerned about the physical and psychological health and well-being of the nursing workforce. Exploring best practices and strategies to support interventions that promote wellness and professional satisfaction are critical to a productive and satisfied workforce (Chesak et al., 2019; Pipe et al., 2012; Virkstis et al., 2018). CNLs are pivotal in connecting frontline workers to holistic practices that foster a spirit of caring and empathy for all involved. The CNL has been described as the "nurses' nurse" focused on creating partnerships through collaboration and fostering a culture of inquiry. CNLs engage frontline workers in meaningful work, and share an appreciation for contributions to positive patient outcomes and quality care across the continuum. CNLs are instrumental in creating a culture of wellness and well-being, fostering joyful work environments.

The IHI purports that burnout in healthcare would be considered epidemic in clinical or public health arenas (Perlo et al., 2017). For example, a study revealed over 50% of physicians' report symptoms of burnout (Shanafelt et al., 2015). All facets of the drive for better health and healthcare outcomes are affected by burnout leading to lower levels of staff engagement. This aligns with lower patient satisfaction with the care experience; lower productivity; lower safe, quality patient care; and an increased risk of workplace accidents. Another study reported that 33% of new RNs seek another job within a year (Lucian Leape Institute, 2013). These all significantly affect the financial viability of an organization (Perlo et al., 2017). Burnout limits providers' empathy, essential to effective person-centered care.

There are several organizational initiatives providing guidelines that facilitate healthy work environments. For example, the American Nurses Association with its Healthy Nurse, Healthy Nation challenge, are encouraging nurses to exert control of individual well-being serving as role models of health, safety, and wellness for their patients. This underscores nurses' roles as educators and advocates (American Nurses Association, 2017). A healthy nurse is described as one who can strike a balance among physical, intellectual, emotional, social, spiritual, personal, and professional well-being (American Nurses Association, 2019). Well-being is a more global perspective offering a holistic lens on a whole-of-life experience. The CDC identifies that well-being is fulfillment, satisfaction with life, positive functioning, the presence of positive emotions, and the absence of negative behaviors (CDC, 2018). CNLs in collaboration and coordination roles within the microsystem seek to facilitate a holistic work environment by maintaining environments that support mental health and well-being. This is particularly critical given frontline nurses' risk for compassion fatigue often brought on by work-related stress. It is not unusual for nurses at the point of care to experience secondary traumatic stress (STS) often compromising well-being and frequently leading to moral distress, burnout, illness, poor satisfaction, and absenteeism (Christodoulou-Fella et al., 2017). Along with frequent illnesses and absenteeism, nurses may also experience presenteeism that has been described as reduced job productivity resultant of health issues. Presenteeism has personal and professional costs, such as frequent mistakes related to poor concentration and focus, which may lead to breaches in safety (Letvak et al., 2012). This alone warrants attention to nurses' mental wellness and well-being, which has created more recent concern due to the reported suicides among nurses (Davidson, Mendis et al., 2018; Davidson, Zisook, et al., 2018; Rizzo, 2018).

Reduced job satisfaction, productivity, quality of care, safety, and job performance that accompany compromised nurse well-being is well known by organizational leaders (Virkstis et al., 2018). We also are aware that burnout among nurses has been significantly associated with patients' poor outcomes, such as urinary tract and surgical site infections. Reduced burnout has also been associated with drops in the rates and costs of hospital infections, with substantial financial savings to healthcare organizations (Cimiotti et al., 2012). Leaving the nursing profession, particularly within the first two years has been reported due to their exposure to pain, suffering, and secondary stress (Flinkman & Salantera, 2015). It is imperative that healthcare systems address turnover and short staffing. Voluntary overtime demands and attrition of nurses in healthcare organizations further aggravates nurse stress because of work overload. While research evidence abounds related to STS, burnout, and compassion fatigue among nurses, there is limited rigorous evidence that inform nurse leaders to the most effective means to enhance resiliency and nurse resistance to stress (Cleary et al., 2018). This supports the business case for addressing health, well-being, and joy in the workplace.

While there is limited research on effective means to enhance a culture of grit and resilience, there are models that can be helpful. For example, Grabee and colleagues (2020) used a randomized controlled trial parallel design to test the effectiveness of a three-hour Community Resiliency Model (CRM) training, a novel set of sensory awareness techniques to improve emotional balance. The research posited that RNs in two urban tertiary-care hospitals were invited to participate in a single three-hour Nurse Wellness and Well-being class; 196 nurses consented and were randomized into the CRM intervention or nutrition education control group. The purpose of the study was to determine if the CRM group would demonstrate improvement in well-being and resiliency, secondary traumatic stress, burnout, and physical symptoms. Pre- and post-data were analyzed for 40 CRM and 37 nutrition group members. Moderate-to-large effect sizes were reported in the CRM group for improved well-being, resiliency, secondary traumatic stress, and physical symptoms. Participants reported using CRM techniques for self-stabilization during stressful work events. Fostering resilience through intentional strategies can mitigate secondary traumatic stress and physical symptoms. Holistic health and well-being can also be notably improved by addressing resiliency. CNLs use evidence-based best practices to advance strategies that support frontline nurse well-being, and create a culture of resiliency. The CNL considers rigorous healthy workplace initiatives that sustain healthy and engaging environments.

National and International Initiatives Supporting Healthy Workplaces

Evidence-based initiatives that support healthy work environments are available and can be useful in assembling resources and when creating resiliency and joyful workplaces. Because CNLs use high levels of evidence to support interventions aimed at quality outcomes of healthy workplaces, they are knowledgeable of initiatives that provide exemplars that can be implemented in microsystems and beyond. A brief description of four models are presented here.

IHI Joy in the Workplace

This IHI white paper provides guidance for healthcare organizations to engage in an interactive, participative process where leaders ask colleagues at all levels of the organization, "What matters to you?" This initiative enables healthcare systems to better understand the barriers and facilitators to joy in work, and cocreate impactful, high-leverage strategies to address these issues. Specifically, the white paper describes the importance of joy in work (the "why"), the four steps leaders can take to improve joy in work (the "how"), and, the IHI Framework for Improving Joy in Work including nine critical components of a system for ensuring a joyful, engaged workforce (the "what"). The white paper also provides key change ideas for improving joy in work as well as exemplars from organizations that helped test them. Measurement and assessment tools are also shared that can assist organizational leaders in gauging efforts to improve joy in work. Specifically, this important IHI work identifies ways to engage staff through getting their input as to what is important to them, and what barriers may hinder ways to achieve greater satisfaction. Working through the lens of improvement science, and being dedicated to a systems focus can create an infrastructure that affords accountability at all levels.

The IHI also provides a framework for improving joy in work focusing on individuals, managers and core leaders, and senior leaders. Nine elements are identified and described in the framework. At the core of the model is happy, healthy, productive, people. Elements surrounding the model's core include physical and psychological safety, meaning and purpose, choice and autonomy, recognition and rewards, participative management, camaraderie and teamwork, daily improvement, wellness and resilience, and real-time measurement. Each of the elements are described and examples are provided. Considering the IHI framework and its elements, senior leaders are responsible for all elements and accountable for cocreating a culture that inspires and fosters trust, improvement, and joy in work. Specifically, senior leaders ensure that improving joy in work is essential at all levels of the organization, beginning with healthy, effective teams and systems. Managers and core leaders, those at the department and clinic levels, are engaged in participative management; developing camaraderie and teamwork; leading and encouraging daily improvement, which includes real-time measurement; and promoting wellness and resiliency through attention to daily practices. Individual members have an essential role in fostering a joyful work environment by committing to doing the best, respecting team members, seeking out opportunities for improvement, and being part of the solution. It is expected that individual members will speak up and take responsibility for personal wellness and resilience. Being a good teammate, role modeling core values of transparency, civility, and respect are individual expectations. Measuring joy in the workplace is also integral to determining successful interventions as part of improvement science. Measurement instruments and tools will be discussed later in this chapter.

American Nurses Association's Healthy Nurse, Healthy Nation Campaign

The American Nurses Association (ANA) in May 2017 launched the Healthy Nurse, Healthy Nation Grand Challenge (HNHN), which is an ongoing national movement created to transform the health of the nation by improving the health of the nation's 4 million RNs. Nursing is one of the most trusted professions and as such nurses have tremendous opportunities to lead healthcare change across the wellness-illness continuum as advocates, role models, and educators. Specifically, nurses work with patients to engage them in living life to its fullest, therefore, modeling wellness, well-being, and a healthy lifestyle goes far in expanding this worthwhile goal. Though this initiative, ANA purports that nurse well-being must be vigilantly guarded, and that unhealthy lifestyles should not be an outcome of dedicated nursing practice. From their research findings, ANA noted from their Health Risk Appraisal that action is needed to improve the health of the nation's nurses. The report revealed that in many of the key indicators, US nurses' health outcomes are worse than that of the average American. That is, nurses have higher levels of stress, get less sleep, and are often overweight notably more so than their non-nurse counterparts. With 24/7 work routines, the demands of shift work worsen the health of the nurse. The work environment can also add to the burden of maintaining a healthy lifestyle considering additional stressors such as workplace violence and musculoskeletal injuries are contributing factors to poorer health (ANA, 2017).

ANA has embarked on this campaign by asking nurses to take the following steps:

1. Register to join Healthy Nurse, Health Nation Connect.
2. Take the health assessment survey and get a heat map of risks.
3. Pick focus area(s), make a commitment, and participate in health challenges. Focus areas include: activity, rest, nutrition, quality of life, and safety.
4. Connect with others for support and advice, and share successes.
5. Repeat the survey annually to measure outcomes and any gains made through the challenge.

The ANA website describing the campaign provides excellent resources, references, tips, and guidelines that can be used to enhance engagement in developing a healthy lifestyle. Additionally, there are exemplars from a variety of state coalitions (Arizona, New York) that used the guidelines to build a culture of health. CNLs can encourage frontline staff to engage in the ANA challenge, and work to improve individual healthy lifestyle choices, which can also have an impact on interprofessional teamwork.

AACN Healthy Work Environments

The AACN's work on creating a healthy work environment (HWE) has been an ongoing, robust effort to support joyful work settings. The AACN in 2001 made a commitment to actively support the creation of healthy work environments in patient care wherever acute and critical care nurses practice. Issued in 2005, *AACN Standards for Establishing and Sustaining Healthy Work Environments: A Journey to Excellence*, took charge by responding to the mounting evidence that untoward outcomes such as ineffective care delivery, medical errors, and conflict among healthcare professionals are associated with unhealthy work environments. Without attention to these stressors and concerns, it is unlikely that individuals and organizations will achieve excellence in patient care. AACN called for the creation and continual fostering of healthy work environments as mandates for ensuring patient safety and optimal outcomes, enhancing staff recruitment and retention, and maintaining healthcare organizations' financial viability. The focus is on the HWE facilities nurses' opportunities to deliver the highest standards of compassionate patient care while working in physical and psychological safe work environments. Specifically, AACN's data consistently revealed units that implemented HWE standards outperform those that did not use the standards. These outcomes included the overall health of the work environment, better nurse staffing and retention, less moral distress, and lower rates of workplace violence. There are six HWE standards (guiding principles) that frame AACN's work in support of a joyful work setting. AACN's six essential standards provide evidence-based guidelines that can be applied for improving critical care work environments. The healthiest work environments integrate all six standards to help produce effective and sustainable outcomes for both patients and nurses. These standards include skilled communication, true collaboration, effective decision-making, appropriate staffing, meaningful recognition, and authentic leadership. Each of the standards is described and an assessment tool has been developed and recommended for use. Specifically, the AACN suggests the following steps:

- Checking out the assessment tool to review for possible unit-level evaluation of their work environment.
- Sending out the HWE survey via e-mail with a link to send an anonymous online survey.
- Download the organization (unit) HWE report. After completing the report, the team can collectively measure their work environment's current health against the HWE standards.
- Take action. The report recommends steps and resources to help the unit start improving the health of their work environment and measure progress.

CNLs do work in critical care units, and as such are concerned about frontline staff's ability to work in possibly toxic environments. Using valid and reliable instruments, and evidence-based guidelines are important to fostering workplaces that afford true collaboration and authentic leadership.

WHO's Healthy Workplace Framework and Model

WHO defines a healthy workplace as one where workers and managers collaborate to use a continual improvement process to protect and promote the health, safety and well-being of workers and the sustainability of the workplace. The following identified needs include health and safety concerns in the physical work environment, health, safety and well-being concerns in the psychosocial work environment including organization of work and workplace culture, personal health resources in the workplace, and ways of participating in the community to improve the health of workers, their families, and other members of the community. The framework includes several intersecting circles at the center of which is ethics and values that is surrounded by leadership engagement and worker involvement. The larger overlapping circles are physical work environment, personal health resources, enterprise community involvement, and psychological work environment. Actions to be taken to move the model forward include mobilize, assemble, assess, prioritize, plan, do, evaluate, and improve. The model makes the business case for concentrating on a multifaceted approach to workplaces that promote psychological and physical safety to allow for greater autonomy in carrying out work responsibilities. This framework and model align with other initiatives presented in this chapter that focus on cocreating work environments that honor the need for frontline workers and organizational leaders to collaboratively partner in meeting job responsibilities, professional development goals, and healthy lifestyles. Building a resilient workforce is an important strategy to this end.

Resiliency

Why is it important to consider resiliency when addressing health and well-being? There are several reasons why it is important to understand resiliency in creating a culture of wellness. Financial uncertainty, mergers, furloughs, layoffs, societal volatilities, COVID-19, and other stressors are reasons to make the business case for facilitating a resilient workforce. Defining resiliency involves a comprehensive approach to the concept and process of coaching for resiliency. For example, resiliency has been described as the process of adaption through experience when facing adversity (Foureur et al., 2013). A person's ability to overcome adverse situations with optimism and self-control is also a quality of being resilient (Lee et al., 2015). Further, resiliency can also be the ability to overcome stress by using external and internal coping strategies (Rushton et al., 2015). There is evidence that high resilience is linked to joy in the workplace. For example, overall health and well-being, staff engagement, staff retention, and reduced burnout can be impacted by coaching for resilience. Psychological health, improved work relations, and increased job satisfaction also improves when resiliency becomes core to the organization's culture (Bernard, 2019; Delgado et al., 2017; Turner, 2014).

Bernard (2019) describes internal and external protective factors of creating a resilient workforce. Specifically, internal protective factors include a sense of security, positive emotions, self-respect, self-efficacy, hope, humor, flexibility, emotional intelligence, autonomy, sense of psychological safety, and morality. External protective factors include social support from peers, positive family relationships, supportive social networks, and job experience and competency. Additional external factors also relate to physical and psychological safety, positive relationships with colleagues, gratitude and appreciation, work-life balance, and a morally aligned work environment fostered by ethical leadership (Bernard, 2019).

Approaches to Building Resiliency

Essentially, nurses are responsible for individual wellness and well-being. Vigilance regarding adequate sleep, good nutrition, regular exercise, and social interaction are necessary elements of building resilience. The CNL encourages (through role modeling) frontline nurses to create feasible, effective practices and habits to support their mental well-being and resiliency. Mindfulness training as a part of yoga and meditation as a strategy have received much attention for stress management and relaxation. Other strategies that promote well-being include self-reflection, gratitude, journaling, prayer, and support groups. Making a commitment to developing an effective daily self-care plan may help counteract emotional exhaustion that comes with nursing. Organizational strategies can also be useful in reducing stressors and by promoting nurses' personal and professional development of tailored self-care strategies. Taylor (2019) states that resiliency training alone has limited efficacy in a stressful work environment in need of significant improvements. Therefore, organizations must be cognizant of and manage variables that contribute to compassion fatigue and emotional distress.

Workplace resilience is an ongoing interactive, engaging process between the nurse and the workplace to promote well-being and healthy responses to emotional distress or adversity (Delgado et al., 2019). Specifically, CNLs and nurse managers have become aware of four gaps in the care environment that include safety threats, compromises in care delivery, traumatic experiences without recovery and technology, responsibilities and protocols that isolate nurses from collaborating with each other as part of daily work (Virkstis et al., 2018). Using a primary framework, Maslow's hierarchy of needs, the organization defines basic human needs. It follows that nurses' basic needs in the workplace will not be addressed if demands of workflow exceed the capacity of the work environment to support nurses' work. Considering basic needs such as safe staffing and ongoing communication of emotionally challenging situations with trained providers are important to address. We know that many of the stress management strategies have been individually focused versus the larger organizational system elements (Chesak et al., 2019). There is clearly a need for creating methods of organizational empowerment for nurses and for strategies of individual resiliency skill training for nurses. Rewards, recognition, policies, and programs to promote well-being and prevent understaffing are workplace mediators. Freedom from bullying, incivility, violence, or other environmental stressors are basic rights of frontline workers and must be addressed. This also impacts other healthcare providers. For example, physicians are noting burnout, depression, early retirement, and suicide (Shanafelt et al., 2017). It has been suggested that physicians often consider personal mental health as a taboo subject and may resist reaching out because of shame, financial, or licensure issues (Reith, 2018). This has also been true for many nurses who often deny mental health issues. Healthcare environments may also unconsciously support a culture of stoicism. It is critical that organizations increase awareness of creating a safe, transparent culture to address the stigma around mental healthcare. One strategy to address this concern is normalizing mental health needs and supporting staff to seek treatment as it is safe to do so (Chesak et al., 2019; Cleary et al., 2018; Mcdonald et al., 2016; Stephens et al., 2017; Tubbert, 2016).

Resiliency can be fostered in the workplace through internal and external approaches. Internal approaches can be related to physical well-being, spiritual well-being, and can embrace self-care. Physical interventions may include getting enough sleep (at least seven hours), exercise, healthy eating, and decompression. Spiritual well-being focuses on mindfulness, communication, and self-awareness. Embracing self-care involves seeking role models and mentors, avoiding negativity (asset-based thinking), and being tolerant and patient when our coworkers are having a stressful day (Bernard, 2019; Wicks & Buck, 2013). Hatler and Sturgeon (2013) provide a variety of approaches to resiliency from assessment, acceptance, adaptation, and action.

Considering *assessment* for resiliency includes being proactive in evaluating the potential for building resiliency through an intentional review of events, environment, and individual characteristics as a starting point. Being mindful of the relationship among feelings, thoughts, and behaviors allows for anticipatory responses from others and consideration of contingencies for dealing with stressors. Additionally, assessment of strengths that exist allows for development of an accurate view of circumstances as well as fostering a greater ability to maximize personal and team strengths. Acceptance focuses on spending less energy resisting, complaining about, or opposing the need for change and being open to new ways to think about and address our situation. Staying focused, centered, poised, and positioned for new opportunities are important mindsets in developing resilience. Changing the way, one speaks about unplanned events, for example, as opportunities for growth and professional development versus ongoing chaos and crises matters in how to approach daily life. Adaptation considers looking for ways to adjust to new circumstances and potential opportunities. Making change works by considering perceptions and attitudes that invite opportunities for professional growth. Developing nurturing professional relationships is important to career growth, and eventually mentoring others in the workplace. Resilient people learn to use cognitive reframing to gain more control of their situations and create teachable moments that have greater compatibility with personal values. Action involves responding to an event by assessing the impact and defining what can be controlled. This can be approached by developing options for handling life situations and seeking out and engaging mentors in finding ways to overcome barriers and cocreating new realities. Mentors can facilitate brainstorming to address possible obstacles and reduce automatic negative thinking such as catastrophizing (this is a disaster), personalizing (why me?), and overgeneralizing (this always happens; Hatler & Sturgeon, 2013).

What is the CNL's role in building resilient workplaces? CNLs ensure that each nurse has access to resources, participates in institutional mechanisms to form and support issues, and develops strategies that foster nurses' resilience. Introducing staff to resiliency tools and measuring resilience are also strategies that CNLs bring to the work environments. Other responsibilities of the CNL involve documenting and studying the impact of individual interventions on staff, supporting strategies to foster clinician well-being, and becoming skilled in recognition, analysis, and action in response to issues that negatively impact staff (ANA, 2017).

Resiliency Tools

There are several resilience tools that can be taught, reinforced for individual practice, and introduced into healthcare systems. Developing resilience can be a personal decision, and reinforced through organizational culture. Resilience is the ability to recover from setbacks and adapt to challenging circumstances and is required to thrive, flourish, and is a foundational tool that empowers effectiveness and capacity when handling uncertainty. Individuals can develop and improve resilience. Identifying resiliency strategies that become part of self-care practice and routines, can foster a more focused and centered life that can add to work-life balance. Mindful and intentional practice combined with self-awareness may be aligned to enhance grit and mental toughness. The resilience tools suggested in this chapter are intended to be a starting point for a primary journey of building resilience and well-being. Through a variety of activities and strategies, these skills can be developed through small, incremental changes. The CNL can be instrumental in introducing a variety of tools to frontline workers and interdisciplinary team members to increase mindfulness, intentional practices, which can foster a culture of gratitude and well-being.

Storytelling Activity

Being able to change the stories told is important to messages that guide individual thinking and eventual actions. This can be viewed as asset-based thinking. Worldviews may be adjusted by re-creating narratives for oneself. Getting stuck in replaying the same stories may not be helpful or productive. By creating a healthier storyline, a sense of control is fostered over our thinking and how one interprets, and possibly reframes, events. Pennebaker and colleagues' (1988) research indicated that individuals who engaged in therapeutic writing experienced more well-being and happiness (i.e., resilience) long after the experience. An example of this activity would involve writing a version of a story that typically produces anxiety and replacing it with a new example with a more positive interpretation. Reflecting on the process and outcomes of this storytelling activity can be useful in learning novel ways of dealing with multiple stressors in daily life.

The Upside of Stress Activity

McGonigal (2015) identifies that there is an upside of stress noting that seeing the good in stress can be valuable. In the book *The Upside of Stress,* McGonigal purports that considering the upside of stress is not an either/or regarding "good" or "bad" experiences, however, it means considering opportunities to stretch self, and use strengths to overcome barriers and obstacles. Reaching out and helping others can facilitate resiliency. McGonigal considers personal situations when individuals use personal crises to help others such as Mothers Against Drunk Drivers (MADD) by turning tragedy into learning ways to address traumatic events.

Perform Acts of Kindness Activities

Lyubomirsky et al.'s (2005) research revealed that one of the best strategies to boost happiness and resilience is to engage in acts of kindness such as mentoring, or expressing gratitude toward others. Activities that support acts of kindness, for example, include volunteering for a program that aligns with your values and selecting one person a day to show extra kindness (a word of thanks and encouragement). There are a number of examples of random acts of kindness including planting a tree, letting someone take your place in line, paying the toll for the car behind you, slowing down so someone can merge in front of you in traffic, giving someone your seat in a crowded bus or subway, and putting coins in an expired parking meter. Being mindful by paying attention, and living intentionally can increase our opportunities to engage in acts of kindness.

Gratitude Activities

Random acts of kindness and gratitude activities are EBPs that enhance resilience (Wood et al., 2010). Emmons and McCullough (2003) found that individuals who kept gratitude journals reported improved well-being. Examples include writing down three to five experiences each day that bring about gratitude, starting a gratitude blog or group text with friends, writing a letter of gratitude to people who are special to you, and intentionally sharing appreciation to those you encounter in your daily work. Journaling these actions can further enhance the positive benefits of experiencing well-being and positivity. Fredrickson (2009) purports to broaden-and-build theory approaches and that positive emotions can be useful in broadening momentary thoughts, actions, and attention to daily experiences. One example of this is to foster positive thoughts and emotions. In the book *Positivity*, Fredrickson recommends ending each day reflecting on and writing down three positive experiences and intentionally describing the experience noting feelings, and what was best about the activity, and lessons learned. The CNL can engage individuals and the team in finding the good in the most stressful situations, thus, this can become a group effort as one checks in with each other in daily work schedules.

Body Scan Activities

Body scan is one example of mindfulness meditation, centered on what we are experiencing at a physical level. It is a technique that focuses attention on different areas of the body to gain awareness of tense areas and optimizing positive sensations. Carmody and Baer (2008) report that practicing body scan techniques correlates with greater well-being and increases resilience. It is recommended that when beginning body scan meditation to start with 30 to 40 minutes and closing your eyes (or lowering or half-closing) for greater focus. The next step is to bring awareness to the body breathing in and out, noticing touch and pressure where it makes contact with the seat or floor. Throughout this practice, allow as much time as needed to experience and investigate each area of the body. When ready, intentionally breathe in, and move attention to whatever part of the body that may be particularly tight and tense. A body scan can be done systematically from head to toe, or in the reverse. When going through a body scan exercise, you may experience several sensations including buzzing, or tingling, pressure, tightness or temperature, or anything else noted. The main point is being curious and open to what one is noticing, investigating the sensations as fully as possible, and intentionally releasing the focus of attention before shifting to the next area to explore. It is not unusual for one's mind to wander when engaging in this intentional activity. Neuroscience implies that noticing drifting attention, and gently returning focus over and over, is how one creates new pathways in the brain. When finishing this exploration of bodily sensations, spend a few moments to expand attention to feeling the entire body breathing freely. If eyes have been closed, open them, and then move mindfully into this moment.

Measuring Resilience

Working to create a culture of resilience and to improve joy in work requires ways to measure progress made, and to guide efforts for sustainability. Self-assessment tools provide data that can provide opportunities for improvement and to direct future changes. These tools are a sampling of instruments that can assess several characteristics of healthy work environments including positive qualities such as resilience and well-being, as well as burnout and stress. As described throughout the chapter, resilience can be defined in several ways, and there is no single agreed on set of characteristics. Optimism, moral compass, humor, meaning or purpose in life, and adaptation are linked to resiliency. These qualities would promote healthy work environments. CNLs are positioned to impact healthy and joyful workplaces guided by competency-based education and immersion experiences. Academic-clinical partnerships underscore educational and practice opportunities. For example, Essential 2, "Organizational and Systems Leadership," considers systems theory in the assessment, design, delivery, and evaluation of healthcare within complex organizations, which also supports collaboration with healthcare professionals, including physicians, advanced practice nurses, nurse managers, and others, to plan, implement, and evaluate an improvement opportunity. Guided by this Essential, CNLs have active involvement in cocreating a resilient workforce to deal with rapid cycle changes for sustainable and innovative outcomes. Another example includes Essential 3, "Quality Improvement and Safety," which promotes using performance measures to assess and improve the delivery of evidence-based practices and outcomes that demonstrate delivery of higher-value care.

Several tools that measure resiliency can be useful when CNLs are focused on creating joyful work environments. The following three instruments are described next.

Connor-Davidson Resilience Scale (CD-RISC)

Windle and colleagues (2011) reviewed 19 resilience measures, and out of these, only 3 received superior psychometric ratings. The Connor-Davidson Resilience Scale (CD-RISC) grew out of this work, which was originally developed by Davidson (2018) as a self-report measure of resilience within the PTSD clinical community (CD-RISC, n.d.). Specifically, it was a validated and widely recognized scale with 2, 10, and 25 items that measured resilience as a function of five interrelated components: personal competence, acceptance of change and secure relationships, trust/tolerance/strengthening effects of stress, control, and spiritual influences. Much research has reported using this tool within a varied range of populations.

The CD-RISC is considered one of the higher scoring scales in the psychometric evaluation of resilience (Windle et al., 2011).

Resilience Scale for Adults (RSA)

Authored by Friborg et al. (2003), the Resilience Scale for Adults (RSA) is a resilience tool highly rated by Windle and colleagues (2011). The RSA is a self-report scale focused on adults and suggested for use in the health and clinical psychology population. Specifically, the RSA examines both the intrapersonal and interpersonal protective qualities that foster adaptation to adversity. Friborg et al. (2003) identify that the key factors contributing to highly resilient individuals are family support and cohesion, external support systems, and dispositional attitudes and behaviors. The scale items are founded on and include: personal competence, social competence, support, family coherence, and personal structure. In their later work, Friborg et al. (2005) used the RSA to measure the relationship among personality, intelligence, and resilience in which many links between personality and resilience factors were aligned. The authors noted a connection between higher personal competence and elevated emotional stability. There was no statistical significance correlated with cognitive ability (Friborg et al., 2005). Windle et al. (2011) reported that the RSA is extremely useful for assessing the protective factors that inhibit or provide a buffer against psychological disorders.

Net Promoter Score (NPS)

Measuring work engagement is important to a resilient workforce. The Net Promoter Score (NPS), originally devised by *Harvard Business Review* in 2003 to assess whether customer engagement is adaptable to measuring internal team members' engagement (Reichheld, 2003). By asking individuals if they would recommend an organization as a place to work (0–10 scale; 0 suggests warning others away from applying and 10 suggesting to apply immediately). Using the NPS, scores of 0 to 6 indicate detractors, 7 and 8 passives, and 9 and 10 promoters. When responses have been collected, calculate the internal NPS (NPS = [# of promoters – # of detractors] / total # of respondents). Results can be shared and provide an excellent opportunity to begin the conversation about engagement. This is a good tool to use when a healthcare system is considering one overall measure of joy in work and could be a good measure to track because it provides a perspective of how employees view organizations.

Brief Resilience Scale (BRS)

Many resilience assessment instruments explore the factors and quality in which to develop resilience. A self-rating questionnaire centered on measuring an individual's ability to manage stress and bounce back is the Brief Resilience Scale (BRS). Smith et al. (2008) developed a scale that has not been used in the clinical population, however, could provide some critical perspectives for individuals with health-related stress. According to Amat et al. (2014), the BRS tool consists of six items, three positively stated questions and three negatively worded questions; however, all six items relate to an individual's ability to bounce back from adversity. Smith et al. (2008) when developing their scale specifically controlled for protective factors such as social support to get a reliable resilience measure. This instrument is also considered to be a highly valid and reliable measure of resilience by Windle et al. (2011) and an effective instrument to measure an individual's ability to deal with adversity.

Daily Visual Measure

Measuring joy in the workplace can be completed in real time. Developed by the IHI, this daily visual measure uses a glass jar placed by the elevator or breakroom in which team members drop one marble each day. A blue marble signifies a good day, where the individual made progress, or a tan marble for a day without progress. The number of blue and tan marbles are tracked for a total count, and a quick glance at the jar provides a visual measure of the daily mood of the unit or microsystem. CNLs can use this data to assess if there is joy in the workplace, particularly over time. This is a quick, real-time measurement that can be used to engage staff in a daily assessment of their work environment. Another simple visual measurement, like the marble jar, can be a whiteboard with two columns (smiling face and frowning face) where staff indicate their joy in work each day by putting a checkmark in the appropriate column. This also provides quick, daily perspective in real time that can provide an excellent way to engage team members in creating healthy work environments (IHI, 2017).

Maintaining Healthy Work Environments During a Pandemic

There has been much reported on the uncertainty, miscommunication, burnout, and overwhelming stress and burnout of frontline workers. Much attention has been given to providing opportunities to build a culture of resiliency and joy at work despite the adversity being experienced. CNLs and nurse leaders are strategically positioned to coach for resiliency by offering tools, strategies, and interventions that focus on individuals' needs as well as engaging the team in positive communication through role modeling and authentic and servant leadership.

Summary

- Joy in the workplace is essential to self-care and quality patient care.
- Resilience is a key concept in healthy work environments.
- It is important that personal and systems strategies align to maintain a culture of health and well-being.
- Authentic leadership is essential to fostering joyful workplaces.
- Organizational leaders can foster resilience by using resiliency tools and measurement strategies to enhance healthy and joyful work environments.
- Evidence-based initiatives that support healthy work environments are available and can be useful in putting together resources in building resiliency and joyful workplaces.
- Identifying resiliency strategies that become part of your self-care practice, and routines can foster a more focused and centered life that can add to work-life balance.

- Mindful and intentional practice combined with self-awareness can be aligned to enhance grit and mental toughness.
- Engaging in resilience activities can foster self-care practices that add to quality of life and work-life balance.
- Measuring resilience through a variety of tools and instruments helps organizational leaders to evaluate levels of joy in work and assess the impact of their improvement efforts in building positive work environments and a resilient workforce.

Reflection Questions

1. Do a scan of your workplace to determine if there are daily practices that support joy in the workplace. Based on your assessment, are you noting a culture of health and well-being? If not, what changes would you make? How would you lead these efforts? How would you measure your improvement efforts?
2. How can CNLs promote healthy work environments? How would you lead this initiative?
3. Describe leadership's role in promoting the healthy nurse.

Learning Activities

1. Using the IHI Framework for Improving Joy in Work, consider step 1: Ask staff, "What matters to you?" How would you prepare for these conversations? What communication skills would you reinforce as you engage staff in understanding primary concerns and potential barriers to joy at work.
2. Consider the ANA's Healthy Nurse, Healthy Nation campaign, how would the CNL use the Nurses Bill of Rights, the seven basic principles concerning workplace expectations and environments, to promote a positive workplace that provides physical and psychological safety?

References

Amat, S., Subhan, M., Jaafar, W. M. W., Mahmud, Z., & Johari, K. S. K. (2014). Evaluation and psychometric status of the Brief Resilience Scale in a sample of Malaysian international students. *Asian Social Science, 10,* 240–245. https://doi.org/10.5539/ass.v10n1

American Association of Colleges of Nursing. (2011). *The essentials of master's education in nursing.* http://www.aacn.nche.edu/educationresources/MastersEssentials11.pdf

American Association of Colleges of Nursing. (2013). *Competencies and curricular expectations for clinical nurse leader education and practice.* https://www.aacnnursing.org/Portals/42/AcademicNursing/CurriculumGuidelines/CNL-Competencies-October-2013.pdf

American Nurses Association. (2017a). *Exploring moral resilience toward a culture of ethical practice.* https://www.nursingworld.org/geinvolved/share-yourexpertise/proissues-panel/moral-resilience-panel/

American Nurses Association (2017b). *A call to action: Exploring moral resilience toward a culture of ethical practice.* https://www.nursingworld.org/~4907b6/globalassets/docs/ana/ana-call-to-action-exploring-moral-resilience-final.pdf

Bajaj, B., & Pande, N. (2015). Mediating role of resilience in the impact of mindfulness on life satisfaction and affect as indices of subjective well-being. *Personality and Individual Difference, 93,* 63–67. https://doi.org/10.1016/j.paid.2015.09.005

Bernard, N. (2019). Resilience and professional joy: A toolkit for nurse leaders. *Nurse Leader, 17*(1), 43–48.

Boyle, P. A., Buchman, A. S., Wilson, R. S., Yu, L., Schneider, J. A., & Bennett, D. A. (2012). Effect of purpose in life on the relation between Alzheimer disease pathologic changes on cognitive function in advanced age. *Archives of General Psychiatry, 69*(5), 499–505. https://doi .org/10.1001/archgenpsychiatry.2011.1487

Brown, S., Whichello, R., & Price, S. (2018). The impact of resiliency on nurse burnout: An integrative literature review. *MedSurg Nursing, 27*(6), 349–378.

Carmody, J., & Baer, R. A. (2008). Relationships between mindfulness practice and levels of mindfulness, medical and psychological symptoms and well-being in a mindfulness-based stress reduction program. *Journal of behavioral medicine, 31*(1), 23–33. https://doi.org/10.1007 /s10865-007-9130-710.1007/s10865-007-9130-7

Centers for Disease Control. (2018). *Well-being concepts: HRQOL.* https://www.cdc.gov/hrqol /wellbeing.html

Chau, J. P. C., Lo, S. H. S., Choi, K. C., Chan, E. L. S., McHugh, M. D., Tong, D. W. K., & Lee, D. T. F. (2015). A longitudinal examination of the association between nurse staffing levels, the practice environment and nurse-sensitive patient outcomes in hospitals. *BMC Health Services Research, 15*, 538. https://doi.org/10.1186/ s12913-015-1198-0

Chesak, S. S., Cutshall, S. M., Bowe, C. L., Montanari, K. M., & Bhagra, A. (2019). Stress management interventions for nurses: Critical literature review. *Journal of Holistic Nursing, 37*(3), 288–295. https://doi.org/10.1177/0898010119842693

Cimiotti, J. P., Aiken, L. H., Sloane, D. M., & Wu, E. S. (2012). Nurse staffing, burnout, and health care associated infection. *American Journal of Infection Control, 40*(6), 486–490. https:// doi.org/10.1016/j.ajic.2012.02.029

Christodoulou-Fella, M., Middleton, N., Papathanassoglou, E. D. E., & Karanikola, M. N. K. (2017). Exploration of the association between nurses' moral distress and secondary traumatic stress syndrome: Implications for patient safety in mental health services. *BioMed Research International, 2017*, 1–19. https://doi.org/10.1155/2017/1908712

Cleary, M., Kornhaber, R., Thapa, D. K., West, S., & Visentin, D. (2018). The effectiveness of interventions to improve resilience among health professionals: A systematic review. *Nurse Education Today, 71*, 247–263. https://doi.org/10.1016/j.nedt.2018.10.002

Cohen, J. K. (2019, August 17). How bad is the nursing shortage? *Modern Healthcare.* https://www .modernhealthcare.com/labor/how-bad-nursing shortage

Connor, K. M., &, Davidson, J. R. (2003). Development of a new resilience scale: The Connor-Davidson Resilience Scale (CD-RISC). *Depression and Anxiety, 18*(2), 76–82. https:// doi.org/10.1002/da.10113

Davidson, J. (2018). *The Connor-Davidson Resilience Scale (CD-RISC).* http://www. connordavidson -resiliencescale.com/faq.php

Davidson, J. E., Zisook, S., Kirby, B., DeMichele, G., & Norcross, W. (2018). Suicide prevention: A healer education and referral program for nurses. *Journal of Nursing Administration, 48*(2), 85–92. https://doi.org/10.1097/NNA.0000000000000582

Davidson, J., Mendis, A. R., Stuck, G., DeMichele, G., & Zisook, S. (2018). Nurse suicide: Breaking the silence. *NAM Perspectives. Discussion Paper.* National Academy of Medicine. https://doi .org/10.31478/201801a

Delgado, C., Roche, M., Fethney, J., & Foster, K. (2019). Workplace resilience and emotional labour of Australian mental health nurses: Results of a national survey. *International Journal of Mental Health Nursing, 29* (1), 35–46. https://doi.org/10.1111/inm.12598

Delgado, C., Upton, D., Ranse, K., Furness, T., & Foster, K. (2017). Nurses' resilience and the emotional labour of nursing work: An integrative review of empirical literature. *International Journal of Nursing Studies, 70*, 71–88. https://doi.org/ 10.1016/j.ijnurstu.2017.02.008

Emmons, R. A., &, McCullough, M. E. (2003). Counting blessings versus burdens: An experimental investigation of gratitude and subjective well-being in daily life. *Journal of Perspectives of Social Psychology, 84*(2), 377–389. https://doi.org/10.1037/0022-3514.84.2.377

Flinkman, M., & Salantera, S. (2015). Early career experiences and perceptions—A qualitative exploration of the turnover of young registered nurses and intention to leave the nursing profession in Finland. *Journal of Nursing Management, 23*(8), 1050–1057. https://doi.org/10.1111 /jonm.12251

Foureur, M., Besley, K., Burton, G., Yu, N., & Crisp, J. (2013). Enhancing the resilience of nurses and midwives: pilot of a mindfulness-based program for increased health, sense of coherence and decreased depression, anxiety and stress. *Contemporary nurse, 45*(1), 114–125. https://doi .org/10.5172/conu.2013.45.1.114

Fredrickson, B. (2009). *Positivity: Groundbreaking research reveals how to embrace the hidden strength of positive emotions, overcome negativity, and thrive.* Crown Publishers/Random House.

Friborg, O., Hjemdal, O., Rosenvinge, J. H., & Martinussen, M. (2003). A new rating scale for adult resilience: What are the central protective resources behind healthy adjustment? *International Journal of Methods in Psychiatric Research, 12,* 65–76. https://doi.org/10.1002 /mpr.143

Friborg, O., Barlaug, D., Martinussen, M., Rosenvinge, J. H., & Hjemdal, O. (2005). Resilience in relation to personality and intelligence. International Journal of Methods of Psychiatric Research, (14) 1, 29–42. https://doi.org/10.1002/mpr.15Grabee, L., Higgins, M. K., Baird, M., Craven, P. A., & Fratello, S. S. (2020). The community resiliency model to promote nurse well-being, *Nursing Outlook, 68*(3), 324–336. https://doi.org/10.1016/j.outlook.2019.11.002

Hamby, S., Grych, J., & Banyard, V. (2018). Resilience portfolios and poly-strengths: Identifying protective factors associated with thriving after adversity. *Psychology of Violence, 8*(2), 172–183. https://doi.org/10.1037/vio0000135

Hatler, C., & Sturgeon, P. (2013). Resilience building: A necessary leadership competence. *Nurse Leader, 11*(4), 32–34, 39.

Lee, K. J., Forbes, M. L., Lukasiewicz, G. J., Williams, T., Sheets, A., Fischer, K., & Niedner, M. F. (2015). Promoting Staff Resilience in the Pediatric Intensive Care Unit. *American journal of critical care: an official publication, American Association of Critical-Care Nurses, 24*(5), 422–430. https://doi.org/10.4037/ajcc2015720

Letvak, S. A., Ruhm, C. J., & Gupta, S. N. (2012). Original research: Nurses' presenteeism and its effects on self-reported quality of care and costs. *American Journal of Nursing, 112*(2), 30. https:// doi.org/10.1097/01.NAJ.0000411176.15696.f9

Lucian Leape Institute. (2013). Through the eyes of the workforce: Creating joy, meaning, and safer health care. *National Patient Safety Foundation.*

Lyubomirsky, S., Sheldon, K. M., & Schkade, D. (2005). Pursuing happiness: The architecture of sustainable change. *Review of General Psychology, 9*(2), 111–131. https://doi.org /10.1037/1089-2680.9.2.111

Mcdonald, G., Jackson, D., Vickers, M. H., & Wilkes, L. (2016). Surviving workplace adversity: A qualitative study of nurses and midwives and their strategies to increase personal resilience. *Journal of Nursing Management, 24*(1), 123–131. https://doi.org/10.1111/jonm.12293

McGonigal, K. (2015). *The upside of stress: Why stress is good for you, and how to get good at it.* Penguin Random House.

Mindfulness. (n.d.). *Body scanning for beginners.* https://www.mindful.org/beginners-body-scan -meditation/

Pennebaker, J. W., Kiecolt-Glaser, J. K., & Glaser, R. (1988). Disclosure of traumas and immune function: Health implications for psychotherapy. *Journal of Consulting and Clinical Psychology, 56,* 239–245.

Perlo, J., Balik, B., Swensen, S., Kabcenell, A., Landsman, J., & Feeley, D. (2017). *IHI Framework for Improving Joy in Work* [White paper]. Institute for Healthcare Improvement. http://www.ihi.org /resources/Pages/IHIWhitePapers/Framework-Improving Joy-in-Work.aspx

Pipe, T. B., Buchda, V. L., Launder, S., Hudak, B., Hulvey, L., Karns, K. E., & Pendergast, D. (2012). Building personal and professional resources of resilience and agility in the healthcare workplace: Building resilience. *Stress and Health, 28*(1), 11–22. https://doi.org/10.1002/smi.1396

Reichheld, F. F. (2003). The one number you need to grow. *Harvard Business Review.* https://hbr .org/2003/12/the-one-number-you-need-to-grow

Reith, T. P. (2018). Burnout in United States Healthcare Professionals: A Narrative Review. *Cureus, 10*(12), e3681. https://doi.org/10.7759/cureus.3681

Rizzo, L. H. (2018). Suicide among nurses: What we do not know might hurt us. *American Nurse Today, 13*(10), 10–15.

Rushton, C. H., Batcheller, J., Schroeder, K., & Donohue, P. (2015). Burnout and resilience among nurses practicing in high-intensity settings. *American Journal of Critical Care, 24*(5), 412–420.

Shanafelt, T. D., Dyrbye, L. N., & West, C. P. (2017). Addressing physician burnout: The way forward. *JAMA, 317*(9), 901–902. https://doi.org/10.1001/jama.2017.0076.

Shanafelt, T. D., Hasan, O., Dyrbye, L. N., Sinsky, C., Satele, D., Sloan, S., & West, C. P. (2015). Changes in burnout and satisfaction with work-life balance in physicians and the general US working population between 2011 and 2014. *Mayo Clinic Proceedings, 90*(12), 1600–1613.

Smith, B. W., Dalen, J., Wiggins, K., Tooley, E., Christopher, P., & Bernard, J. (2008). The brief resilience scale: assessing the ability to bounce back. *International Journal of Behavioral Medicine, 15*(3), 194–200.

Stephens, T. M., Smith, P., & Cherry, C. (2017). Promoting resilience in new perioperative nurses. *AORN Journal, 105*(3), 276–284. https://doi.org/10.1016/j.aorn.2016.12.019

Taylor, R. A. (2019). Contemporary issues: Resilience training alone is an incomplete intervention. *Nurse Education Today, 78,* 10–13. https://doi.org/10.1016/j.nedt.2019.03.014.

Taylor, S. E., Klein, L. C., Lewis, B. P., Gruenewald, T. L., Gurung, R. A. R., & Updegraff, J. A. (2000). Biobehavioral responses to stress in females: Tend-and-befriend, not fight-or-flight. *Psychological Review, 107,* 411–429.

Tubbert, S. J. (2016). Resiliency in emergency nurses. *Journal of Emergency Nursing, 42*(1), 47–52. https://doi.org/10.1016/j.jen.2015.05.016

Turner, S. (2014). The resilient nurse: An emerging concept. *Nurse Leader, 12*(6), 71–73, 90.

Virkstis, K., Herleth, A., & Langr, M. (2018). Cracks in the foundation of the care environment undermine nurse resilience. *The Journal of Nursing Administration, 48*(12), 597–599. https://doi.org/10.1097/NNA.0000000000000687

Wicks, R. J., & Buck, T. C. (2013). Riding the dragon: Enhancing resilient leadership and sensible self-care in the healthcare executive. *Frontiers in Health Services Management, 30*(2), 3–13.

Windle, G., Bennett, K. M., & Noyes, J. (2011). A methodological review of resilience measurement scales. *Health Quality of Life Outcomes, 4*(9), 8. https://doi.org/10.1186/1477-7525-9-8

Wood, A. M., Froh, J. J., & Geraghty, A. W. (2010). Gratitude and well-being: A review and theoretical integration. *Clinical Psychology Review, 30*(7), 890–905. https://doi.org/10.1016/j.cpr.2010.03.005

EXEMPLAR

The CNL's Role in Building Resilience

Linda A. Roussel

Within healthcare, individuals have faced adversity in a variety of forms such as a pandemic, limited resources, long work hours, and situations that cause moral distress. How individuals deal with that adversity impacts not only psychological health, overall health, and well-being, but also one's joy or satisfaction in work. Resiliency is needed to be able to overcome stress using both internal and external coping strategies. Without resiliency, individuals may experience increased psychological stress, job dissatisfaction, breakdowns in relationships, and burnout.

Working with CNLs, it is evident that they are pivotal to healthy work environments within systems for sustainable effectiveness. The CNL is frequently key in identification of stress and lack of resiliency through coordinating and collaborative roles with nursing staff and patients. The CNL may be tasked with the implementation of strategies that could reduce such stress and build resilience. As such, it is essential the CNL understands this phenomenon and the impact a lack of resiliency has on both nursing and the healthcare environment. Evidence-based strategies to build resilience are essential in improving well-being of nurses, including the CNL, as well as the care delivery for patients.

Index

Note: Page numbers followed by b, f, or t indicate material in boxes, figures, or tables respectively.

A

AACN. *See* American Association of Colleges of Nursing
ACA. *See* Affordable Care Act
access, 348, 350
accountability, 141, 143
accountable care team (ACT), 207
ACT. *See* accountable care team
acute care setting, health promotion in, 268–269
acute delirium interventions, 249
Adult Stem Cell Transplant, 85
advanced master's-prepared generalist, 60
Advanced Practice Providers (APP), 60
advanced practice registered nurse (APRN), 31
advocacy, 347
    defined, 173–174, 385
    in health policy, 392–393
Affordable Care Act (ACA), 44–45, 48, 95
Agency for Healthcare Research and Quality (AHRQ), 41
AGREE II. *See* Appraisal of Guidelines Research and Evaluation II
AHRQ. *See* Agency for Healthcare Research and Quality
algorithm, 295
AMA. *See* American Medical Association
ambulatory care, 171–172
ambulatory heart failure clinic, 377–378
American Association of Colleges of Nursing (AACN)
    assumptions for CNL practice, 2
    assumptions for preparing CNLs, 21, 39–40
    healthy work environment, 412
American Medical Association (AMA), 234
American Society for Healthcare Risk Management (ASHRM), 68
AMSTAR. *See* Assessment of Multiple Systematic Reviews
antibiotic stewardship program (ASP), 97

APP. *See* Advanced Practice Providers
Appraisal of Guidelines Research and Evaluation II (AGREE II), 234
apprentice, 196
APRN. *See* advanced practice registered nurse
ASHRM. *See* American Society for Healthcare Risk Management
ASP. *See* antibiotic stewardship program
assessment
    5 P, 255–258, 256–257f
    microsystem, 254–255
Assessment of Multiple Systematic Reviews (AMSTAR), 238, 239–240t
at-the-elbow, 83
attitude, 397
authentic leadership, 412
autonomy, 410, 413

B

bachelor's degree in nursing (BSN), 172
bar chart, 284
bed safety alarms, 163
bedside handoff, 53–54
Behavioral Pain Scale (BPS), 89–90
Better Outcomes for Older Adults through Safe Transitions (BOOST), 175, 321–322
big data, 272–273, 278
body scan, 417–418
BOOST. *See* Better Outcomes for Older Adults through Safe Transitions
BPS. *See* Behavioral Pain Scale
break buddy system, 339–340
Bridge Model, 175
Brief Resilience Scale (BRS), 419–420
The British Journal of Clinical Pharmacology, 57
BRS. *See* Brief Resilience Scale
BSN. *See* bachelor's degree in nursing
building alliances, 130–132
business models, 220–221, 221t

C

California Maternal Quality Care
     Collaborative Toolkit (CMQCC), 99
capability beliefs, 229
care
   coordination, 317
     CNL role in, 326–329
     defined, 314
     reuniting families, 329–331
   improvement and timely implementation,
     273–274
care transition, 316. *See also* transitional
     care
   models
     Better Outcomes for Older Adults
       through Safe Transitions, 321–322
     Interventions to Reduce Acute Care
       Transfers, 322–323
     Project Re-Engineered
       Discharge, 322
     nursing initiative to improve patient's,
       332–333
     re-admission reduction, 333–335
Care Transitions Intervention (CTI), 175
Carolinas Medical Center (CMC), 61
case management, 317
Catheter-associated urinary tract infections
     (CAUTI), 82–83
causation, 274
CAUTI. *See* Catheter-associated urinary tract
     infections
CDS. *See* clinical decision support
Centers for Medicare and Medicaid Services
     (CMS), 4–5, 95–96
central line associated bloodstream infection
     (CLABSI), 84, 91, 92
certification, 396–397
CFIR. *See* consolidated framework for
     implementation research
change
   in insulin delivery, 357–358
   types of, 385–386
chaos, 362
character, 397
charts, types of, 284–285
CHG. *See* chlorhexidine gluconate
chlorhexidine gluconate (CHG), 91, 92
CICI framework. *See* Context and
     Implementation of Complex
     Interventions framework
CLABSI. *See* central line associated
     bloodstream infection
clinical decision support (CDS), 132,
     297–298
clinical engagement, 367

clinical immersion
   data and resources to craft meaningful,
     217–219, 218*t*, 220*f*
   examples of, 206–207
   impact on healthcare system, 206–207
   intention of, 216–217
   performance contract, 222, 223*f*
   portfolios, usefulness of, 221–222
   projects, developing meaningful and
     sustainable, 200–206
     developing step-by-step time line,
       205–206
     identifying and selecting plan, 201–204
     setting measurable and attainable goals,
       204–205
     summarize findings and results, 206
   success, measurement of, 222–223
clinical leadership
   behaviors, 365–366
   need for, 364–365
   through team science, 371
Clinical Nurse Leader (CNL)
   in action, 371
   as advocate in end-of-life care delivery,
     191–192
   ambulatory care, 171–172
   certification, 396–397
   clinical immersions, applying business
     model to, 220–221, 221*t*
   CNLA, 403–404
   and CNS, 210–211, 308
   community networks, 171–172
   competencies to community, 331–332
   curriculum framework, 398*f*, 399*t*
   for diabetes, 310
   effective communication, 338–339
   engagement in health policy, 383–393
   improvement and timely implementation,
     273–274
   informatics competencies, 295–296
     clinical decision support, 297–298
     communicating and disseminating
       healthcare information, 298–299
     understanding and evaluating data, 298
     use of technology to support patient
       care, 297
   lateral integration, 338–339
   learning environment, 199–200
   less is not always more, 210
   lifelong learning, 199–200
   as mentor, 211–212
   and microsystem assessment, 266–268
     on trauma unit, 379–381
   in networking and advocacy, tools and
     models for
     discharge planning, 174

epidemiological triad, 175–176
interprofessional team building, 175
mind maps, 177, 178f
natural history of disease model,
    176–177
transition care model, 175
nurse empowerment through, 405–406
partnerships for patient quality and safety,
    309–310
as patient and family advocate, 190–191
performance contract, 222, 223f
preceptor role satisfaction on dedicated
    education unit, 212–213
preceptorship, 209–210
preparation of, 171
professional development, 402–403
professionalism, 397–398
in public health practice, 356–357
requirements for successful immersion
    experience, 197–199
role, 39–40
    advocate, 60
    in ambulatory heart failure clinic,
        377–378
    in building resilience, 424
    care coordination, 326–329
    catalyst, 60
    CMC, 61
    decreasing CAUTI in the ICU, 156–158
    in optimizing care, 327–328
    outcomes manager, 60
    PTN, 58
    risk anticipator, 60
    supply management, 50
    in transitions of care, 314–315
simulation exercise, 305–306
success, measurement of, 222–223
system-wide implementation of mobility
    program, 381–382
tools of trade (case study), 183–184
transition to practice, 398–402,
    400–402t
using informatics and healthcare
    technologies to guide, 307–308
utilizing informatics to improve patient
    outcomes, 306–307
Clinical Nurse Leader Association (CNLA),
    206, 403–404
clinical nurse specialist (CNS), 2
    and CNL, 2, 210–211
clinical project, selling your idea for, 226
CMC. See Carolinas Medical Center
CMQCC. See California Maternal Quality
    Care Collaborative Toolkit
CMS. See Centers for Medicare and Medicaid
    Services

CNL. See Clinical Nurse Leader
CNL clinical immersion experience, 77
CNL education, future implications, 5–6
CNL practice
    AACN assumptions, 2
    actionable result, 4
    defining aspects, 3
    disruptive forces, 3–4
    fundamental aspects of, 25–26,
        27–28t
    future implications, 5–6
    healthcare technologies, 24
    model, developing of, 9–10
    peaceful revolution of, 6–7
    role transitions, 10–11
    stroke and, 11–17
    Wakefield's statement of, 4
CNL praxis, 24–25, 25f
CNL skill set/pandemic, 137–138
CNLA. See Clinical Nurse Leader
    Association
CNS. See clinical nurse specialist
coaching, 413
Coleman's model, 175
collaboration, 20, 24, 32–34, 36, 219, 408,
    409, 412, 418
collaboration team improvement
    description, 140–141
    multidisciplinary, 150–151
    in obstetrics, 160–162
    patient outcomes, impact on, 149–150
    and safety, 163
column chart, 284
communication
    and conflict management, 137
    SBAR, 142
    wireless, 158
community assessment, 179, 180b
community-based wound care integration,
    184–186
community network, 171–173
Community Resiliency Model (CRM),
    409–410
competency, 397
complex adaptive system, 124
complex care, pain and, 337
complex medical care, 355–356
complexity, 173, 362
comprehensive assessment, 319
computerized provider order entry (CPOE),
    299
conduct, 397
Connor-Davidson Resilience Scale (CD-RISC),
    418–419
consolidated framework for implementation
    research (CFIR), 116, 118

contemporary leadership theories, 367
  servant leadership, 367–369
    awareness, 368
    building community, 369
    commitment to growth of people, 369
    conceptualization, 368
    empathy, 368
    foresight, 368
    healing, 368
    listening, 368
    persuasion, 368
    stewardship, 369
  transactional leadership, 369–370
  transformational leadership, 369–370
Context and Implementation of Complex
    Interventions (CICI) framework, 26
continuum of care, 160–162
core competencies, for evidence-based
    practice, 229–230
correctional healthcare facility, 163
correlation, 280–282
cost-savings initiative, 244
COVID-19 pandemic, 22, 24, 35, 137–138,
    294, 351, 413
CPOE. *See* computerized provider order entry
CRM. *See* Community Resiliency Model
cross-continuum care, need for, 336–337
CTI. *See* Care Transitions Intervention
culture of quality, safety, and value, CNLs
    creating
  aim or purpose, definition of, 71
  closing the loop, 101–102
  CNL role, 69–70
  counting on moms, 99–100
  critically Ill oncology patient, pressure
    ulcers in, 87–88
  culture of safety, 67
  design thinking, 72–73
  ED, 90–91
  electrolyte boluses, 88–89
  evidence-based practice, 69–70, 82–83
  facilitate improvement, resources to, 72
  hourly rounding initiative, 92–93
  ICU, evidence-based practice in, 89–90
  improving fall outcomes, 100–101
  innovation/collaboration, 84–85
  interleukin (IL-2), 86
  literature, review of, 71
  looking for risk, 84
  mapping current processes, 72
  measures and metrics, 73–74
  microsystems, 74–75
    assessment of, 75
  philosophical elements of quality
    improvement, 70–71
  quality improvement, 69–71, 77–78, 83–84

    initiatives, systematic and purposeful
        identification of, 75–76
    projects, 76
  rapid cycle review, 74
  reducing readmissions, 95–97
  risk anticipation, 68–69
  risk assessment, 68–69
  risk management, 68–69
  root-cause analysis (RCA), 73
  secretarial daily rounding, 93–94
  sepsis, 97–99
  spectrum of value, 78
  stem cell transplant (SCT), 91–92
  team, hardwiring hourly rounding, 85–86
  team leader tools for success, 76–77
  tools, 73
  trauma tracheostomy patients, 94–95
  VTE prevention and *outcomes*, 82
culture of safety, 67, 102
customer obsession, 363

D

daily visual measure, 420
data, 298
  additional consideration, 276–277
  analysis, 278
    correlation, 280–282, 281*f*, 282*t*
    presentation, 283–284, 283–284*f*
    statistical significance, tests of,
        278–280, 279*f*
    to craft meaningful clinical immersions,
        217–219, 218*t*, 220*f*
    process and solution, 274–276, 275–276*f*
    uses of, 276
deep-tissue injury (DTI), 87
define, measure, analyze, improve, control
    (DMAIC), 153
delivery model, transformation and quality
    improvement in, 359
destination, 170
discharge planning, 174, 317
discipline of nursing, 106
disease management, 317
DMAIC. *See* define, measure, analyze,
    improve, control
DTI. *See* deep-tissue injury

E

EBM. *See* evidence-based medicine
Ebola, 22, 23
EBP. *See* evidence-based practice
EBP core competency

assemble evidence resources from multiple sources on selected topics into reference management software, 240–241

critically appraise evidence summaries for practice implications, 234–240, 235–238*t*, 239–240*t*

exhaustive search for external evidence to answer clinical questions, 230–231, 231*f*

locate evidence summary reports for practice implications, 231, 232–233*t*

ED. *See* emergency department

effective communication, 128–130, 135–136

EHR. *See* electronic health record

electrolyte imbalance, 88

electronic health record (EHR), 89, 291
maturity, 293

emergency department (ED), 52, 98, 137
communication and handoff in, 338
post-discharge calls in, 264–266

Emergent change, 386

emotional intelligence, 140–141, 145, 387

empathy, 145

end-of-life care, 187–188

end-of-life care delivery, 191–192

engagement
defined, 385
in health policy, 392–393

enterprise risk management (ERM), 68

entrepreneur, 170

epidemiological triad, 175–176

ERM. *See* enterprise risk management

Essential 3, 272

Essential 4, 272

Essential 8, 315

Essentials of Master's Education in Nursing, 105

evaluation, of improvement plan, 262

evidence-based medicine (EBM), 42–43

evidence-based practice (EBP), 22, 23, 39, 40, 71, 112, 116, 118, 245–246, 255, 362, 364, 367, 371, 387, 388
early referral to palliative care, 353–354
improving patient medication education using, 247–248

excellence, 397

experimental failure, 363

F

falls and interdisciplinary team, 153–154

fiscal year to date (FYTD), 49–50

5 P assessment, 216, 255–258, 256–257*f*

Food and Drug Administration, 65

FYTD. *See* fiscal year to date

G

gap analysis, 219

gastroparesis, 84

geriatric population, 152–153

Geriatric Resources for Assessment and Care of Elders (GRACE), 175

GLIA. *See* GuideLine Implementability Appraisal v.2.0

global community, clinical nurse leaders
best practice, challenges of, 22
CNL competencies, 25–28, 26*f*, 27–28*t*
CNL praxis, 24–25, 25*f*
digital health, 24
engaging with international partners, 36
humanitarian and health crisis, 22–23
international partners, microsystem-macrosystem interfaces, 32–34
Japanese nurses, 31–32
CNL certification of, 34–35
models and frameworks, 23–24

glycemic control, 166–167
improving, 269–270

GRACE. *See* Geriatric Resources for Assessment and Care of Elders

GRADE approach. *See* Grading of Recommendations Assessment, Development and Evaluation approach

Grading of Recommendations Assessment, Development and Evaluation (GRADE) approach, 234–235

gratitude, 417

Guided Care, 175

GuideLine Implementability Appraisal v.2.0 (GLIA), 234

H

HAIs. *See* healthcare-associated infections; hospital-acquired infections

HAPUs. *See* hospital-acquired pressure ulcers

HCAHPS. *See* Hospital Consumer Assessment of Healthcare Providers and Systems

Health Care at the Crossroads: Guiding Principles for the Development of the Hospital of the Future, 65

health disparities, 22

Health Information Technology for Economic and Clinical Health (HITECH) Act, 292

health IT, 291
  barriers to adoption, 291–292
  emerging tools and applications
    algorithms/machine-learning
      models, 295
    mobile health, 294
    patient education and engagement, 294
    tablets, 293–294
    telehealth, 294
health literacy-language barrier, 358–359
health of communities, 348–350
health policy
  advocacy, 392–393
  defined, 384–385
  engagement, 392–393
  trends and impacts of, 388–390
  unintended consequences of, 387–388
health promotion
  in acute care setting, 268–269, 360
  overview, 347
healthcare-associated infections (HAIs),
      155–156
Healthcare Environment Job Satisfaction
      Survey (HES), 33
Healthcare Information and Management
      Systems Society (HIMSS), 293
healthcare information, communicating and
      disseminating, 298–299
healthcare technology, 366
  IT role in, 291
  for safe and cost-effective care, 310–311
Healthy Nurse, Healthy Nation Grand
      Challenge (HNHN), 411–412
Healthy People 2020, 348
Healthy People 2030, 348
Healthy People initiative, 347–348
healthy work environments, 408–409
  AACN's work on, 412
  defined, 413
  national and international initiatives, 410
  during pandemic, 420
HES. See Healthcare Environment Job
      Satisfaction Survey
high-reliability and value-added outcomes,
      CNL microsystem leadership for
  CNL vs. advanced practice provider, 60–61
  CNL's role, 39–40
  evidence-based practice, 42–43
  healthcare economics, 44–45
  high-reliability organizations, 40–42
  hospital-acquired vancomycin-resistant
      enterococcus, 54–55
  intensive care unit, resource management
      in, 48–50
  medication administration errors, 57–58
  microsystem, 61–62

patient handoff, 51–54
predictive assessment tool, 55–56
process excellence, 42
  training, 43–44
risk management, 45–46
sustaining heart success education
  compliance, 56–57
visible teamwork, 58–59
high-reliability organizations (HROs), 39, 40
HIMSS. See Healthcare Information and
      Management Systems Society
HITECH Act. See Health Information
      Technology for Economic and
      Clinical Health Act
HMC. See Hunterdon Medical Center
HNHN. See Healthy Nurse, Healthy Nation
      Grand Challenge
horizontal chart, 284
hospital-acquired infections (HAIs), 91
hospital-acquired pressure ulcers (HAPUs), 92
Hospital Consumer Assessment of Healthcare
      Providers and Systems (HCAHPS),
      93, 94, 151
Hospital Readmissions Reduction Program
      (HRRP), 95
HROs. See high-reliability organizations
HRRP. See Hospital Readmissions Reduction
      Program
Hunterdon Medical Center (HMC), 54
hypoglycemic episodes, 83

I

i-PARIHS model, 116, 117
ICC. See interdisciplinary care conferences
illness prevention, 347
immersion
  business models, 220–221, 221t
  intention of, 216–217
  project, identifying meaningful, 226
improvement, and implementation science
  complexity change theory, 124–125
  evidence-based quality improvement, 120
  importance of, 105–108
  overriding goal of improvement and
      implementation sciences, 108–109
  priorities in, 109–111, 110–111t
  research priorities in, 111, 112t, 113f
    discovery research, 113
    evaluation, 118–120, 119t
    evidence summary, 114, 114b
    integration, 115–118
    translation to guidelines, 114–115,
      115b, 116t
infectious messages, 363

informatics competencies, 295–296
information management, 228
information technology (IT), role in
        healthcare, 291
innovation, 141, 143, 346
    defined, 362
    science of, 362–364
institutional review board (IRB), 33
insulin delivery, leading change in, 357–358
intentional destruction, 363
INTERACT framework. *See* Interventions
        to Reduce Acute Care Transfers
        framework
interdisciplinary care conferences (ICC), 152
interdisciplinary team, 141, 149, 151
    building, 172–173
    falls, reducing, 153–154
International Organization for Migration
        (IOM), 64–65, 105–106, 108, 136
International Scholarly Research Network
        (ISRN), 110, 110–111*t*
interoperability, 299
Interprofessional Collaborative Practice
        Competencies (IPEC), 144
interprofessional team, 384–385
    building, 175
    improvement
        competency development, 144–145
        emotional intelligence, 145
        synergistic, 141–143
        value and, 143–144
Interventions to Reduce Acute Care Transfers
        (INTERACT) framework, 322
intravenous fluids (IVF), 88–89
IOM. *See* International Organization for
        Migration
IPEC. *See* Interprofessional Collaborative
        Practice Competencies
IRB. *See* institutional review board
ISRN. *See* International Scholarly Research
        Network
IT. *See* information technology
IVF. *See* intravenous fluids

J

JHNEBPM. *See* Johns Hopkins Nursing
        Evidence-Based Model
Johns Hopkins Nursing Evidence-Based
        Model (JHNEBPM), 99

K

kindness, 416–417

L

lateral integration, 20, 31, 36, 82, 154–155,
        314, 338–339, 396
lateral integrator, 172
leadership, 172–173
Lean, 42, 51
Lean management system, 342–344
Lean methodology, 95
learning environments, 199–200
lifelong learning, 199–200
Likert scale, 160
line charts, 284
linear change, 124

M

machine-learning models, 295
macrosystem, 23, 25, 26
MADD. *See* Mothers Against Drunk Drivers
Maine Medical Center, 5
MAR. *See* medication administration record
massive transfusion protocol (MTP), 100
MD Anderson Cancer Center (MDACC), 58
MDACC. *See* MD Anderson Cancer Center
meaningful use program, 292–293
medication administration record (MAR), 57
medication administration, technology to
        support, 299
medication error, 57
Melanoma/Sarcoma unit, 86
mentor, CNL as, 211–212
mesosystem, 23, 25, 26
messages, infectious, 363
meta-networking, 173
methicillin-resistant *Staphylococcus aureus*
        (MRSA), 54
metrics, 219, 222, 223
    measurement, 64, 74
MEWS. *See* modified early warning system
mHealth (mobile health), 294
Microsoft Office, 283
microsystem, 23, 25, 26, 41–43, 66, 82, 84,
        107, 120, 384–388
    assessments, 254–255, 256–257*f*
    defined, 341
    partnerships, 371
mind maps, 177, 178*f*
mindfulness, 414–417
mobile health. *See* mHealth
modified early warning system (MEWS), 100
Mothers Against Drunk Drivers (MADD), 416
MRSA. *See* methicillin-resistant
        Staphylococcus aureus
MTP. *See* massive transfusion protocol
multidisciplinary communication, 374–375

N

National Cancer Institute (NCI), 56
National Database of Nursing Quality
        Indicators (NDNQI), 90
National Patient Safety Goals, 163
National Quality Forum, 71
National Translations of Care Coalition
        (NTCC), 314
natural history of disease model, 176–177
NCI. *See* National Cancer Institute
NDNQI. *See* National Database of Nursing
        Quality Indicators
needs assessment, 226
neonatal intensive care unit (NICU), 161
Net Promoter Score (NPS), 419
networking, 175
    defined, 170–171
NI. *See* nursing informatics
NICHE Steering Committee. *See* Nurses
        Improving Care for Health System
        Elders Steering Committee
NICU. *See* neonatal intensive care unit
NPS. *See* Net Promoter Score
NTCC. *See* National Translations of Care
        Coalition
Nurses Improving Care for Health
        System Elders (NICHE) Steering
        Committee, 61
nursing informatics (NI), 290
nursing profession, on medical-surgical unit,
        375–377

O

obstetrics, 160–162
organizational learning, 67
outcomes, 367
outcomes manager, 170

P

pain management, 159–160, 335–336
    patient satisfaction with, 355
palliative care, 187–188
pandemic, maintaining healthy work
        environments during, 420
PAPR hoods. *See* powered air-purifying
        respirators hoods
parking lot, 71
partnership, 346–347, 349–350
pathogenesis period, 176
patient care
    through improved multidisciplinary
        communication, 374–375

    use of technology to support, 297
patient engagement, 315, 320, 321
Patient Protection and Affordable Care Act
        (PPACA), 48, 349
patient safety
    CNI's approach to, 164–165
    CPOE, 299
    technology to support medication
        administration, 299
patient satisfaction, 367
    with pain management, 355
patient service coordinators (PSCs), 57
PDCA cycle. *See* plan-do-check-act cycle
performance contract, 222, 223*f*
personal protective equipment (PPE), 22, 24
physical and psychological safety, 410, 414
pie charts, 284–285
plan-do-check-act (PDCA) cycle, 74
planning, 216, 218, 219
population health, 315–317, 346–347
    promoting foundational capabilities of,
        350–351
portfolio, 217, 219
    usefulness of, 221–222
postdischarge calls, in ED, 341–342
postpartum hemorrhage (PPH), 99
powered air-purifying respirators (PAPR)
        hoods, 137
PPACA. *See* Patient Protection and Affordable
        Care Act
PPE. *See* personal protective equipment
PPH. *See* postpartum hemorrhage
practice, translating and integrating
        scholarship into, 248
preceptee, 196–197
preceptor, 194–196
    portfolios, for career advancement,
        213–214
    role of, 212–213
Preferred Reporting Items for Systematic
        Reviews and Meta-Analyses
        (PRISMA), 235, 235–238*t*
prepathogenesis period, 176
primary care, 317
primary team nursing (PTN), 58
PRISMA. *See* Preferred Reporting Items
        for Systematic Reviews and
        Meta-Analyses
privacy, 300
problem, defined, 273
problem identification, 273
professional development, 196, 402–403
professional membership, 396
professionalism, 397–398
project management, 251–270
    5 P framework, 255–258, 256–257*f*

conducting microsystem assessments, 254–255, 256–257*f*
defined, 252
evaluation of improvement plan, 262
improvement plan, evaluation of, 262
interprofessional and organizational team leaders in, 253, 253*f*
tool selection for, 259–261, 260–262*f*
Project Re-Engineered Discharge (RED), 175, 322
Projectable change, 386
PSCs. *See* patient service coordinators
PTN. *See* primary team nursing
public health, context for, 348–350
public health practice, 356–357

Q

quadruple aim, 133
quality, CNL's approach to, 164–165
quality improvement
tool selection for, 259–261, 260–262*f*
quality of healthcare, 112

R

recognition and rewards, 410
RED. *See* Project Re-Engineered Discharge
reference management, 230, 240–241
registered nurses (RNs), 57, 59, 172
research-effectiveness-adoption-implementation-maintenance (RE-AIM) framework, 118
research, to improve patient outcomes, 246–247
residency program, 399
resilience, 413–414
assessment for, 415
building
approaches, 414–415
CNL's role in, 424
measuring, 418
tools, 416
Resilience Scale for Adults (RSA), 419
responsiveness of staff, 93
RNs. *See* registered nurses
RSA. *See* Resilience Scale for Adults

S

SACN. *See* Saint Anthony College of Nursing
safe insulin infusion dosing, 310
Saint Anthony College of Nursing (SACN), 31

SBAR. *See* situation, background, assessment, recommendations
scatter charts, 285
science of change, 106
science of innovation, 362–364
SCIP. *See* Surgical Care Improvement Project
SCT. *See* stem cell transplant
SDGs. *See* Sustainable Development Goals
security, 300
self-awareness, 145
self-care, 315, 339–340
self-efficacy beliefs. *See* capability beliefs
self-management, 320–321
self-regulation, 145
servant leadership, 367–369
awareness, 368
building community, 369
commitment to growth of people, 369
conceptualization, 368
empathy, 368
foresight, 368
healing, 368
listening, 368
persuasion, 368
stewardship, 369
Silver Beacon Award for Excellence, 58
situation, background, assessment, recommendations (SBAR), 142
Six Sigma, 42
social determinants of health, 20, 351, 384–385, 389
social skill, 145
SPD. *See* sterile processing departments
stakeholders, 254, 256–257, 259, 260, 262
stem cell transplant (SCT), 91, 92, 151–152
sterile processing, CNL's approach to, 164–165
sterile processing departments (SPD), 164–165
Stevens Star Model of Knowledge Transformation, 112, 113*f*, 120
storytelling, 416
stress, upside of, 416
stroke, 11–17
success, measurement of, 222–223
Surgical Care Improvement Project (SCIP), 166
sustainability value, 254, 262
Sustainable Development Goals (SDGs), 20
sustainable value, 203
SWOT analysis, 255–258, 256*f*
examples of, 258–259*f*
systems analyst and risk anticipator, 170
systems life cycle, 299–300
systems thinking, 35, 36

T

Tablets, 293–294
TCM. *See* Transitional Care Model
TDM. *See* Team Development Measure
team building, 142
team cohesion, 141
team collaboration
    messages to innovate, 177, 179
Team Development Measure (TDM), 142
team synergy, 140–141
Team Training for Enhancement of
        Performance and Patient Safety
        (TeamSTEPPS), 118
teams, 367
TeamSTEPPS. *See* Team Training for
        Enhancement of Performance and
        Patient Safety
TEFCAS model. *See* trial, event, feedback,
        check, adjust, and success model
telehealth, 294
Texas Health Resources, 82
TIGER Initiative, 295
*To Err Is Human: Building a Safer Health
        System*, 64
total quality management (TQM), 42
TQM. *See* total quality management
transactional leadership, 369–370
transferring patient care, 186–187
transformational leadership, 369–370
transformative change, 386
transition care model, 175
transitional care
    defined, 314, 316–317
    quality and safe patient outcomes, impact
        on, 318–320
    root causes of ineffective, 320–321
    vs. transitions of care, 318
Transitional Care Model (TCM), 175
translational science, 106
transparency, 200
trauma tracheostomy patients, 148
trend hunting, 363

trial, event, feedback, check, adjust, and
        success (TEFCAS) model, 177
triple aim, 38, 133

U

unintended consequences, of health policy,
        384, 387–388
unit-acquired pressure ulcers, 378–379
US Preventive Services Task Force, 115

V

VA Tennessee Valley Healthcare System, 5
vaccination rates, 354
Value Analysis Team (VAT), 87
value, and interprofessional team
        collaboration, 143–144
value of communication, 136
vancomycin-resistant *Enterococcus* (VRE), 54,
        91, 92
VAT. *See* Value Analysis Team
vertical chart, 284
Veterans Health Administration (VHA), 5
VHA. *See* Veterans Health Administration
VRE. *See* vancomycin-resistant *Enterococcus*
vulnerable patients, changing system for,
        287–288

W

wellness, 349
wicked healthcare problems, 21
workplace
    IHI joy in, 410–411
    national and international initiatives, 410

Z

Zika virus, 22